PARKINSON'S DISEASE

Edited by

Dr. Neda Nikolovski

ALLIED HEALTH PRESS

Parkinson's Disease

Editor: **Dr. Neda Nikolovski**

Allied Health Press
4164 Lakeshore Road
Burlington ON L7L 1A4
Canada
www.alliedhealthpress.com
Email: orders@arclereducation.com

ISBN: 978-1-77956-258-6

Allied Health Press publishes wide variety of books and eBooks. For more information about Allied Health Press and its products, visit our website at www.alliedhealthpress.com

ABOUT THE EDITOR

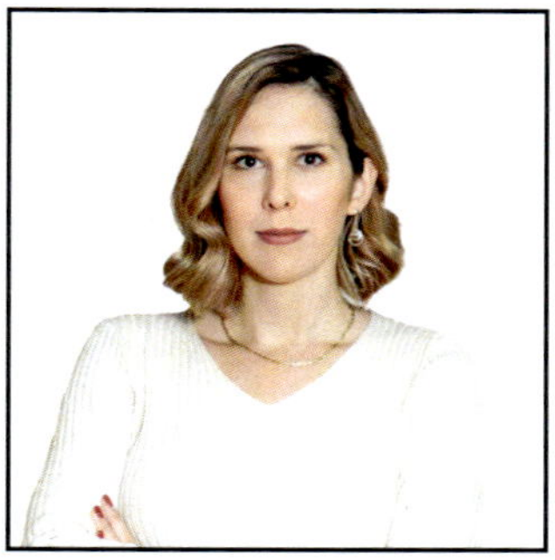

Dr. Neda Nikolovski, a Molecular Biologist and Physiologist holding a PhD in Immunology, has been dedicated to scientific research since 2015 at the Institute for Biological Research, Belgrade University, Belgrade, Serbia. Her primary areas of expertise encompass immunology, autoimmunity, neurodegenerative diseases, multiple sclerosis and its animal models, dendritic cells, and cell-based immunotherapy in autoimmune conditions. She is author of 27 research papers published in esteemed international journals and has contributed her expertise as a reviewer for numerous international publications.

Word Roots, Prefixes, and Suffixes by Chapter

Chapter 1 Parkinson's Disease Facts and Figures

cerebr-: the brain
cyt-: cell
fron-: pertaining to the forehead
hypo-: below
inter-: between, among
intra-: within

Chapter 2 Clinical Diagnosis of Parkinsonism and Tremor

abdomin/o: abdomen
-acusis: hearing
aden/o: gland
-algia: pain
cardi/o: heart

Chapter 3 Diagnostic Testing and Neuroimaging

Neuro-: "related to the nervous system."
Imaging: process of producing images.
Graphy: "process of recording" or "writing."
Tomography: process of creating tomographic images.
Cerebro-: "related to the brain."
Scopy: process of examination or observation.

Chapter 4 Drug Treatment of Parkinson's Disease

Onco: mass/tumor
Histio: tissue
sten: narrowing
para-: beside, beyond, around, abnormal
pre-: before

Chapter 5 Non-Motor Features of Parkinson's Disease

cervic/o: neck; cervix (neck of uterus)
gastr/o: stomach
-paresis: weakness
pector/o: chest
pharmac/o: drug
ur/o: urine; urinary tract
vesic/o: urinary bladder

Chapter 6 Surgical Therapy for Parkinson's Disease

poly-: many, much
cat-: down
-lepsy: seizure
-oma: tumor
-plasty: surgical repair

Chapter 7 The Role of the Nurse Practitioner/Physician Assistant

–ology, meaning 'the study of'
hyp(o)-:below normal
dys-: abnormal, painful.
-somn(o): sleep
-mimia: refers to the act of mimicry or imitation
-kinesia: refers to movement or motion

Chapter 8 The Role of the Speech Language Pathologist

brady-: slow
-lysis, -lyso: destruction
-oid: resembles
-osis: pathologic condition
patho-: diseased state
psych-: the mind, mental

Chapter 9 Malnutrition and Related Disorders

-trophy: nutrition, growth
neuro-: nerve
para-: alongside, near
endo-: inside
epi-: upon

Chapter 10 Complementary Medicine and PD

"-therapy" (treatment, healing)
"Holos" (whole, entire)
"Alter-" (other, different)
"Integr-" (together, whole)
"Tradit-" (handing down, delivering)
"Heal" (to make whole, to restore)

Table of Contents

5 Non-Motor Features of Parkinson's Disease 173

6 Surgical Therapy for Parkinson's Disease 213

LIST OF FIGURES

LIST OF TABLES

PREFACE

The neurodegenerative disorder known as Parkinson's disease (PD) is a complicated condition that is characterized by a clinical syndrome that is easily identifiable and typically presents itself in later life. The condition is characterized by a collection of symptoms, some of which include rigidity, resting tremor, and bradykinesia, which is characterized by delayed movement. It is common for these motor symptoms to be accompanied by a variety of non-motor manifestations, such as a loss of smell, sleep disturbances, mood disorders, excessive salivation, constipation, and periodic limb movements while the individual is sleeping. There is no infectious agent that is responsible for this disease; rather, it is the result of a number of underlying factors, such as genetic predispositions and environmental influences.

Parkinson's disease is becoming more prevalent all over the world, which is a reflection of the fact that it is one of the most significant public health concerns globally. Although only a small percentage of cases, approximately three to five percent, can be directly attributed to genetic causes that involve specific genes (monogenic Parkinson's disease), a significant portion of the risk is associated with genetic variants that collectively contribute to the heritable risk of the disease (non-monogenic Parkinson's disease). Constipation, a history of Parkinson's disease or tremor in one's family, and the fact that one does not smoke are all items that have been identified as factors that increase the likelihood of developing the condition.

The presence of bradykinesia in conjunction with rest tremor, rigidity, or both is essential for the diagnosis of Parkinson's disease. The clinical assessment is the primary method upon which the diagnosis is based. It is possible that cases with atypical presentations require additional testing to make a diagnosis. Because the progression of the disease can vary greatly from person to person, it is necessary to provide personalized prognostic counseling that is based on the identification of various disease subtypes before beginning treatment. It is important to note that Parkinson's disease frequently presents with a prodromal period that lasts for a considerable amount of time before clinical symptoms manifest. During this time, the identification of prodromal symptoms may have potential implications for future treatments that modify the disease.

At the moment, the treatment for Parkinson's disease is aimed at reducing the severity of symptoms and enhancing the patient's quality of life. As the most effective medication for the management of motor symptoms, levodopa continues to be the cornerstone of pharmacological therapy. It is strongly recommended that those who are experiencing disability as a result of the disease receive treatment for their symptoms without delay. There are a variety of non-pharmacological interventions that are used in conjunction with pharmacotherapy. Management approaches are multidisciplinary and include these interventions.

There is currently no treatment that can stop or slow the progression of Parkinson's disease, despite the fact that research efforts against the disease are still ongoing. On the other hand, research currently being conducted into the genetic underpinnings and mechanisms of neuronal death is continuing to investigate potential avenues for disease modification. This evolving understanding highlights the significance of taking a holistic approach to the management of Parkinson's disease. This approach should incorporate the latest developments in pharmacological and non-pharmacological interventions, while also preparing for future breakthroughs in treatment strategies.

This book maintains a focus on the perspective of individuals with Parkinson's disease, serving as a guiding theme to demonstrate the optimization of personalized disease management. It aims to provide a comprehensive overview of the condition, focusing on both the medical aspects and the personal experiences of those living with Parkinson's. It is intended for a wide readership, including healthcare professionals, caregivers, patients, and anyone interested in gaining a deeper understanding of Parkinson's disease.

The book covers topics like the underlying causes of the disease, current treatment options, and the latest research in the field. It will also examine the daily challenges faced by individuals with Parkinson's and offer practical advice on managing symptoms and improving quality of life. By combining medical expertise with practical tips, this book seeks to educate, inspire, and empower readers to better understand and cope with Parkinson's disease.

Chapter 1

PARKINSON'S DISEASE FACTS AND FIGURES

Contents

Introduction

Parkinson's disease (PD) is a complex neurodegenerative disease that worsens over time and is characterized by bradykinesia, tremor, and rigidity. As the disease worsens, some patients may also experience postural instability. We are still learning more about PD, which was initially identified by James Parkinson in 1817 and later further defined by Jean-Martin Charcot. After Alzheimer's disease (AD), PD is the second most prevalent neurodegenerative disease. Its prevalence ranges from 0 to 1% in people 65 to 69 years old to 1–3% in people 80 years of age and above. The prevalence and incidence of PD are predicted to rise by over 30% by 2030 due to an aging population. This will have an impact on society and the economy overall, both directly and indirectly.

The loss of nigrostriatal dopaminergic innervation is the pathological hallmark of PD; however, neurodegeneration affects cells throughout the neural network, not just the nigral dopaminergic neurons. PD is a very heterogeneous disorder due to its widespread pathology, and there is currently no reliable diagnostic test for the condition. Diagnoses are made based on clinical symptoms, and two of the following clinical features must be present to make a diagnosis: rigidity, bradykinesia, resting tremor, and/or postural instability. However, based solely on clinical criteria, a diagnosis of probable PD can only be made; histopathological evaluation and the detection of Lewy bodies (LBs) or Lewy neurites containing α-synuclein are necessary for a definitive diagnosis.

Drugs designed to either act on striatal post-synaptic dopamine receptors or restore dopamine levels in the striatum are used primarily to relieve symptoms. However, since dopamine is not the only neurotransmitter implicated in PD, a variety of other medications are also being used to address different symptoms, like dementia or depression. However, research on new treatments to slow down the rate of neurodegeneration or even to replace lost dopaminergic cells is still ongoing, with some of them in the early phases of clinical trials. The prospect for the creation of disease-modifying treatments appears bright as we learn more about the pathophysiology of Parkinson's disease and discover new therapeutic targets.

Orientation and Directional Terms

Term	Definition	Illustration
Genetics	Genetics is the study of genes. Our genes carry information that gets passed from one generation to the next.	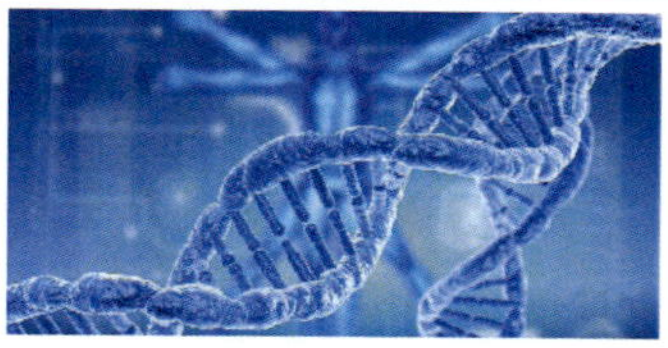
Traumatic brain injury	A TBI (traumatic brain injury) is a major cause of death and disability in the U.S. TBIs happen after the head trauma.	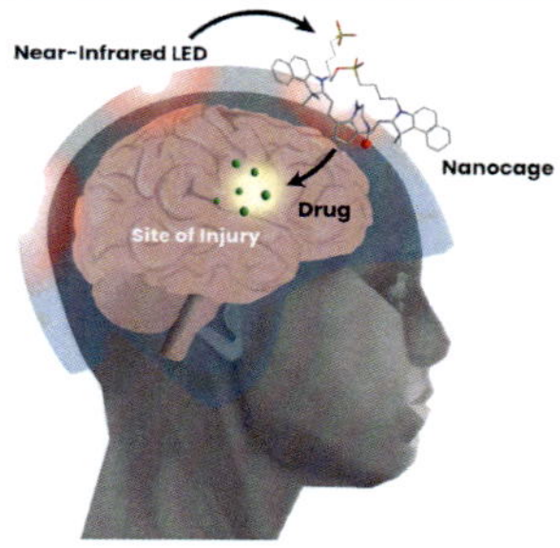
Pesticides	Pesticides kill, repel, or control forms of animal and plant life considered to damage or be a nuisance in agriculture and domestic life.	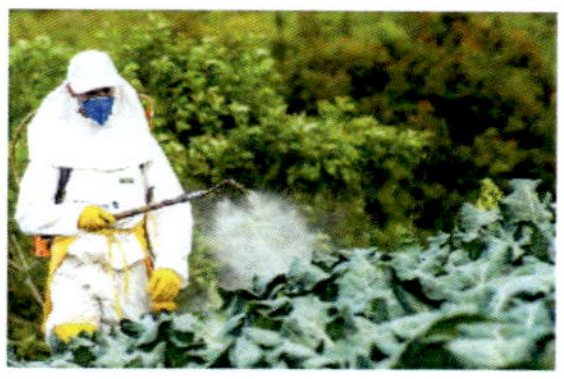
Trichloroethylene	Trichloroethylene (TCE) is a volatile, colorless liquid organic chemical. TCE does not occur naturally and is created by chemical synthesis. It is used primarily to make refrigerants and other hydrofluorocarbons and as a degreasing solvent for metal equipment.	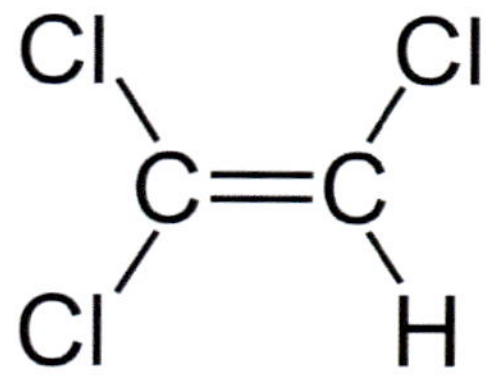
Probiotics	Probiotics are live microorganisms that are intended to have health benefits when consumed or applied to the body. They can be found in yogurt and other fermented foods, dietary supplements, and beauty products.	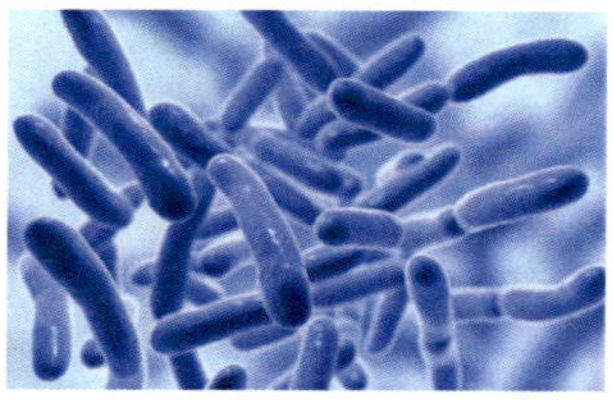

1.1. History of Parkinson's Disease

The British apothecary James Parkinson published An Essay on the Shaking Palsy in 1817, and that is when the history of Parkinson's disease began. Fast forward to the present day. Parkinson's disease had been previously described by others, and the 20th century saw a significant advancement in our understanding of the condition and its therapies. Back then, PD was referred to as paralysis agitans, or shaking palsy in English. The French neurologist Jean-Martin Charcot popularized the term "Parkinson's disease," which was first used by William Sanders in 1865 (Goetz, 2011).

1.1.1. Early Descriptions

Many ancient sources mention symptoms that are similar to Parkinson's disease. A 12th-century B.C. Egyptian papyrus references a king who is drooling with age, and the Bible makes several references to shaking. An ancient 10th-century B.C. Ayurvedic medical treatise. D. characterizes a condition that progresses with Parkinson's disease symptoms, such as tremor, immobility, and drooling. Furthermore, mucuna family medicines, which are high in L-DOPA, were used to treat this illness. Galen described tremors that only happen at rest, postural abnormalities, and paralysis in his writing about a condition that was most likely Parkinson's disease.

Unambiguous references to PD are not known to exist after Galen until the 17th century. Before Parkinson's description, some writers discussed various aspects of the disease in this and the century that followed. Similar to Galen, Franciscus Sylvius distinguished tremor at rest from other tremors, and Johannes Baptiste Sagar and Hieronymus David Gaubius talked about festination, the term for the distinctive gait associated with Parkinson's disease. Parkinson's idea to gather and characterize patients with "paralysis agitans" may have originated from John Hunter's detailed description of the illness. Last but not least, several descriptions of aberrant movements and rigidity resembling those observed in Parkinson's disease were included by Auguste François Chomel in his pathology treatise, published contemporaneously with Parkinson's essay.

1.1.2. 19th Century

James Parkinson wrote an essay in 1817 detailing six instances of what he termed paralysis agitans. The characteristic resting tremor, abnormal posture and gait, paralysis and decreased muscle strength, and the disease's progressive nature were all detailed in an essay on shaking palsy. He also praised the numerous writers who were already mentioned for their contributions to our knowledge of Parkinson's disease. Over the forty years that followed, the article attracted little attention, despite being later recognized as the seminal work on the disease. Additionally, any condition characterized by a loss of motor activity and convulsions was occasionally referred to as paralysis agitans. In fact, the word "paralysis" itself covered deficiencies in both motor and sensory functions. Taking note of this, William Sanders proposed in 1865 that the diagnosis of Parkinson's disease—previously known as paralysis agitans festinia, -senilis, or Parkinsonii—be applied to the onset of symptoms in the elderly.

Neurologists Trousseau, Gowers, Kinnier Wilson, Erb, and most notably Charcot, whose research between 1868 and 1881 was a turning point in our understanding of the disease, are among those who contributed to our understanding of the condition. Among his many contributions was the differentiation he made between bradykinesia, weakness, and rigidity. Additionally, he supported renaming the illness in Parkinson's honor.

1.1.3. 20th Century and Beyond

Eighty years after Parkinson's essay, Édouard Brissaud made the first conjectures regarding the anatomical basis of PD, speculating that it may be caused by an ischemic lesion and that it originated in the subthalamus or cerebral peduncle. "Lewy bodies" were subsequently named after Frederic Lewy, who reported a pathologic finding in affected brains in 1912. The main cerebral structure affected, according to Konstantin Tretiakoff's 1919 report, was the substantia nigra. However, Rolf Hassler's 1938 publication of additional studies confirmed this finding, which was not widely accepted. The work of Oleh Hornykiewicz on the neurotransmitter dopamine and Arvid Carlsson on its role in PD helped identify the underlying biochemical alterations in the brain in the 1950s. In the end, Carlsson's efforts earned him a Nobel Prize.

PD's genetic component was identified by Alice Lazzarini et al. in 1994. A few years prior, the neurology clinic at Robert Wood Johnson Medical School (RWJMS) identified an Italian family with at least 400 members spanning five generations, including at least 60 individuals with PD. The family's ancestors were found to be in the small Italian village of Contursi. In an attempt to identify the gene causing PD in the Contursi family, the RWJMS team teamed up with the National Center for Human Genome Research at the National Institutes of Health in 1995. This allowed them to utilize the laboratory resources provided by the NIH. The group discovered the first mutation in the brain protein alpha-synuclein that causes Parkinson's Disease (PARK1). Alpha-synuclein was found to be the primary component of Lewy bodies within PD patient brain cells within days of the PARK1 findings being published. As stated in the UMDNJ magazine, "This discovery changed the direction of research into PD by providing scientists with an entirely new protein whose manufacture, function, or breakdown could be the key to the disease." Spillantini, Trojanowski, Goedert, and others discovered in 1997 that the primary constituent of Lewy bodies is synuclein proteins. 1998 saw the discovery of parkin gene mutations in autosomal recessive juvenile Parkinsonism. Finally, between 2002 and 2005, mutations in the DJ-1, PINK1, and LRRK2 genes were found in both European and Japanese families. Heiko Braak published a description of the pathological staging of Parkinson's disease in 2003.

1.1.4. History of Treatments

During the 19th century, Charcot, Erb, and other researchers reported the beneficial, if mild, effects of anticholinergic alkaloids derived from the belladonna plant on tremor. The lesioning of certain basal ganglia structures was the first attempt at modern tremor surgery in 1939, and it was refined over the next 20 years. Surgery performed before this date involved lesioning the corticospinal pathway, which resulted in paralysis as opposed to tremor. Up to the introduction of levodopa, which significantly decreased their use, the only available treatments were anticholinergics and surgery. Levodopa was first synthesized by Casimir Funk in 1911, but until the middle of the 20th century, not much was known about it. It was first used in clinical settings in 1967. In 1968, a sizable study was published that detailed the benefits of levodopa treatment for individuals with Parkinson's disease. The treatment of Parkinson's disease was revolutionized by levodopa. Deep brain stimulation was first proposed by Alim-Louis Benabid and team in Grenoble, France, in the late 1980s and was eventually approved for clinical use by the FDA in 1997.

1.2. Epidemiology

At any given time, 1-2 people out of every 1000 are affected by PD. 1% of people over 60 are affected by PD, and the prevalence of PD rises with age. The primary neuropathological observation is the presence of Lewy bodies containing α-synuclein and a decrease in dopaminergic neurons in the substantia nigra, which results in a decreased ability to facilitate voluntary movements. Lewy body pathology extends to cortical and neocortical areas as Parkinson's disease progresses. The three main symptoms of PD are bradykinesia, rigidity, and tremor. A recent update to the diagnostic criteria defines absolute exclusion criteria, red flags, and supportive criteria while eliminating postural instability as a fourth hallmark. As non-motor symptoms in PD have drawn more attention, both motor and non-motor signs are now considered part of the supporting criteria. In most cases, PD has no known cause. There are known genetic risk factors, such as rare monogenetic causes in unselected populations. 5-10% of the patients have some genetic component identified. Several environmental factors are linked to a higher chance of Parkinson's disease. According to autopsy studies, a sizable percentage of patients have their clinical diagnosis of PD ruled out at autopsy. It is anticipated that updated diagnostic standards will increase a clinician's precision in PD diagnosis. As our understanding of the genetic and environmental risk factors for PD grows, the etiology of this illness will likely become clearer soon.

1.2.1. Prevalence

The percentage of current patients in a population who have PD at any given time is measured by the prevalence. According to door-to-door surveys, the crude prevalence of PD varies from 15 (per 100,000 population) in China to 657 (per 100,000 population) in Argentina, and from 100 to 250 in North America and Europe. For similar populations, the prevalence estimates obtained using this method are higher than those obtained using other techniques. Socioeconomic and survival rate-related factors can readily impact prevalence.

1.2.2. Incidence

A more accurate measure of frequency is incidence, which counts the number of new PD cases in a population of people at risk in a specific time period. It remains largely unaffected by factors that impact the survival of diseases. However, it can be challenging to determine the precise incidence of PD due to the possibility of a protracted latent stage preceding the clinical manifestations and a slow clinical progression. The crude annual incidence rates of PD over the past forty years have varied from 1.5 per 100,000 people in China in 1986 to 14.8 in Finland in 1968–1970. The variation may be partially explained by variations in study design, including case ascertainment techniques and diagnostic criteria.

1.2.3. Age Distribution

There are significant differences in PD incidence and prevalence among age groups. PD is less common in people under 50 and increases gradually in older people up to the ninth decade of life.

There are probably not many people in this age group, which contributes to the decline among the oldest people observed in some studies. Diagnostic and ascertaining challenges may also be to blame.

According to a recent study, Yonago City, Japan saw an increase in prevalence from 80.6 (per 100,000 people) in 1980 to 117.9 in 1992; however, the prevalence fell from 103.9 per 100,000 to 99.5 when age and sex were taken into account.

Although the age-adjusted incidence in people under 55 in 1992 was lower than in people under 55 in 1980, there was no discernible change in incidence between 1980 and 1992. According to this study, the population's aging may be the primary cause of the rising prevalence.

1.2.4. Gender Differences

While gender-specific differences show greater variability than age-related associations, most studies indicate that PD is slightly more common in men than in women, typically between a 1.2:1 and a 1.5:1 ratio.

1.2.5. Ethnic Distribution

Different countries have different rates of PD prevalence and incidence, which is partially due to differences in the racial makeup of the populations surveyed. White people are more prevalent in Europe and North America overall, accounting for 100 to 350 of every 100,000 population. Less than one-fifth to one-tenth of white people have higher rates than black Africans and Asians from China and Japan. In Mississippi, USA, door-to-door screening revealed no statistically significant difference in age-adjusted PD prevalence between Whites and Blacks.

Meanwhile, two studies found that the incidence of PD was comparable to that of European-American Americans in Asian-American men and African-American women. Furthermore, PD prevalence was found to be 119 per 100,000 for the entire population of the Taiwanese islet of Kinmen, according to a door-to-door survey. This figure is significantly higher than previous studies on Asian populations and is comparable to that of a white population. Rather than being a result of racial factors, these observations might instead be the result of environmental exposure. For PD prevalence estimates in populations of African descent, however, the confounding effects of low case ascertainment and high selective mortality should be taken into account.

1.2.6. Time Trends

In terms of the incidence of PD, a population-based study conducted from 1935 to 1988 in Olmsted County, Minnesota, revealed that the annual incidence of PD increased from 9.2 per 100,000 for the years 1935 to 1944 to 16.3 per 100,000 for the years 1975 to 1984. In contrast, Zhang and Roman conducted a meta-analysis in which they adjusted reported data using a single standard population and came to the conclusion that over the previous 40 years, the prevalence and incidence of PD appear to have stayed constant. It is currently difficult to reliably evaluate changes in time trends of PD because there are very few longitudinal data for PD incidence, and the data may lack consistency for diagnostic criteria and study methods over time.

1.2.7. Geographic Distribution

Geographic differences in Parkinson's disease frequency have been documented. As an example, door-to-door surveys in China, India, Mississippi, USA, and Argentina have found that crude prevalence is 15 per 100,000, 328 per 100,000, and 657 per 100,000, respectively. The mortality rates for White individuals, irrespective of gender, exhibited robust north-to-south decreasing gradients in a recent study that looked at geographic variation in PD mortality reporting in the US; however, no discernible west-to-east gradient was shown. The information on prevalence seems to be in line with the geographic distribution of incidence. While there have been reports of significant regional differences with northwest to southeast gradients in both Canada and the United States contributing to PD, this may indicate that environmental factors also play a role.

1.2.8. Mortality

Only 37% of patients had PD coded as the underlying cause of death in all cases where PD was diagnosed during life, although the mortality rate is a unique population-based statistic that has been used to investigate both the temporal trends and the geographic distribution of PD. This is because PD is not a major or direct cause of death. Between 1962 and 1984, the average annual age-adjusted death rate from PD in the United States was estimated to be 2 deaths per 100,000 white men and 1 death per 100,000 non-white men, 1 death per 100,000 white women, and less than 1 death per 100,000 non-white women. For those 75 years of age and older, mortality went up, but it went down for those under 70. In general, PD death rates went up for older age groups but down for younger ones.

1.2.9. Survival

Even though PD patients now have a longer life expectancy, their lifespan is still somewhat shorter than that of the general population. The lower mortality rate among younger adults may be partially explained by improved survival following the introduction of effective symptomatic therapy and decreased or postponed mortality from other disorders.

The survival rate for individuals diagnosed with PD before the age of 60 is comparable to the general population but decreases for those diagnosed at an older age. A study in Japan found that pneumonia was the leading cause of death amongst PD patients of all ages, indicating a need for more aggressive treatment of PD-related conditions in addition to better anti-Parkinsonian therapy.

Developing a novel etiologic hypothesis for PD may be aided by epidemiological studies. Due to variations in case ascertainment techniques, diagnostic standards, classification guidelines, healthcare facilities, and population age distribution, the majority of published research cannot be compared. Difficulties in determining appropriate controls and assessing exposure limit research on risk factors. According to recent research, Parkinson's disease is a diverse illness. A small percentage of cases —between 10 and 15% —are familial, and among them are a few patients who have a strong family history that suggests autosomal dominant inheritance; these patients typically present at a younger age. Although drinking coffee and smoking have been identified as protective factors, the exact mechanism is still unknown.

1.3. Causes

PD is thought to be caused by a confluence of environmental and genetic factors. PD is a very broad disorder. Even though every person with Parkinson's disease experiences the disease differently, there are some commonalities Parkinson's affects about one million people in the U.S. and 10 million worldwide. The primary characteristic of PD patients' brains is the loss of dopaminergic neurons in the substantia nigra, a region of the brain important for movement regulation and Parkinson's disease progression.

1.3.1. Genetics

About 10 to 15% of cases of Parkinson's are genetically based. Scientists have compared the genes of patients with Parkinson's disease by analyzing their DNA over time. Numerous gene mutations connected to Parkinson's disease were found.

1.3.2. Environmental Factors

Parkinson's disease development has been linked to exposure to metals, pesticides, solvents, and other toxicants. As of yet, no clear-cut cause and effect relationship has been found. Additionally, mild head injuries, or concussions, have been linked to an increased risk of developing the disease, according to recent studies.

1.3.3. Genetic and Environmental Interactions

While a number of genetic mutations have been linked to an increased risk of PD, these genetic variations are not present in the majority of the population. However, most people do not clearly have any exposure to head traumas or pesticides, despite the fact that these environmental factors are linked to Parkinson's disease. Parkinson's disease is brought on by a confluence of lifestyle, environmental, and genetic factors. Parkinson's disease propensity is determined by the interplay of these three factors. To learn more about how these factors interact to cause PD and how to prevent it, research specific to the disease is essential.

1.4. Risk Factors

PD is a common neurodegenerative disorder affecting the elderly population. It is predicted that between 2015 and 2040, the prevalence of PD will double to 12.9 million, placing a significant burden on healthcare systems. The contribution of biologic and environmental factors to the risk of PD has been increasingly recognized over the past few decades. Toxins, traumatic brain injury (TBI), cancer, illegal substances, and cardiovascular risk factors are known risk factors linked to PD. PD-related protective factors include nutrition, medication, exercise, and smoking. The goal of many current epidemiologic studies is to identify environmental risk factors that are modifiable and could be addressed with preventative measures. Because study designs differ and conclusions are inconsistent, interpreting the studies can be difficult. We offer a succinct overview of the data supporting both biologic and environmental risk factors and protective factors against Parkinson's disease (Suraj Rajan, 2022).

1.4.1. Environmental Risk Factors

- **Pesticides:** Numerous environmental pollutants, such as rotenone, paraquat, and organochlorine pesticides, have been linked to an increased risk of PD. Recently, there has been a lot of discussion about paraquat. The Environmental Protection Agency (EPA) has reaffirmed the drug's safety following lawsuits from several public health and agriculture organizations due to growing worries about its link to PD. Furthermore, residing in rural regions and areas with high farming and well-water consumption rates may lead to elevated pesticide exposure and a corresponding elevated risk of Parkinson's disease.
- **Trichloroethylene:** The industrial chemical trichloroethylene (TCE), which is frequently used as a degreaser, to decaffeinate tea and coffee, and in dry cleaning, has been linked to a 500% higher risk of PD.
- **Dairy Intake:** Dairy consumption and PD risk have been linked in many studies, with higher dairy intake associated with a higher risk.
- **Air Pollution:** Air pollution has often been mentioned as a possible factor that could increase the risk of Parkinson's disease, as well as other neurodegenerative conditions like Alzheimer's disease and amyotrophic lateral sclerosis. The ways in which these pollutants could elevate risk include toxicity to neurons, inflammation in the central or systemic nervous system, and changes to the gut microbiome. Due to the fact that exposure to multiple pollutants commonly happens at once, it has been challenging to pinpoint specific factors that contribute to these disorders.

1.4.2. Biologic Risk Factors

- **Traumatic Brain Injury:** Following the early 1980s diagnosis of early-onset PD in professional boxer Muhammad Ali, research interest in the connection between traumatic brain injury (TBI) and PD increased. According to systematic reviews, former American football and soccer players have a markedly increased risk of Parkinson's disease. There is no agreed-upon definition of head trauma among the studies that exist, and the majority of TBI research focuses on risk following a single severe head injury. Despite these drawbacks, there appears to be a link between PD risk and head trauma. Potential secondary causes of the pathophysiology include disruptions to the blood-brain barrier, inflammation in the brain, impaired mitochondrial function, elevated glutamate release, or accumulation of α-synuclein in the brain.
- **Cancer:** Multiple epidemiological studies have indicated a lower risk of smoking-related cancers in individuals with PD, although it is uncertain if this is due to biases in cancer screening following a PD diagnosis. Some studies have found a higher risk of melanoma, skin, breast, and prostate cancer in people with PD. The connection between PD and melanoma is well-established, with individuals having an increased likelihood of developing both conditions. Research suggests that melanoma and PD share genetic susceptibility factors, environmental risks like exposure to pesticides, and embryonic origins, as levodopa plays a role in the synthesis of dopamine and melanin.
- **Illicit Substance Use:** Cocaine, methamphetamine, and amphetamine use are linked to an increased risk of PD. The use of stimulants similar to amphetamines increases the risk of PD by three times, according to epidemiologic studies. There are several theories explaining the connection between methamphetamine use and PD, including increased dopamine release from neurons and neurotoxicity from long-term use. Substance abusers may not live to older ages, when Parkinson's disease is more prevalent because it raises the risk of dying young. Though there aren't enough clinical studies to support this theory, cocaine has also been linked to a higher risk of PD by downregulating postsynaptic dopamine neurons.
- **Cardiovascular Risk Factors**

a. **Body Mass Index:** Meta-analyses and observational studies on the relationship between PD and body mass index (BMI) have produced inconsistent findings. A lower body mass index (BMI) has been linked to a higher risk of PD, while a higher risk of Parkinson's disease has been linked to obesity. These findings are consistent with previous research on the subject. It's unclear if the disparity in the data is related to variations in racial or ethnic backgrounds, the distribution of fat, or other related metabolic conditions.

b. **Diabetes and Metabolic Syndrome:** Diabetes's connection to Parkinson's disease is still debatable. Numerous cohort studies have demonstrated that diabetes and prediabetes raise the risk of PD by 27–37%. Case-control research, however, has not discovered this correlation. Among the hypothesized mechanisms are the exposure of neurons to elevated metabolic stress, neuronal dysfunction, and hyperglycemia-induced neuronal death. Because of this potential link, the Movement Disorder Society now views diabetes as a risk factor for PD. Cohort studies have linked metabolic syndrome to an increased risk of PD; however, more research is required to confirm this association.

1.4.3. Protective Factors

- **Smoking:** Research shows that smoking is linked to a decreased risk of developing PD. One study found that current smokers had a 30% to 40% lower risk of PD compared to those who did not smoke, depending on the survey used to gather smoking habits. This information is now informing research on potential neuroprotective approaches that could replicate the benefits of nicotine without the risks associated with smoking.
- **Exercise:** The link between exercise and a lower risk of PD is becoming more widely acknowledged. The highest levels of total or moderate-to-intense physical activity (relative risk 0.79 and 0.71, respectively) were found to significantly reduce PD risk in men more than in women, according to a systematic review and meta-analysis of 8 studies with over 500,000 participants. Improved autophagy, reduced neuroinflammation, elevated neurotrophic factors, and improved mitochondrial function are some of the hypothesized processes underlying this protective effect.
- **Medications:** Drugs that increase glycolysis, statins, ibuprofen, and inhibitors of the renin-angiotensin system are among the medications that have been studied in relation to Parkinson's disease. Exposure to non-sterodial anti-inflammatory drugs (NSAIDs) has been linked to a lower incidence of PD, according to some meta-analyses, but not all of them have found this link. Regarding the correlation between statin therapy and the risk of PD, there are also notably contradictory data. A single observational study revealed a higher risk of PD in conjunction with statin use, while other studies found no correlation between statin use and PD risk. Few studies have demonstrated that renin-angiotensin receptor blockers and medications that increase glycolysis reduce the risk of PD.
- **Nutrition:**

a. ***Diet:*** Numerous cohort and cross-sectional studies have shown that the Mediterranean diet is linked to a reduction in the age at which PD onset, a slower rate of progression, an improvement in motor symptoms, and a lower prodromal risk of PD progression. According to a randomized controlled trial (RCT) with thirty-five PD participants, following a Mediterranean diet improved cognitive function. The Mediterranean diet decreases oxidative stress, α-synuclein aggregation, and early neuronal degeneration, and has an anti-inflammatory effect on gut microbiota. A different RCT revealed that the ketogenic diet lessened Parkinson's disease symptoms. But because this was a brief study, care must be taken in interpreting the findings. Six PD patients' motor symptoms were shown to improve when they followed a low-protein diet.

b. ***Probiotics:*** Dysbiosis of the gut microbiota has been linked to the etiology of Parkinson's disease. This has sparked curiosity about whether PD patients could benefit from improved microbiota. Twelve weeks of probiotic consumption improved Unified Parkinson's Disease Rating Scale scores, according to a randomized controlled trial. However, over the course of a person's life, their microbial environment varies depending on a variety of factors, such as nutrition, hygiene, location, and diet. Thus, generalizing this study is not possible.

c. ***Vitamins:*** A growing field of research examines the function of vitamins in preventing oxidative stress and neuroinflammation in Parkinson's disease. Numerous meta-analyses have demonstrated that deficiency in vitamin D, B6, or B12 increases the risk of PD; however, there is currently no evidence to support the benefits of vitamin D and B12 supplementation. High dietary thiamine intake was linked to a lower risk of PD in a cohort study involving over 5000 PD participants. Since people with PD have lower plasma levels of vitamin C, vitamin C has been suggested as a potential biomarker for the disease; however, it is unclear if supplementing with vitamin C improves results. A vitamin E deficiency has been linked to an increased risk of PD, and supplementation with the vitamin showed clinical benefits in an RCT involving sixty PD participants. While vitamin levels have been linked to Parkinson's disease pathogenesis, there is ongoing debate regarding the advantages of vitamin replacement therapy. Iron has been the most studied mineral, but more research is needed because the data are not entirely clear.

d. ***Urates:*** Numerous factors, such as sex, diet, physical activity, and medications, influence the levels of uric acid. Both the onset of PD and the advancement of the illness are linked to low uric acid levels. Although uric acid was once believed to be an antioxidant, new research indicates that low uric acid levels may be a consequence of the disease rather than its cause, linked to changes in the gut microbiome, decreased physical activity, and mitochondrial dysfunction. Oral inosine has been tested in interventional studies to raise uric acid levels, but the results did not demonstrate any clinical benefit.

The most prevalent PD risk factors and protective factors are outlined in this succinct summary. Targeting disease mechanisms after the onset of the disease may not be as effective as optimizing risk factors during the prodromal phase of PD. High-quality research and exposome analysis are desperately needed as the prevalence of PD rises to clarify possible causes and bolster the data in support of more potent preventative strategies (Figure 1.1).

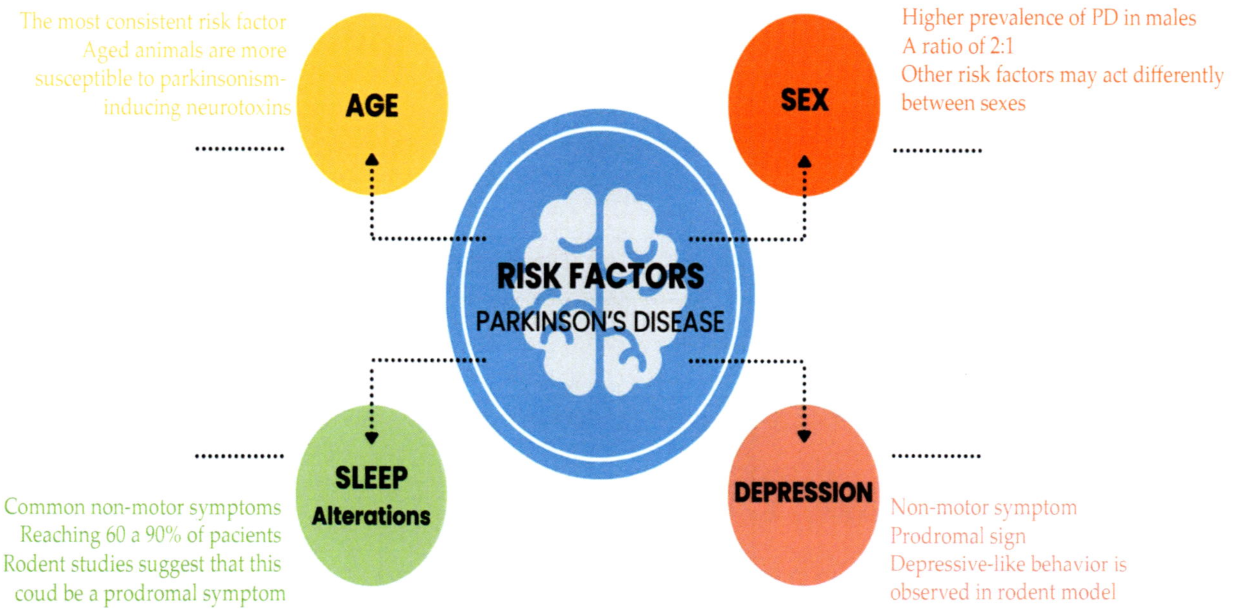

Figure 1.1. *Risk factors for PD.*

Source: Silva RH, Lopes-Silva LB, Cunha DG, Becegato M, Ribeiro AM, Santos JR. Animal Approaches to Studying Risk Factors for Parkinson's Disease: A Narrative Review. Brain Sciences. 2024; 14(2):156. https://doi.org/10.3390/brainsci14020156.

1.5. Genetic Factors

For a long time, it was believed that the majority of Parkinson's disease subtypes had no genetic origin. However, by the late 1990s, research in a number of patient populations showed that first-degree relatives of an afflicted person have a 2–14 times higher risk of developing Parkinson's disease than the general population. Genetic linkage maps have significantly improved as genome technologies have become more accurate and affordable, opening up new avenues for studying the genetic basis of disease. Individual patients can now have whole genome sequence analyses done at a cost that is both affordable and steadily declining.

Some genes are likely to raise the risk of Parkinson's disease without actually causing it, and a small number of genes have been linked to up to 6% of all cases of Parkinson's disease. A direct family member with PD may account for up to 15% of cases (Simo et al., 2020) (Table 1.1).

Table 1.1. *Summary of Monogenic Variants Associated with Parkinson's Disease*

	Gene (HGNC Approved Name)	Alternative Gene Names	Inheritance	Pathogenicity	PD Phenotype	Function
High penetrance	*SNCA*	*PARK1, PARK4, NCAP*	AD	Pathogenic	Early-onset	Uncertain (encodes α-synuclein)
	VPS35	*PARK17, MEM3*	AD	Pathogenic	Typical	Retromer and endosomal trafficking
	PINK1	*PARK6*	AR	Pathogenic	Early-onset	Mitochondrial
	PARK7	*DJ-1*	AR	Pathogenic	Early-onset	
	PRKN	*PARK2, PARKIN*	AR	Pathogenic	Early-onset	
	PLA2G6	*PARK14, IPLA2*	AR	Pathogenic	Early-onset, atypical	Cell membrane
	ATP13A2	*PARK9*	AR	Pathogenic	Early-onset, atypical	Lysosomal
	FBXO7	*PARK15, FBX7*	AR	Pathogenic	Early-onset, atypical	Mitochondrial
	POLG	*POLG1, POLGA*	AD	Pathogenic	Early-onset, atypical	Mitochondrial DNA maintenance
	DNAJC6	*PARK19, DJC6*	AR	Likely pathogenic	Early-onset	Synaptic vesicle formation and trafficking
	DNAJC13	*PARK21, RME8*	AD	Conflicting reports	Typical	
	TMEM230	*C20ORF30*	AD	Conflicting reports	Typical	
	SYNJ1	*PARK20*	AR	Pathogenic	Early-onset, atypical	
	VPS13C	*PARK23*	AR	Pathogenic	Early-onset	Mitochondrial
	CHCHD2	-	AD	Pathogenic	Typical	Uncertain
	DCTN1	-	AD	Pathogenic	Atypical	Microtubule

	Gene (HGNC Approved Name)	Alternative Gene Names	Inheritance	Pathogenicity	PD Phenotype	Function
Variable penetrance	*LRRK2*	*PARK8, DARDARIN*	AD	Pathogenic	Typical	Lysosomal, mitochondrial, microtubule
	GBA	*GBA1*	AD	Pathogenic	Typical	Lysosomal
Associated with PD but unlikely to be pathogenic	*HTRA2*	-	AD	Uncertain/likely benign	-	Mitochondrial
	UCHL1	*PARK5*	AD	Uncertain/likely benign	-	Ubiquitin-proteasome
	GIGYF2	*PARK11*	AD	Uncertain/likely benign	-	Uncertain
	EIF4G1	-	AD	Benign	-	mRNA translation
	LRP10	*LRP9*	AD [1]	Uncertain	-	Uncertain

Source: Day JO, Mullin S. The Genetics of Parkinson's disease and Implications for Clinical Practice. Genes. 2021; 12(7):1006. https://doi.org/10.3390/genes12071006.

[1] AD = autosomal dominant, AR = autosomal recessive, HNGC = HUGO Gene Nomenclature Committee.

1.5.1. PARK Family of Genes

A gene family is a collection of genes that have significant traits in common. Research on the PARK gene family has been particularly interesting and is being conducted widely. PARK gene mutations impact the survival and functionality of nerve cells necessary for proper balance, coordination, and movement.

Families with dominant inheritance have been found to have mutations in three known genes (SNCA, UCHL 1, and LRRK 2). Affected people who had siblings with the illness but whose parents did not have Parkinson's disease (recessive inheritance) have mutations in three additional genes (PARK 2, PARK 7, and PINK 1). These genes may also play a role in dominantly inherited Parkinson's disease or early-onset Parkinson's disease, which is diagnosed before the age of thirty, according to some evidence, but it is too early to say for sure. The genes in the PARK family are listed in the following table, with their approved symbol in the first column and their previous names in the middle (Table 1.2).

Table 1.2. *PARK Genes That are Linked with Mitochondrial Function*

Locus	Genes	Mutation	No. of cases reported	Mean age at onset	Disease progression/ disease duration	Initial signs and symptoms (Top 5 whenever available)	L-Dopa response (out of PD patient tested)	α-synuclein pathology	Brain region M vs Y Up-regulated (≥2 folds)	Brain region M vs Y Down-regulated (≥2 folds)
Autosomal dominant inheritance										
PARK1/PARK4	*SNCA*	Missense (A30P^, E46K^, H50Q^, G51D^, A53E^, A53T^, A32V) or multiplication^#	146	40s	Rapid (<10 years)	Bradykinesia; Rigidity; Depression	Good (50/103)	Yes	ATZ, BLA, Pu	BMA, 10, RaM
PARK8	*LRRK2*	Missense (R1441G^, Y1699C^ G2019S, I2020T, G2385) or gain of function	724	50s	Rapid (15–20 years)	Tremor; Bradykinesia; Rigidity	Good (276/476)	Yes	CgGf,10, RaM, LC, Rpn, FuG	ATZ, BLA, BMA, Dt, CgGr, Rpn, Acb, VT
PARK17	*VPS35*	Missense (D620N#)	67	50s	Slow	Bradykinesia; Postural instability; Rigidity	Good (8/45)	Yes	BLA, Pu	BMA, PrG, RPN, FuG
Autosomal recessive inheritance										
PARK2	*PRKN*	Missense (K161N#, R256C#, R275W^, T415N#, 202–203 delAG#, 255delA# and 321–322insGT#, W453STOP#), multiplication, deletion ^#, or loss of function	1,000	30s	Slow (27–50)	Tremor; Bradykinesia; Dystonia; Tremor at rest; Rigidity;	Good (192/427)	Yes	Dt	BMA, VTA
PARK6	*PINK1*	Missense (G411S#, Q456X#), deletion ^# or loss of function	151	30s	Median (6–28)	Tremor; Bradykinesia; Rigidity; Dystonia; Tremor at rest	Good (84/113)	Yes	Dt,CA4,	ATZ, BMA, CgGr, SN,10, RaM, RPn, Pu, VT
PARK7	*DJ1*	Missense (A104T, M26I, L10P#, L166P#, L172Q^, and P159DEL#) or loss of function	33	20s	Slow	Bradykinesia; Dystonia; Tremor;	Good (5/25)	Yes	Crus II, CgGf, SN	BMA, CgGr, 10, RaM, RPn, Acb
Atypical Parkinsonism										
PARK9	*ATP13A2*	Missense (F182L, G504R, G877R, T12M#, G533R#, A746T#) or loss of function	36	10s	Slow	Bradykinesia; Intellectual development disorder; Cognitive decline; Gait difficulties; Rigidity	Good (9/30)	Yes (*in vitro*)	ATZ, BLA, BMA, CA4, VT	CgGf, CgGr, SPL, RPn, FuG, STG
PARK14	*PLA2G6**	Missense (G31A, D331Y/M3581IfsX) or loss of function	7	20–30s	Rapid (1–15)	Bradykinesia; Rigidity; Spasticity; Hyperreflexia	Moderate	Yes	CgGf, CA2, SPL, Acb, Pu, FuG, STG	BMA, Dt, VTA, RaM, RPN,
PARK15	*FBXO7*	Missense (R378G#, R498X#, and T22M#)	26	10–20s	Rapid	Bradykinesia; Tremor; Gait difficulties; Rigidity; Behavioral abnormalities	Good (6/18)	Yes	CgGf	10, SPL, Pu, STG
PARK22	*CHCHD2**	Missense (T61I#^)	19	50s	Long	Bradykinesia; Resting tremor; Posture instability;	Good	Yes	Dt, VTA, LC	BMA, PrG,10, SPL, RPn, Pu, FuG, STG
PARK23	*VPS13C*	Missense (A269S, W395C^, A444P#^, G1389R#^, Q1593L, and E3109STOP and deletion (V452-K3035)	4	20–30s	Rapid	Bradykinesia; Rigidity; Dystonia; Depression	Moderate	Yes	CgGf, VTA, LC	CgGr, SPL, RPn, Acb

*Information for SNCA, LRRK2, VPS35, PRKN, PINK1, DJ1, ATP13A2, PLA2G6, FBXO7, and VPS13C in this table were extracted from MDS gene, International Parkinson and Movement Disorder Society (http://msdgene.org). MDSGene currently collects data on 1651 different mutations in 6628 movement disorder patients extracted from 1250 publications (Klein et al., 2018). *Information for PLA2G6 and CHCHD2 gene extracted from Online mendelian Inheritance in Man® (http://omim.org). #Mutations were shown to affect mitochondria function. ^Mutations were shown to involve in the formation of α-synuclein pathology. Abbreviations: Y-Young age (age of 24, 31, and 39), M-Middle age (age of 49, 55, and 57). M vs Y up-regulated: up-regulated gene expression with a fold change of greater or equal to 2. M vs Y down-regulated: down-regulated genes expression with a fold change of greater or equal to 2 (M vs Y).*

Source: Li W, Fu Y, Halliday GM and Sue CM (2021) PARK Genes Link Mitochondrial Dysfunction and Alpha-Synuclein Pathology in Sporadic Parkinson's Disease. Front. Cell Dev. Biol. 9:612476. doi: 10.3389/fcell.2021.612476.

1.5.2. Dominant Genes in PD

Alpha-synuclein is the main component of these pathologic protein aggregates, which are typically caused by dominantly transmitted mutations in a group of genes that encode LRRK 2 and alpha-synuclein. These mutations typically result in Lewy body pathology. Genetic testing can identify the LRRK 2 mutation, but it is not possible to diagnose PD with certainty using these tests alone.

- **SNCA:** The first indication of a genetic basis for PD was the finding of mutations in the SNCA gene. Alpha-synuclein, the primary constituent of Lewy bodies and a recognized pathology marker in autopsy slides of Parkinson's disease patient brains, is encoded by this gene. About 2% of familial cases are caused by mutations in the SNCA gene, which include nucleotide changes, duplications, triplications, and extra copies of the SNCA gene. However, not all individuals with these changes have developed PD. For those with mutations in this gene, the average age of onset is 46 years old.

Alpha-synuclein controls neurotransmitter release at the presynaptic terminal, according to recent research. Furthermore, alpha-synuclein's interactions with proteins that control dopamine synthesis and uptake appear to modulate intracellular dopamine concentration.

- **LRRK2 (PARK8):** A signaling protein called LRRK 2 (previously PARK8) can become toxic when it mutates. The dardarin protein is encoded by the LRRK 2 gene. Leucine is an amino acid that is present in high concentration in one area of the dardarin protein. Leucine-rich proteins seem to be involved in processes that need for interactions with other proteins, like signal transmission or the building of the cytoskeleton, which is the structural framework of cells. It is believed that other regions of the dardarin protein are engaged in interactions between other proteins.

The LRRK 2 gene has been found to have almost a dozen distinct mutations. The most frequently known cause of both familial and sporadic PD is mutations in LRRK 2, which affects roughly 5% of people with a family history of the condition and 3% of sporadic cases. One of the two well-known Google co-founders, Sergey Brin, has a known mutation in this autosomal dominant PD gene, which increases his risk of developing PD by 20–80%. At the age of 50, his mother Genia Brin, who also carried the same mutation, was given a PD diagnosis in 1998.

1.5.3. Recessive Genes in PD

Parkinson's disease that develops slowly due to mutations in PARK2 (parkin), PINK1 (PARK 6), and DJ-1 (PARK 7) causes a variable pathology that frequently leaves the remaining neurons without the recognizable Lewy bodies. Remarkably, new research indicates that these genes are involved in mitochondrial function, pointing to a potential shared molecular route for recessive Parkinson's disease.

- **PARK2(Parkin):** One of the biggest human genes, PARK2, codes for the production of a protein called parkin, which aids in the digestion of extraneous proteins. It accomplishes this by attaching molecules known as ubiquitin to both damaged and excess proteins. Unneeded proteins are transferred into specialized cell structures called proteasomes by ubiquitin, where they are broken down.

The ubiquitin-proteasome system eliminates excess, ill-formed, and damaged proteins, functioning as the cell's quality control mechanism. Additionally, this system controls the availability of proteins involved in some vital cell functions, including the timing of cell growth and division. Parkin is a member of the E3 ubiquitin ligases protein family due to its involvement in the ubiquitin-proteasome system.

Parkin seems to play a role in the upkeep of mitochondria, which are the cells' energy-producing organelles. Over the past ten years, research in genetics and cell biology has revealed the critical functions of parkin and PINK1 in the regulation of mitochondrial quality. When PINK1 detects damaged mitochondria, parkin is activated and brought in to break down and recycle the damaged mitochondria. PD may be brought on by flaws in this pathway, according to a wealth of evidence.

The Parkin gene has been extensively studied. The identification of parkin's crystal structure early in 2013 was a major discovery that shed light on the role of this crucial gene. One of the researchers who contributed to the discovery of parkin's crystal structure, Jennifer Johnson, claims that the structure serves as a kind of manual for parkin's functionality. Scientists can precisely observe how it functions, start creating drugs to target dysfunctional areas, and then more accurately determine whether drugs administered to trouble spots are having an impact.

Parkin may play a number of additional roles, according to research on the protein's structure and function. Parkin has the potential to function as a tumor suppressor protein, which means it stops cells from proliferating and dividing uncontrollably or too quickly. Additionally, Parkin may control the release and influx of synaptic vesicles from nerve cells.

The parkin type of juvenile-onset Parkinson's disease, which was first identified in Japan, is distinguished by the typical features of Parkinson's disease and manifests itself between the ages of 20 and 40. The disease progresses slowly, and lower-limb dystonia—a condition in which muscles contract and spasm uncontrollably—is frequently observed. Levodopa response is sustained, and early, frequently serious dopa-induced side effects (e.g., variations, and dyskinesias.

- **PINK1(PARK6):** The PINK1 (PARK6) gene has more than seventy mutations that have been linked to Parkinson's disease. It's interesting to note that giving vitamin K2 to fruit flies with PINK1 mutations improved the insects' ability to produce energy for flight and partially restored energy production in their mitochondria. Because vitamin K2 had improved electron transport in the mitochondria, researchers were able to determine that energy production had been restored. Better adenosine triphosphate (ATP) and energy production for flight resulted from this. Defective mitochondria produce energy in part through the action of vitamin K2. Vitamin K2 may hold out hope for a novel Parkinson's treatment because some Parkinson's patients also have damaged mitochondria.
- **DJ-1(Park7):** The DJ-1 protein is made according to instructions provided by the PARK7 gene. The brain is one of the many tissues and

organs that contain this protein. The protein may have a role in defending against oxidative stress in cells, especially brain cells. When unstable molecules known as free radicals build up to amounts that can harm or even kill cells, oxidative stress takes place. Furthermore, the DJ-1 protein may function as a chaperone molecule, aiding in the proper three-dimensional folding of newly produced proteins as well as the refolding of damaged proteins.

The DJ-1 protein may also help deliver specific proteins to cell structures called proteasomes, which degrade unnecessary molecules. The DJ-1 protein may also be involved in processes that generate and handle RNA, DNA's chemical cousin, according to research.

1.5.4. Genetic Testing

Analyzing human DNA, RNA, and protein is just one of the many methods included in the broad category of genetic testing. Genetic tests are used for nonclinical purposes like paternity testing and forensics, as well as to identify gene variants linked to a particular disease or condition. Genetic testing can be done in a clinical context to:

- Verify a suspected diagnosis
- Anticipate the likelihood of another illness in the future
- Identify carriers (whose children may be at risk)
- Anticipate how a treatment will work.

Genetic tests can be conducted to screen fetuses, newborns, or embryos used in *in vitro* fertilization for genetic defects. Recent advancements have made testing available for the parkin and PINK1 genes. However, testing for parkin can be challenging due to its size. Generally, genetic testing is most informative for individuals who develop the condition before the age of 30. PINK1 is a rare cause of inherited Parkinson's disease, with about 2% of those affected at an early age carrying mutations in the gene. Additionally, genetic testing for the DJ-1 (PARK7), SNCA, and LRRK2 genes is also an option.

By getting in touch with a genetics specialist, people and families interested in genetic testing can find out more about their risk of developing Parkinson's disease as well as the availability and precision of genetic testing. Genetics specialists can talk about the advantages, disadvantages, and restrictions of the various genetic testing options for Parkinson's disease. They can also offer support and information to people or families who may be at risk for inherited diseases or who have genetic disorders.

1.5.5. Gene Therapy

Gene therapy, also known as "the use of genes as medicine," is the process of introducing a functional or therapeutic copy of a gene into particular cells to correct a malfunctioning gene or grant the cell a new function. The most efficient carrier or vector of a therapeutic gene is a tiny virus that elicits no immune response or inflammation.

The viral genetic material of a gene is removed and replaced with the therapeutic gene before the therapeutic gene is implanted into a patient. After that, the modified virus is injected into a particular region of the brain, where its genetic material is deposited. Once inside the brain, it releases its gene and infects the target cells. In Parkinson's disease, which is associated with a dopamine deficiency and is managed with an oral medication, gene injection into a specific region of the brain may enable the cells there to produce more of the neurotransmitter that is lacking. Compared to oral medications, gene therapy offers two advantages:

a. It lessens the negative effects of dopamine replacement therapy, which, when taken orally, activates dopamine receptors throughout the brain and causes undesirable side effects.

b. Compared to an oral tablet, whose levels rise when the medication is taken and then fall as the medication wears off, it may offer a consistent supply of the missing neurotransmitter.

- **Surgical Insertion of Inhibitory Neurotransmitters:** A study at the University of California, San Francisco (UCSF) focused on the subthalamic nucleus, the part of the brain affected by deep brain stimulation in PD. In this gene therapy study, an inhibitory neurotransmitter was surgically implanted into the subthalamic nucleus to reduce its overactivity. Initial tests in animals and a small group of PD patients showed promising results, with significant and lasting improvements. Critics suggested the improvements may have been due to the placebo effect, but the study confirmed the feasibility and safety of gene therapy for PD.
- **AADC Enzyme: Converting Levodopa to Dopamine:** An enzyme that changes levodopa into dopamine has been the subject of other gene therapy experiments. It has long been known by researchers that the reason dopamine replacement therapy becomes less effective after a few years is not because the drug stops working, but rather because the substantia nigra is gradually losing its capacity to produce the enzyme that changes levodopa into dopamine. The second gene therapy study conducted for Parkinson's disease patients was conducted at UCSF, and it centered on the enzyme aromatic acid decarboxylase (AADC), which is responsible for converting levodopa into dopamine.

By introducing a virus that contained the AADC enzyme into a gene, the study participants' brains were injected with the virus in an attempt to restore the brain's capacity to convert levodopa to dopamine. Ten fairly severe Parkinson's disease patients who would have been excellent candidates for deep brain stimulation instead chose to take part in the AADC clinical trial. Several scales were employed by researchers to assess the effectiveness of treatment, such as the United Parkinson's Disease Rating Scale (UPDRS), which demonstrated a roughly 30% improvement after six months. Additionally, there was a reduction in "off" times and an improvement in "on" times for medication fluctuations. It also seemed that enzyme activity increased.

- **Neurturin Gene Therapy:** By injecting a growth/trophic factor, a third gene therapy method based on neurturin aims to "rescue" damaged dopaminergic nerve cells. The intention is to facilitate the self-healing of injured nerve cells. The genes needed to produce neurturin were inserted and the viral genes were eliminated in this gene therapy study. The study participants' brains were then injected with the modified virus.

Twelve patients participated in the phase 1 study and were tracked for a full year. After a year, their UPDRS demonstrated a notable improvement. While the patient's symptoms appeared to improve in the phase 1 trial, the positive outcomes could not be repeated in a larger, phase 2 study, according to the researchers.

1.6. Disease Progression

The presence of specific identifiable symptoms is indicative of Parkinson's disease, also known as Parkinsonism. These include uncontrollable shaking or trembling, disorientation, and trouble speaking. On the other hand, as the illness worsens, the symptoms might change.

Parkinson's disease primarily manifests as uncontrollable shaking and trembling, slowed movement (bradykinesia), trouble balancing, and eventually trouble standing up due to stiffness in the limbs.

1.6.1. Stages of Parkinson's Disease

The "Hoehn and Yahr" stages refer to the five phases of Parkinson's disease. The phases outline Parkinson's disease's movement (motor) symptoms. However, they don't deal with the other symptoms, which include constipation and disturbed sleep. These could manifest years in advance of the movement symptoms. Later on, additional symptoms such as hallucinations and memory issues are more common. Remembering that not everyone goes through every stage is also crucial. Further, every person may experience each stage in a unique way. They serve as a broad guide for what to anticipate when the illness worsens (Hoehn & Yahr,1998).

- **Stage 1:** The mildest stage of Parkinson's is called stage 1. There may be symptoms at this point, but they aren't severe enough to get in the way of everyday activities or way of life in general. In fact, at this point, the symptoms are so slight that they are frequently overlooked. However, your walk, posture, and facial expressions might change, and your family and friends might notice. One characteristic of Parkinson's disease that is unique to stage 1 is that tremors and other movement issues usually only affect one side of the body. At this point, prescribed drugs can effectively minimize and reduce symptoms.
- **Stage 2:** Parkinson's disease is thought to be in a moderate stage at which stage 2 symptoms are significantly more pronounced than those in stage 1. There may be more obvious stiffnessand trembling, as well as changes in facial expressions. Stage 2 does not affect balance, but muscle stiffness makes tasks take longer to complete. Walking difficulties might appear or get worse, and the person's posture might start to shift. At this point, a person may have minimal symptoms on one side of the body and occasionally have trouble speaking. They also experience symptoms on both sides of the body. Most individuals with stage 2 Parkinson's disease are still able to live alone, though they might find that some tasks take longer to finish. Stage 1 to stage 2 development can happen over the course of months or even years. Furthermore, it is impossible to forecast a person's progress.

- **Stage 3:** The third stage of Parkinson's disease is a significant turning point in the disease's course. Numerous symptoms are similar to those in stage 2. But now, a patients have a higher chance of losing their balance and having slower reflexes. They start to move more slowly all around. For this reason, stage 3 falls become more frequent. Even though people can still perform daily tasks, Parkinson's disease has a significant impact on them at this point. Occupational therapy and medication together may help reduce symptoms.
- **Stage 4:** Stage 3 Parkinson's disease differs from stage 4 Parkinson's disease in terms of independence. In stage 4, standing up without support is feasible. But getting around might call for the use of a walker or other assistive technology. At this point in their Parkinson's disease, many people are unable to live alone due to severe reductions in movement and reaction times. Living alone can be risky and may make many daily tasks impossible if one reaches stage 4 or later.
- **Stage 5:** The most advanced stage of Parkinson's disease is called stage 5. It can also be impossible to stand or walk due to freezing when standing due to advanced leg stiffness. At this point, people frequently need wheelchairs and are unable to stand without falling. Assistance is needed around-the-clock in order to prevent falls. Up to 50% of individuals in stages 4 and 5 report having delusions, hallucinations, and confusion. When you see things that aren't there, you experience hallucinations. When you hold false beliefs despite being shown evidence to the contrary, you are said to be delusional. According to the Alzheimer's Association, between 50 and 80% of Parkinson's patients also have dementia. In these later stages, the risks associated with medication often exceed the benefits.

1.6.2. Alternative Rating System

The Hoehn and Yahr rating system is criticized for concentrating only on movement symptoms. Other kinds of symptoms, like intellectual impairment, are linked to Parkinson's disease. As a result, the MDS—Unified Parkinson's disease Rating Scale—may also be used by numerous physicians. Fifty detailed questions about both motor and nonmotor symptoms are included in this rating system. It enables them to rank cognitive issues that could interfere with daily activities and the efficacy of therapy. Although this scale is far more intricate, it is also more comprehensive. It enables medical professionals to consider a more comprehensive picture that looks at the patient's overall health rather than just their motor symptoms.

1.6.3. Non-Motor Symptoms

Parkinson's disease progression is most commonly assessed using motor symptoms, such as tremors and muscle stiffness. Non-motor symptoms are also frequent, though. These symptoms can appear years before Parkinson's disease in some people, and years later in others. The majority of Parkinson's patients also have nonmotor symptoms.

The following are examples of nonmotor symptoms: mood disorders (e.g., anxiety, depression), sleep disorders (e.g., insomnia), fatigue, constipation, vision problems, speech and swallowing difficulties, difficulties with memory or planning, or slowing of thought. For many people, additional treatment may be necessary for nonmotor symptoms. The illness may worsen these symptoms as it goes on. PD can progress in different ways over a period of years or decades. This is dependent in part on when the initial symptoms appear. For instance, it can take 20 years or more for PD symptoms to appear in people who get the disease before the age of 50. This condition is also referred to as "young onset Parkinson's disease (YOPD)."

The condition might advance more quickly if it appears after the age of 50. However, getting to the later stages still frequently takes years. The PD subtype is another factor influencing the course of the condition. Individuals who primarily experience movement symptoms, for instance, might advance more slowly. However, some people may not respond as well to medicine if they have both severe movement and non-movement symptoms from the beginning. Also, PD might advance more quickly in these individuals.

1.7. Pathophysiology

Cell death in the brain's basal ganglia—which, by the end of life, affects up to 70% of the dopamine-secreting neurons in the substantia nigra pars compacta—is the primary pathological feature of PD. Alpha-synuclein gets misfolded and clusters with other alpha-synuclein in Parkinson's disease. The alpha-synuclein turns cytotoxic and damages the cells because the cells are unable to get rid of these clumps. These aggregates, known as Lewy bodies, are visible in neurons when viewed under a microscope. In the substantia nigra, the loss of neurons is correlated with the death of astrocytes, or star-shaped glial cells, and an increase in microglia, another type of glial cell. Braak staging can be used to gauge the degree to which the PD-affected brain regions are progressing. This staging suggests that PD first affects the medulla and olfactory bulb, then progresses to the rest of the midbrain/basal forebrain and the substantia nigra pars compacta. The substantia nigra pars compacta is affected by the disease first, which is when movement symptoms first appear.

The brain's five main pathways link the basal ganglia to other regions of the brain. The motor, oculomotor, associative, limbic, and orbitofrontal circuits are the names given to these. Each circuit's primary projection area is indicated by its name. All are impacted by PD, and their disturbance results in symptoms related to learning, movement, and attention. The motor circuit has undergone the most extensive scientific analysis.

Since 1980, a specific conceptual model of the motor circuit and how it changes with PD has been influential; however, some limitations have been identified, prompting changes. According to this model, the basal ganglia typically have a continuous inhibitory effect on a variety of motor systems, keeping them from activating at the wrong moments. The inhibition for the necessary motor system is decreased when a decision is made to carry out a specific action, freeing it up for activation. Because dopamine helps release inhibition, high dopamine function tends to encourage motor activity, whereas low dopamine function, as in Parkinson's disease, requires more effort for every movement. Dopamine deficiency causes hypokinesia, which is characterized by a general decrease in motor output. On the other hand, medications used to treat PD may cause excessive dopamine activity, which could cause motor systems to fire inappropriately and result in dyskinesias.

1.7.1. Brain Cell Death

One mechanism leading to the death of brain cells is the aberrant build-up in damaged cells of the protein alpha-synuclein bound to ubiquitin. Lewy bodies, or accumulations of this insoluble protein, are found inside neurons. The olfactory bulb, medulla oblongata, and pontine tegmentum are where these bodies initially appear. At this stage, people may not exhibit any symptoms at all or may exhibit early nonmotor symptoms (like loss of smell, difficulty sleeping, or malfunctioning automatically). Lewy bodies appear in the substantia nigra, parts of the midbrain and basal forebrain, and ultimately the neocortex as the disease worsens. The primary locations of neuronal degeneration in PD are these brain regions; however, Lewy bodies may protect against cell death by sequestering or walling off the aberrant protein. Further variations of alpha-synuclein (e.g., oligomers) may actually be the harmful protein forms if they do not congregate into Lewy bodies and Lewy neurites. Lewy bodies are frequently seen throughout cortical regions in dementia patients. Alzheimer's disease-related neurofibrillary tangles and senile plaques are rare unless the patient has dementia. Additional mechanisms include decreased activity of the mitochondria and malfunctions of the lysosomal and proteasomal systems. Protein inclusions are usually seen in conjunction with iron accumulation in the substantia nigra. The mechanisms are unknown, but they may be connected to protein aggregation, oxidative stress, and neuronal death.

1.7.2. Neuroimmune Interaction

In PD pathology, the neuroimmune interaction is strongly implicated. Genetic variants and molecular pathways are shared by PD and autoimmune disorders. As much as 33% higher chance of Parkinson's disease has been linked to certain autoimmune diseases. PD is associated with autoimmune diseases that are connected to the protein expression profiles of monocytes and $CD4^+$ T cells. Alpha-synuclein-related autoimmune reactions can be brought on by herpes virus infections, possibly as a result of molecular mimicry of viral proteins. Microglia can bind to alpha-synuclein and its aggregate form, known as Lewy bodies. Alpha-synuclein binding to MHC receptors on inflammasomes can cause microglia to proliferate and become hyperactivated, which in turn releases proinflammatory cytokines such as TNFα, interferon-γ (IFNγ), and IL-1β.

The activation of astrocytes is influenced by activated microglia, which changes their neuroprotective phenotype to a neurotoxic one. In a healthy brain, astrocytes guard the connections between neurons. Astrocytes are unable to shield the striatal dopaminergic connections in Parkinson's disease. T cells are exposed to antigens by microglia through MHCI and MHCII. This process activates $CD4^+$ T cells, enabling them to cross the blood-brain barrier (BBB) and release more pro-inflammatory cytokines, such as IL-1β, TNFα, and IFNγ. The BBB breakdown in Parkinson's disease is linked to mast cell degranulation and the release of proinflammatory cytokines that follow. Peripheral monocytes, another immune cell linked to PD, are discovered in the substantia nigra of PD patients. These monocytes may cause additional disruption of dopaminergic connections. Furthermore, through vasodilation, monocytes isolated from PD patients express higher levels of the PD-associated protein, LRRK2, than do non-PD patients. Furthermore, elevated levels of pro-inflammatory cytokines, like IL-6, can cause the liver to produce C-reactive protein, another protein that is frequently detected in PD patients, which can exacerbate peripheral inflammation. The gut-brain axis, a region of the body strongly linked to Parkinson's disease, can be impacted by peripheral inflammation. Years before motor difficulties manifest, people with PD have altered gut microbiota and colon issues. The gut produces alpha-synuclein, which can move from there to the brainstem and substantia nigra through the vagus nerve.

1.8. Neuropathology

In idiopathic Parkinson's disease, the brain is typically unremarkable macroscopically, showing mild frontal cortex atrophy and occasionally ventricular dilatation. In transverse sections of the brainstem, where nearly all cases present with loss of the darkly pigmented area in the substantia nigra pars compacta (SNpc) and locus coeruleus, the main distinctive morphological change in the PD brain is observed. The death of noradrenergic neurons in the locus coeruleus and dopaminergic (DA) neuromelanin-containing neurons in the SNpc is directly correlated with this loss of pigmentation. Other neuronal and glial cell types in the SNpc are mainly spared, with cell death primarily confined to a subset of neuromelanin-containing dopaminergic neurons, known as the A9 neurons (Figure 1.2) (KouliA,TorsneyKM; 2018Dec21).

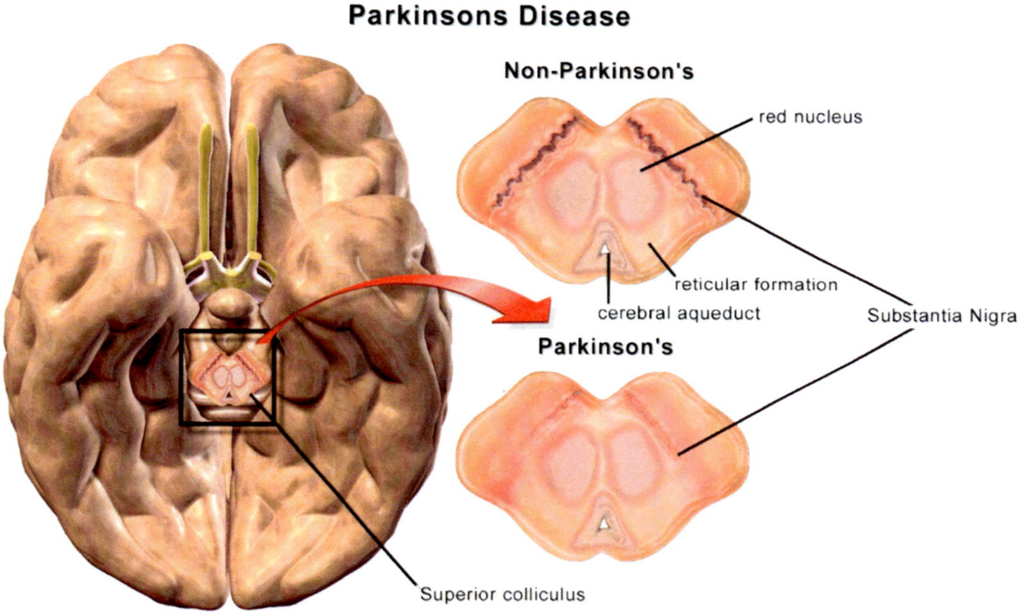

Figure 1.2. *Parkinson's Disease.*

Source: By BruceBlaus. When using this image in external sources it can be cited as:Blausen.com staff (2014). "Medical gallery of Blausen Medical 2014." WikiJournal of Medicine 1 (2). DOI:10.15347/wjm/2014.010. ISSN 2002-4436. – Own work, CC BY 3.0, https://commons.wikimedia.org/w/index.php?curid=27924394.

After controlling for age, quantitative morphometric studies in postmortem Parkinson's disease brains have estimated that, by the time motor symptoms start, there will be about 30% less DA neurons in the SNpc. The degree of motor feature severity and the length of the disease are closely correlated with the increase in nigral DA neuron loss, which can reach 60% or more after the onset of motor symptoms. The nigrostriatal pathway is denerved as a result of this extraordinary cell loss, which lowers dopamine levels in the striatum. The emergence of the cardinal motor symptoms in PD is thought to be caused by a decrease in dopaminergic signaling. Recent research has demonstrated that the loss of axon terminals that project to the striatum occurs prior to nerve cell death in the SNpc. Mechanistically, the early loss of neurons and axon terminals seen in PD points to a significant preclinical stage that occurs several years before symptoms manifest.

In addition to the SNpc, many subcortical nuclei exhibit extensive cell loss: the locus coereleus, the Meynert nucleus basalis, the vagus nerve's dorsal motor nucleus, the pedunculopontine nucleus, the raphe nuclei, the hypothalamus, and the olfactory bulb. There is an impact on several non-dopaminergic neurotransmitter systems, including the glutamatergic, cholinergic, adenosinergic, GABAergic, noradrenergic, serotonergic, and histaminergic systems. It is believed that some of the non-motor symptoms of PD that do not improve with dopamine replacement therapy are caused by degeneration in those systems. It is still not entirely clear, though, what specific pathological mechanisms underlie the non-motor symptoms of Parkinson's disease.

1.8.1. Lewy Body Pathology

The presence of aberrant cytoplasmic deposits within neuronal cell bodies that are immunoreactive for the protein α-synuclein is the pathological hallmark of PD under a microscope. Lewy bodies (LBs) are pathological protein aggregates that are frequently accompanied by dystrophic neurites (Lewy neurites), which are primarily axonal.

Intracytoplasmic inclusions known as LBs have a granular and fibrillar core encircled by a halo. An LB's diameter can range from 5 to 30 μm, and multiple LBs can be present within a single neuron. The literature has described two types of LBs: cortical and classical brainstem LBs. The primary morphological differences are that cortical LBs are typically smaller, lack the halo, and have less definite outlines. Sometimes referred to as "pale bodies," structures in the SN that resemble cortical LBs are thought to be LB precursors.

Filamentous α-synuclein is a protein that is widely expressed in the brain and is the main structural element of leukemia bodies. It develops an amyloid-like filamentous structure, becomes aberrantly phosphorylated, and aggregates in PD and other synucleinopathies. The main component of an LB's halo is α-synuclein. Proteins like ubiquitin, tau, parkin, heat shock proteins (HSPs), oxidized/nitrated proteins, cytoskeletal proteins (like neurofilaments, MAPs, and tubulin), proteasomal and lysosomal elements, and others are among the molecular components of an LB, aside from α-synuclein.

1.8.2. Braak Staging

PD pathology's primary staging system was first presented by Braak and team in 2003. This was predicated on a large autopsy series' semiquantitative postmortem evaluation of the LB distribution. This research demonstrated that LB pathology propagates in a chronologically predictable manner rostrocaudally throughout the brain. LB lesions are primarily seen in the reticular formation, anterior olfactory nucleus, and dorsal motor nucleus (IX/X) at Braak stages 1 and 2. Patients are regarded as asymptomatic or presymptomatic at these stages, despite the possibility that they may exhibit some early non-motor symptoms, primarily autonomic (e.g., constipation), smell-related, and sleep-associated disorders. The SNpc becomes involved as the disease worsens (Stage 3), and melanized neurons show signs of LB pathology and neuronal loss. At this point, the pathology also affects the amygdala and the locus coeruleus. At Stage 4, it eventually reaches the temporal limbic cortex or transentorhinal region. The typical clinical motor features start to show during stages 3 and 4. The involvement of the entire neocortex and high-order areas, such as the prefrontal cortex and primary sensory and motor areas, is the crucial characteristic during stages 5 and 6. Clinically, this is believed to result in dementia and severe Parkinson's disease with major gait abnormalities. The Braak hypothesis was later modified to suggest that the olfactory bulb and the enteric cell plexuses, which are nasal and intestinal mucosal sites, may actually be the initial sites of α-synuclein-associated pathology (also known as the "dual-hit hypothesis"). The Braak staging system has generated debate ever since it was introduced in 2003. A fraction of PD brains, according to later research, do not seem to fit this pattern, and attempts to link Braak staging to clinical dysfunction have also proven fruitless. One more critique of the Braak system is that its foundation is the distribution of Lewy-related pathology rather than the loss of neurons.

1.8.3. α-Synuclein and Lewy Body Distribution Outside the Brain

There have also been observations of phosphorylated α-synuclein histopathology outside of the brain. It is specifically located in the cervical and thoracic sympathetic ganglia as well as the spinal cord. Additionally, α-synuclein deposition is seen in several peripheral organs, such as the uterus, skin, retina, bladder, and heart ventricles, as well as portions of the cardiovascular system and the gastrointestinal tract, specifically the stomach, bowels, and submandibular gland. This suggests that the peripheral nervous system is heavily involved in PD and begs the question of where the pathology caused by α-synuclein originates—in the periphery or in the brain? A full truncal vagotomy is linked to a lower risk of developing PD in the future, according to a Danish epidemiological study. This finding has sparked interest in the potential involvement of the gut-brain axis in the pathophysiology of PD.

1.8.4. Interaction of α-Synuclein with Other Proteins

One common characteristic of many neurodegenerative diseases, including AD and PD, is protein misfolding within specific brain regions. Thus, "proteinopathy" is a general term that is frequently used to describe these illnesses. The important characteristic that distinguishes each proteinopathy is the type of protein and the distinctive distribution of the pathology. However, it is now becoming more and more obvious that the various diseases frequently overlap with one another and that the pathogenic, misfolded forms of proteins interact with one another. Aging may be a factor in this phenomenon, as it is well known that aberrant protein accumulation can happen with aging even in the absence of neurodegenerative disease. Growing evidence now indicates that distinct aggregated forms of proteins with different molecular pathways clearly interact with one another in the context of PD.

Tau, which is encoded by the MAPT gene, is one such protein. Tau can become abnormally hyperphosphorylated in pathological circumstances, resulting in intracytoplasmic inclusions known as neurofibrillary tau tangles (NFTs). These aggregates, along with amyloid-β plaques, are indicative of AD. But aberrant tau protein has also been connected to Parkinson's disease. Particularly, in the striatum of patients with PD and PD dementia, postmortem investigations have shown a marked increase in tau hyperphosphorylation at Ser262 and Ser396/404. Additional evidence supporting this comes from studies on animals, which demonstrate that tau hyperphosphorylation can be induced *in vivo* and *in vitro* by elevated α-synuclein expression. Moreover, genome-wide association studies revealed a robust association between MAPT and the risk of PD, and later longitudinal research demonstrated that the MAPT H1/H1 haplotype is a powerful predictor of the early onset of PD dementia.

It has also been reported that amyloid-β and α-synuclein interact. In a subset of Parkinson's disease patients, cortical deposition of α-synuclein has been linked to the development of amyloid-β plaques. Furthermore, in some PD patients who develop cognitive dysfunction and dementia, but not all of them, NFTs and amyloid-β senile plaques are widespread at postmortem (Barker et al, 2015).

1.9. Causes of Neuron Death

The primary cause of neuronal loss in Parkinson's disease is apoptosis, as demonstrated by postmortem studies that found apoptotic chromatin alterations and DNA fragmentation in the dopaminergic neurons of patients with the disease. Additionally, postmortem and *in vitro* studies that demonstrated elevated activity of caspase-3 and increased expression of active caspase-3 in the substantia nigra pars compacta confirmed the role of apoptosis in the pathogenesis of Parkinson's disease. Moreover, in cell models of Parkinson's disease, overexpression of anti-apoptotic proteins like Bcl-2 inhibits dopaminergic neuronal death. The idea that apoptosis is the primary mechanism of neuronal death in Parkinson's disease is further supported by the discovery that caspase inhibitors can prevent neurons in cell models of the disease from dying. In postmortem brain tissue from Parkinson's disease patients, there have also been observed increased levels of proapoptotic proteins, including Bax.

Although there is evidence to suggest that Parkinson's disease may involve the extrinsic apoptotic pathway, its exact function is still unknown. An underlying theory of neuronal death is that the intrinsic apoptotic pathway is involved. In Parkinson's disease, mitochondria-mediated apoptosis has been thoroughly investigated. It involves a series of events that include activation of caspase-9 and caspase-3, release of cytochrome c, increased generation of reactive oxygen species, and depletion of ATP. How various pathogenic processes of PD, like α-synuclein aggregation and mitochondrial dysfunction, interact to lead to apoptotic cell death are still unknown. Some of the potential causes of apoptosis in Parkinson's disease are covered in the remaining sections of this article. α-synuclein's interaction with the mitochondrial membrane, nuclear DNA mutations, the accumulation of mitochondrial DNA deletions, and other mechanisms leading to mitochondrial dysfunction are among them.

The central nervous system exhibits high levels of α-synuclein expression, especially in presynaptic regions. It has a propensity for fibrillar aggregation, which contributes significantly to the formation of Lewy bodies, the pathological hallmark of Parkinson's disease. In the brains of patients with Parkinson's disease, rodents treated with mitochondrial toxins, and cells treated with α-synuclein, aggregates and inclusions form. When dopaminergic neurons accumulate wild-type α-synuclein, mitochondrial complex I activity is reduced and reactive oxygen species production is elevated. This effect is accentuated when the aggregation-prone mutant A53T α-synuclein is expressed. Additionally, α-synuclein has been demonstrated to localize to the mitochondrial membrane in isolated rat brain mitochondria and SHSY cells overexpressing wild-type or A53T mutant α-synuclein. *in vitro* systems, this interaction has been suggested to cause oxidative stress and release cytochrome c into the cytosol. Cytochrome c is released into the cytoplasm where it interacts with antiapoptotic, pro-survival proteins to cause mitochondria-mediated apoptosis.

In fact, mitochondrial dysfunction may manifest as early symptoms of Parkinson's disease in both humans and animal models. Patients with Parkinson's disease have been found to have substantia nigra defects related to defects in mitochondrial complex I activity. Reactive oxygen species are produced as a result of dopamine metabolism, and this may reduce the threshold for apoptotic cell death. Monoamine oxidase (MAO) breaks down dopamine enzymatically to produce H_2O_2, which is then converted to reactive oxygen species. Dopamine degradation products experience autoxidation, which increases the production of reactive oxygen species. Because of this, nigral dopaminergic neurons are especially vulnerable to mitochondrial complex I dysfunction, which is thought to be one of the main causes of reactive oxygen species in Parkinson's disease.

Therefore, the generation of reactive oxygen species could be a significant mechanism influencing the apoptosis of dopaminergic neurons. It has been suggested that deficiencies in the function of mitochondrial complex I may heighten the vulnerability of dopaminergic neurons to degeneration by reducing the threshold for the activation of the intrinsic apoptotic pathway.

Dopaminergic nigral neurons selectively degenerate through apoptosis in response to several mitochondrial toxins, supporting the notion that these neurons are especially vulnerable to mitochondrial dysfunction. These include rotenone, 6-hydroxydopamine (6-OHDA), 1-methyl-4-phenyl-1,2,3,6-tetrahydropyridine (MPTP), and 6-hydroxydopamine (6-OHDA), which block mitochondrial complex I, resulting in mitochondrial dysfunction and reactive oxygen species production.

It has been proposed that dopamine itself inhibits mitochondrial complex I, causing dysfunction in the mitochondria.

It experiences autoxidation, which results in an overabundance of toxic metabolites being produced. This causes oxidative stress, mitochondrial swelling, and the opening of the mitochondrial transition pore, which releases factors that are pro- and antiapoptotic. Consequently, the intrinsic apoptotic pathway is triggered by the release of cytochrome c into the cytosol. Moreover, there is a noteworthy rise in p53 phosphorylation linked to it, which may trigger apoptosis. Antioxidants reinforce the idea that reactive oxygen species play a key role in dopamine-induced apoptosis by preventing the activation of caspase-9 and caspase-3 and preventing apoptosis in response to dopamine exposure.

Furthermore, dopamine-induced apoptosis can be somewhat attenuated by overexpressing the antiapoptotic factor Bcl2.

A selective dopaminergic neurotoxin, MPTP targets neurons in the substantia nigra pars compacta. Lipophilic in nature, MPTP actively penetrates the blood-brain barrier to reach the central nervous system, where it is converted to MPP+ (1-methyl-4-phenylpyridinium), its active metabolite. The glial cells' own MAO is responsible for this conversion. MPP+ accumulates in the mitochondria of dopaminergic neurons after being reabsorbed by the dopamine transporter. This inhibits the mitochondrial complex I, which causes ATP depletion and a rise in reactive oxygen species production.

Consequently, caspase-mediated apoptotic pathways cause the death of nigrostriatal dopaminergic neurons. Reactive oxygen species generation, cytochrome c release, p53 expression, caspase-3 cleavage, DNA fragmentation, and other morphological characteristics typical of apoptosis are the hallmarks of MPTP-induced apoptosis. Overexpression of Bcl-2 attenuates MPTP-induced apoptosis.

In a similar vein, rotenone inhibits mitochondrial complex I, which causes oxidative stress and an excess of reactive oxygen species. Consequently, ATP levels are depleted, which causes caspase-dependent apoptosis mediated by the mitochondria to selectively degenerate nigrostriatal dopaminergic neurons.

6-OHDA inhibits mitochondrial complex I, activates caspase-3 and caspase-9, and induces

Bax.Caspase-6 inhibitors reduce the amount of dopaminergic neuronal degeneration caused by OHDA. Moreover, 6-OHDA triggers apoptosis through a mechanism that is dependent on mitochondria. These nigral toxin models provide information about the vulnerability of nigral neurons to mitochondria-mediated apoptosis, even though they may not be entirely representative of the pathogenic mechanisms that are present in patients.

Genes linked to the health and function of mitochondria cause mutations that give rise to several inherited forms of Parkinson's disease.

These include, for instance, mutations in DJ-1, PINK1, LRRK2, Parkin, and LRRK2. These mutations provide some supporting evidence that nigral neurons are vulnerable to mitochondrial damage and mitochondria-mediated apoptosis and that these processes may be relevant in idiopathic Parkinson's disease, even though they are uncommon in the population with Parkinson's disease.

Numerous roles that parkin plays may be important in the etiology of Parkinson's disease. It can encourage, for instance, the transcription of mitochondrial genes, mtDNA replication, and mitochondrial biogenesis.

For mitochondrial respiration and function, Parkin is therefore essential. Furthermore, as an E3 ubiquitin protein ligase, Parkin selects specific substrates—such as the glycosylated form of α-synuclein—for ubiquitin-proteasome system degradation.

Parkinson's disease-causing toxic protein aggregates are believed to be partly built up by the loss of Parkin activity. It's interesting to note that Parkin functions downstream of PINK1, a mitochondrial kinase related to early-onset Parkinson's disease that can result from mutations in an autosomal recessive familial form.

Overexpression of Parkin can compensate for PINK1 mutations, which serves as evidence for this. The PINK1-Parkin pathway may contribute to a person's vulnerability to mitochondria-mediated apoptosis, although it is unclear how these mutations cause Parkinson's disease pathology. PINK1 of the wild-type, for instance, is upregulated, which decreases caspase activation and cytochrome C release.

Parkinson's disease with an early onset can be brought on by mutations in DJ1, which is found in the intermembranous space and mitochondrial matrix. When wild-type DJ1 is overexpressed, it can protect against free radical-associated injury, but DJ1 deficiency increases vulnerability to such harm.

Increased oxidative stress is a consequence of DJ1 mutations. Furthermore, the antiapoptotic protein mitochondrial Bcl-XL is bound very tightly by mutant DJ-1. This causes Bax to separate from Bcl-XL and enrich it in the outer mitochondrial membrane, which in turn causes dopaminergic neuronal degeneration through mitochondria-mediated apoptosis.

Research conducted *in vitro* has indicated that Parkinson's disease is caused by a toxic gain of function caused by mutations in the LRRK2 gene. A mutation in LRRK2 can result in abnormal dynamics and morphology of the mitochondria and raise the production of reactive oxygen species within cells. It has been proposed that dopaminergic neurons die due to mitochondria-mediated apoptosis brought on by LRRK2 mutations after mitochondrial dysfunction. Overexpression of mutant LRRK2 can cause apoptosis *in vitro*, while caspase inhibitors and genetic ablation of Apaf1 can stop cell death.

Mitochondrial DNA deletions have been found in aging and Parkinson's disease patients, particularly in nigrostriatal dopaminergic neurons. This may make these neurons more prone to apoptosis triggered by mitochondria. The exact mechanisms leading to mitochondrial DNA deletions are not fully understood, but oxidative stress could be a contributing factor. When both mitochondrial DNA depletion and deletion occur (without changes in overall mitochondrial mass), it can lead to impaired mitochondrial function and integrity, raising the chances of cytochrome c release and apoptosis. There is also a rare form of inherited Parkinson's disease caused by mutations in the nuclear gene encoding DNA polymerase G (POLG), which is crucial for the expression of several genes in mitochondrial DNA. (Hoehn et al, 1998; Barker et al, 2015; Simon et al, 2020)

A Closer Look

Histopathology

In Parkinson's disease patients, dopamine pigment loss in the substantia nigra is readily apparent. Histologically, PD is distinguished by alpha-synuclein neuronal inclusions in Lewy bodies and Lewy neurites, which are neuronal cell processes. Lewy-related pathology is the term sometimes used to describe the combination of Lewy bodies and Lewy neurites. Selective loss of neurons is a defining feature of all neurodegenerative diseases, and in Parkinson's disease, this loss is most prominent in the substantia nigra pars compacta. However, it has long been known that Lewy bodies in PD extend well beyond the substantia nigra. Braak and colleagues have proposed a PD staging scheme based on the distribution of alpha-synuclein pathology. According to this plan, neuronal pathology starts early in the anterior olfactory nucleus in the olfactory bulb and the dorsal motor nucleus of the vagus in the medulla. As the illness worsens, dopaminergic neurons in the substantia nigra and locus ceruleus neurons in the pons are impacted. Later stages of the pathology affect the medial temporal lobe structures, the amygdala, and the basal forebrain; convexity cortical areas are affected in the final stages. It has since been suggested that the involvement of the central nervous system (CNS) may have an impact on autonomic neurons in the peripheral nervous system. This has led to the realization that PD is a multiorgan disease process rather than just a CNS disorder. Furthermore, it has fueled discussions about the possibility of unknown transmissible agents traveling from the gut to the brain via the vagus nerve's retrograde transmission.

Summary

- PD affects 1–2 per 1000 of the population at any time. PD prevalence is increasing with age and PD affects 1% of the population above 60 years. The main neuropathological finding is α-synuclein-containing Lewy bodies and loss of dopaminergic neurons in the substantia nigra, manifesting as reduced facilitation of voluntary movements.
- Although gender-specific differences reveal more variability than association with increasing age, PD appears to be slightly more common in men than in women in most studies, usually ranging from a 1.2:1 ratio up to a 1.5:1 ratio.
- Geographic variations in the frequency of PD have been reported. For instance, in door-to-door surveys, crude prevalence is 15 per 100,000 in China, 328 per 100,000 in India, 131 per 100,000 in Mississippi, USA, and 657 per 100,000 in Argentina.
- Scientists believe a combination of genetic and environmental factors are the cause of PD. PD is an extremely diverse disorder. While no two people experience Parkinson's the same way, there are some commonalities.
- Known risk factors associated with PD include toxins, traumatic brain injury (TBI), cancer, illicit substances, and cardiovascular risk factors. Protective factors associated with PD include smoking, exercise, medication, and nutrition.
- A gene family is a group of genes that share important characteristics. The PARK gene family has been of particular interest and is the focus of widespread research. Mutations in PARK genes affect the function and survival of nerve cells critical for normal movement, balance, and coordination.
- The main pathological characteristics of PD are cell death in the brain's basal ganglia (affecting up to 70% of the dopamine-secreting neurons in the substantia nigra pars compacta by the end of life). In Parkinson's disease, alpha-synuclein becomes misfolded and clump together with other alpha-synuclein.
- Macroscopically, the brain in idiopathic PD is often unremarkable with mild atrophy of the frontal cortex and ventricular dilation in some cases. The main distinctive morphological change in the PD brain is observed in transverse sections of the brainstem, where almost all cases present with loss of the darkly pigmented area in the substantia nigra pars compacta (SNpc) and locus coeruleus.
- Apoptosis is the main mechanism of neuronal loss in Parkinson's disease, as evidenced by the identification of DNA fragmentation and apoptotic chromatin changes in dopaminergic neurons of Parkinson's disease patients in postmortem studies.

References

1. Abbott, R. D., Petrovitch, H., White, L. R., Masaki, K. H., Tanner, C. M., Curb, J. D., Grandinetti, A., Blanchette, P. L., Popper, J. S., & Ross, G. W. (2001). Frequency of bowel movements and the future risk of Parkinson's disease. *Neurology, 57*(3), 456–462.

2. Aharon-Peretz, J., Rosenbaum, H., & Gershoni-Baruch, R. (2004). Mutations in the glucocerebrosidase gene and Parkinson's disease in Ashkenazi Jews. *New England Journal of Medicine, 351*, 1972–1977. https://doi.org/10.1056/NEJMoa033277.

3. Alves, G., Muller, B., Herlofson, K., Hogen Esch, I., Telstad, W., Aarsland, D., Tysnes, O. B., & Larsen, J. P. (2009). Incidence of Parkinson's disease in Norway: The Norwegian ParkWest study. *Journal of Neurology, Neurosurgery & Psychiatry, 80*(8), 851–857. https://doi.org/10.1136/jnnp.2008.168211.

4. Barker, R. A., Drouin-Ouellet, J., & Parmar, M. (2015). Cell-based therapies for Parkinson disease—past insights and future potential. *Nature Reviews Neurology, 11*, 492–503. https://doi.org/10.1038/nrneurol.2015.123.

5. Bellou, V., Belbasis, L., Tzoulaki, I., Evangelou, E., & Ioannidis, J. P. (2016). Environmental risk factors and Parkinson's disease: An umbrella review of meta-analyses. *Parkinsonism & Related Disorders, 23*, 1–9. https://doi.org/10.1016/j.parkreldis.2015.12.008.

6. Bereczki, D. (2010). The description of all four cardinal signs of Parkinson's disease in a Hungarian medical text published in 1690. *Parkinsonism & Related Disorders, 16*, 290–293. https://doi.org/10.1016/j.parkreldis.2009.11.006.

7. Braak, H., Del Tredici, K., Rüb, U., de Vos, R. A., Jansen Steur, E. N., & Braak, E. (2003). Staging of brain pathology related to sporadic Parkinson's disease. *Neurobiology of Aging, 24*, 197–211. https://doi.org/10.1016/S0197-4580(02)00065-9.

8. Brandt-Christensen, M., Kvist, K., Nilsson, F. M., Andersen, P. K., & Kessing, L. V. (2006). Use of anti-Parkinsonian drugs in Denmark: Results from a nationwide pharmacoepidemiologic study. *Movement Disorders, 21*, 1221–1225.

9. Brundin, P., Barker, R. A., & Parmar, M. (2010). Neural grafting in Parkinson's disease: Problems and possibilities. *Progress in Brain Research, 184*, 265–294. https://doi.org/10.1016/S0079-6123(10)84014-2.

10. Freed, C. R., Greene, P. E., Breeze, R. E., Tsai, W. Y., DuMouchel, W., Kao, R., et al. (2001). Transplantation of embryonic dopamine neurons for severe Parkinson's disease. *New England Journal of Medicine, 344*, 710–719. https://doi.org/10.1056/NEJM200103083441002.

11. Gilks, W. P., Abou-Sleiman, P. M., Gandhi, S., Jain, S., Singleton, A., Lees, A. J., Shaw, K., Bhatia, K. P., Bonifati, V., Quinn, N. P., Lynch, J., Healy, D. G., Holton, J. L., Revesz, T., & Wood, N. W. (2005). A common LRRK2 mutation in idiopathic Parkinson's disease. *Lancet, 365*(9457), 415–416. https://doi.org/10.1016/S0140-6736(05)17830-1.

12. Goetz, C. G. (2011). The history of Parkinson's disease: Early clinical descriptions and neurological therapies. *Cold Spring Harbor Perspectives in Medicine, 1*(1), a008862. https://doi.org/10.1101/cshperspect.a008862.

13. Guo, J. L., & Lee, V. M. (2014). Cell-to-cell transmission of pathogenic proteins in neurodegenerative diseases. *Nature Medicine, 20*, 130–138. https://doi.org/10.1038/nm.3457.

14. Hoehn, M. M., & Yahr, M. D. (1998). Parkinsonism: Onset, progression, and mortality. *Neurology, 50*(2), 318.

15. Horsfall, L., Petersen, I., Walters, K., & Schrag, A. (2013). Time trends in incidence of Parkinson's disease diagnosis in UK primary care. *Journal of Neurology, 260*, 1351–1357.

16. Hristova, D., Zachariev, Z., Mateva, N., & Grozdev, I. (2010). Incidence of Parkinson's disease in Bulgaria. *Neuroepidemiology, 34*, 76–82.

17. Kouli, A., Torsney, K. M., & Kuan, W. L. (2018). Parkinson's disease: Etiology, neuropathology, and pathogenesis. In T. B. Stoker & J. C. Greenland (Eds.), *Parkinson's Disease: Pathogenesis and Clinical Aspects* [Internet]. Codon Publications. https://doi.org/10.15586/codonpublications.parkinsonsdisease.2018.ch1 (accessed on 12 July 2024).

18. Kyrozis, A., Ghika, A., Stathopoulos, P., Vassilopoulos, D., Trichopoulos, D., & Trichopoulou, A. (2013). Dietary and lifestyle variables in relation to incidence of Parkinson's disease in Greece. *European Journal of Epidemiology, 28*, 67–77.

19. Le, W. D., Xu, P., Jankovic, J., Jiang, H., Appel, S. H., Smith, R. G., et al. (2003). Mutations in NR4A2 associated with familial Parkinson disease. *Nature Genetics, 33*, 85–89. https://doi.org/10.1038/ng1066.

20. Leentjens, A. F., Vanden Akker, M., Metsemakers, J. F., & Troost, J. (2003). The incidence of Parkinson's disease in the Netherlands: Results from a longitudinal general practice-based registration. *Neuroepidemiology, 22*, 311–312.

21. Liu, B., Fang, F., Pedersen, N. L., Tillander, A., Ludvigsson, J. F., Ekbom, A., et al. (2017). Vagotomy and Parkinson disease: A Swedish register-based matched-cohort study. *Neurology, 88*, 1996–2002. https://doi.org/10.1212/WNL.0000000000003961.

22. Mao, X., Ou, M. T., Karuppagounder, S. S., Kam, T. I., Yin, X., Xiong, Y., et al. (2016). Pathological α-synuclein transmission initiated by binding lymphocyte-activation gene 3. *Science, 353*, pii: aah3374.

23. Morioka, S., Sakata, K., Yoshida, S., et al. (2002). Incidence of Parkinson disease in Wakayama, Japan. *Journal of Epidemiology, 12*, 403–407.

24. Nalls, M. A., Pankratz, N., Lill, C. M., Do, C. B., Hernandez, D. G., Saad, M., et al. (2014). Large-scale meta-analysis of genome-wide association data identifies six new risk loci for Parkinson's disease. *Nature Genetics, 46*, 989–993. https://doi.org/10.1038/ng.3043.

25. Nutt, J. G., Burchiel, K. J., Comella, C. L., Jankovic, J., Lang, A. E., Laws, E. R., Jr, et al. (2003). Implanted intracerebroventricular glial cell line-derived neurotrophic factor. Randomized, double-blind trial of glial cell line-derived neurotrophic factor (GDNF) in PD. *Neurology, 60*, 69–73. https://doi.org/10.1212/WNL.60.1.69.

26. Przedborski, S. (2017). The two-century journey of Parkinson disease research. *Nature Reviews Neuroscience, 18*, 251–259. https://doi.org/10.1038/nrn.2017.25.

27. Rajan, S., & Kaas, B. (2022). Parkinson's disease: Risk factor modification and prevention. *Neurology, 42*(5), 626–638. https://doi.org/10.1055/s-0042-1758780.

28. Raudino, F. (2012). The Parkinson disease before James Parkinson. *Neurological Sciences, 33*, 945–948. https://doi.org/10.1007/s10072-011-0816-9.

29. Simon, D. K., Tanner, C. M., & Brundin, P. (2020). Parkinson disease epidemiology, pathology, genetics, and pathophysiology. *Clinical Geriatrics Medicine, 36*(1), 1–12. https://doi.org/10.1016/j.cger.2019.08.002.

30. Tan, L. C., Venketasubramanian, N., Jamora, R. D., & Heng, D. (2007). Incidence of Parkinson's disease in Singapore. *Parkinsonism & Related Disorders, 13*, 40–43.

31. Tang, B., Xiong, H., Sun, P., Zhang, Y., Wang, D., Hu, Z., et al. (2006). Association of PINK1 and DJ-1 confers digenic inheritance of early-onset Parkinson's disease. *Human Molecular Genetics, 15*, 1816–1825. https://doi.org/10.1093/hmg/ddl104.

32. Van Den Eeden, S. K., Tanner, C. M., Bernstein, A. L., et al. (2003). Incidence of Parkinson's disease: variation by age, gender, and race/ethnicity. *American Journal of Epidemiology, 157*, 1015–1022.

33. Vives-Bauza, C., Zhou, C., Huang, Y., Cui, M., de Vries, R. L., Kim, J., et al. (2010). PINK1-dependent recruitment of Parkin to mitochondria in mitophagy. *Proceedings of the National Academy of Sciences of the United States of America, 107*, 378–383. https://doi.org/10.1073/pnas.0911187107.

34. Winter, Y., Bezdolnyy, Y., Katunina, E., et al. (2010). Incidence of Parkinson's disease and atypical parkinsonism: Russian population-based study. *Movement Disorders, 25*, 349–356.

35. Zhang, Z. X., Roman, G. C., Hong, Z., Wu, C. B., Qu, Q. M., Huang, J. B., et al. (2005). Parkinson's disease in China: prevalence in Beijing, Xian, and Shanghai. *Lancet, 365*, 595–597. https://doi.org/10.1016/S0140-6736(05)70801-1.

36. Zhang, Z., Dong, Z., & Roman, G. C. (2006). Early descriptions of Parkinson disease in Ancient China. *Archives of Neurology, 63*, 782–784. https://doi.org/10.1001/archneur.63.5.782.

Chapter

2

CLINICAL DIAGNOSIS OF PARKINSONISM AND TREMOR

Contents

Introduction

Clinical diagnosis of tremor disorders and Parkinsonism requires a detailed process that incorporates physical examination, medical history, and occasionally additional testing. Parkinsonism is a term used to describe a group of motor symptoms that includes bradykinesia, tremor, rigidity, and postural instability. It also includes PD and related syndromes. Different from Parkinsonism, tremor disorders can only manifest with tremor as the main characteristic. Making the distinction between these conditions is essential for the proper course of action.

Examining the patient's entire medical history is the first step in the diagnostic process. Doctors ask about the beginning, course, and contributing variables, including family history, drug use, and exposure to toxins. Differentiating Parkinsonism from other tremor disorders is made easier by having an understanding of the temporal sequence of symptoms. Furthermore, the existence of non-motor symptoms like autonomic dysfunction or cognitive impairment may offer more diagnostic hints. A physical examination is essential for determining the characteristics of tremor and motor symptoms. A tremor's resting, postural, or kinetic observations aid in identifying the underlying pathology. A standardized method for measuring symptom severity and tracking the course of Parkinsonism is the Unified Parkinson's Disease Rating Scale (UPDRS).

Moreover, structural abnormalities and dopaminergic function can be assessed using neuroimaging studies such as magnetic resonance imaging (MRI) and dopamine transporter (DAT) scans. These tests help to confirm the diagnosis and rule out other possible causes of tremor or Parkinsonism. Laboratory tests may be performed in addition to clinical evaluations to screen for conditions such as metabolic or inflammatory disorders that may mimic tremor disorders or Parkinsonism. Additionally, genetic testing might be necessary, especially in situations where there is a family history of movement disorders or early-onset symptoms.

Comprehensive management requires a multidisciplinary approach involving allied health professionals, neurologists, and movement disorder specialists. The goal of treatment is to manage symptoms, and methods that may be used to achieve this goal include medication, deep brain stimulation (DBS), physical therapy, and supportive care. Clinical diagnosis of tremor disorders and Parkinsonism requires a methodical approach that incorporates examination, history, and auxiliary investigations. Tailored management strategies that maximize patient outcomes and quality of life are made possible by accurate diagnosis. Our knowledge and treatment of these intricate neurological disorders are constantly being improved by ongoing research and developments in diagnostic techniques.

Orientation and Directional Terms

Terms	**Definition**	**Illustration**
Clinical diagnosis	A clinical diagnosis is a process of identifying and detecting the nature of a disorder or illness.	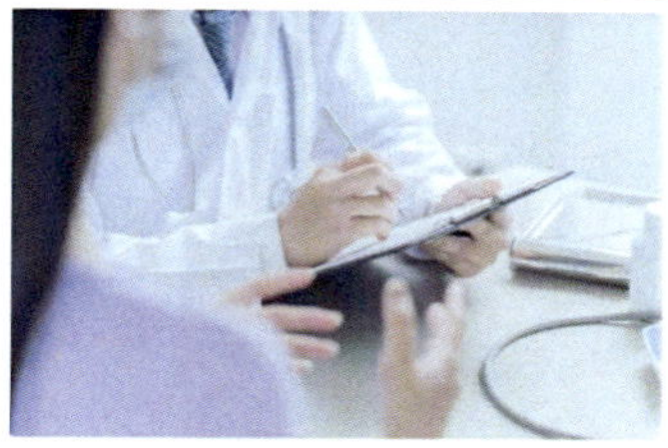
Tremor	It is a neurological condition that includes shaking or trembling movements in one or more parts of the body, most commonly affecting a person's hands.	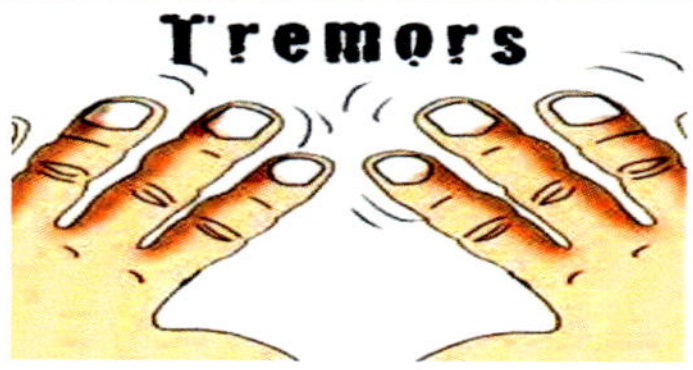
Dopamine transporter	The dopamine transporter (DAT) is a presynaptic monoamine transporter that mediates dopamine reuptake from the synapse.	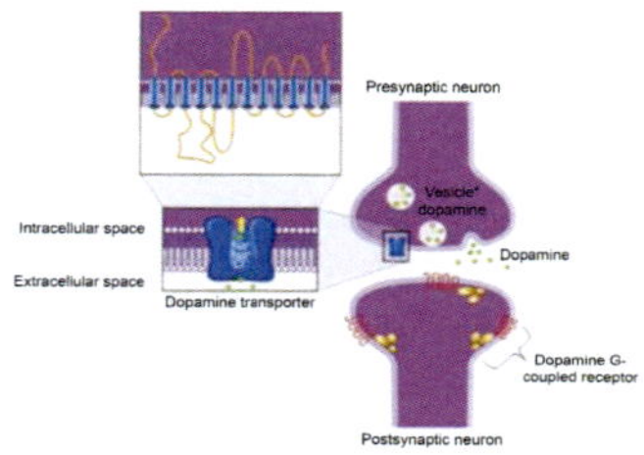
Lewy bodies	Lewy bodies are clumps of abnormal protein particles that, for reasons that are not fully understood, accumulate in the brain.	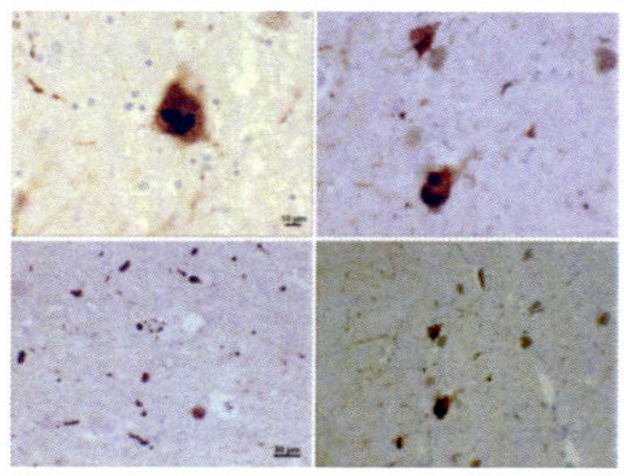
Akinesia	Akinesia is a term for the loss of the ability to move your muscles voluntarily. It's most often described as a symptom of PD.	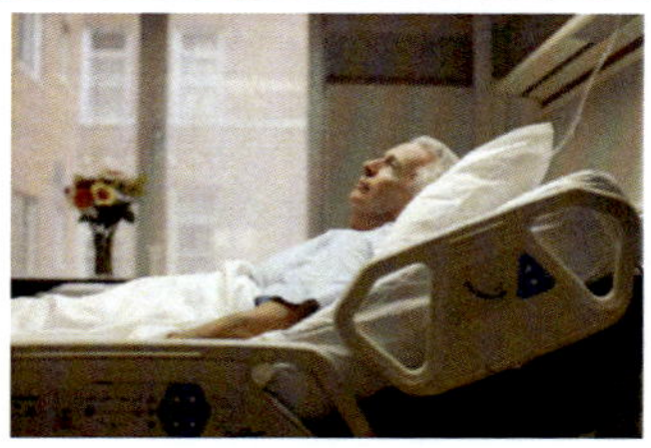

2.1. Clinical Diagnosis of Parkinsonism

A collection of neurological conditions known as Parkinsonism are distinguished by a mix of deviant movements, including tremors, rigidity, bradykinesia (slowness of movement), and postural instability. PD is the most common cause of Parkinsonism, but other conditions known as atypical Parkinsonism or Parkinson-plus syndromes can also cause similar symptoms. To determine whether motor symptoms are present and how severe they are, a physical examination is essential. In addition to evaluating the patient's posture, gait, and coordination, the clinician will check for bradykinesia, rigidity, and tremor.

A standardized instrument for assessing the intensity of motor symptoms and monitoring the course of the disease over time is the Unified Parkinson's Disease Rating Scale (UPDRS). Tremor is most frequently felt when at rest. It is commonly described as a rhythmic shaking and usually affects the hands, though it can also affect the jaw or legs. The term "rigidity" describes limb stiffness or resistance to passive movement, which can result in a restricted range of motion. Bradykinesia causes slowness of movement, which makes even easy things like walking and buttoning shirts difficult. Postural instability frequently develops later in the course of the illness, impairing balance and coordination. Parkinsonism frequently presents non-motor symptoms as well as motor symptoms. These can include mood swings, autonomic dysfunction, cognitive impairment, and sleep difficulties. These non-motor symptoms may occasionally occur before motor symptoms do, and they can have a major negative influence on a patient's quality of life. A thorough evaluation of symptoms, a medical history, exposure to toxins or medications, and the existence of other medical conditions that may exacerbate symptoms will all be questioned by the clinician.

Even though a clinical evaluation is essential, more research might be required to confirm the diagnosis of Parkinsonism and distinguish it from other disorders with comparable symptoms. The dopamine system is frequently linked to Parkinson's disease, so neuroimaging studies like magnetic resonance imaging (MRI) or dopamine transporter (DAT) scans may be carried out to check for structural abnormalities or changes in the system. Furthermore, laboratory tests may be conducted to rule out other potential causes of Parkinsonism, including blood tests to assess thyroid function, vitamin B12 levels, and markers of inflammation. When a person has early-onset symptoms or a family history of Parkinsonism, genetic testing may also be taken into consideration.

Clinical findings, medical history, and, in certain situations, supportive laboratory or imaging studies are used to diagnose Parkinsonism. To maximize patient outcomes and quality of life, appropriate treatment and management strategies must be started as soon as possible. Furthermore, it is essential to provide multidisciplinary care and continuous monitoring to meet the complex and changing needs of people with Parkinsonism.

2.1.1. How Parkinson's Disease is Diagnosed?

It can be difficult to make a precise diagnosis of Parkinson's disease. To reach a decision, doctors must carefully consider symptoms, family history, and other variables. According to specialists at the Johns Hopkins Parkinson's Disease and Movement Disorders Center, the current standard diagnosis of Parkinson's disease is clinical. This indicates that no test, like a blood test, can provide a definitive result. Rather, a person's condition must meet specific physical criteria in order to be classified as

Parkinson's disease. Patients with very early Parkinson's disease may not meet the clinical diagnosis criteria because there is no definitive screening or test. Conversely, because of this lack of specificity, it is possible to receive a Parkinson's disease diagnosis and then learn that you actually have a condition that looks similar to the disease (Figure 2.1).

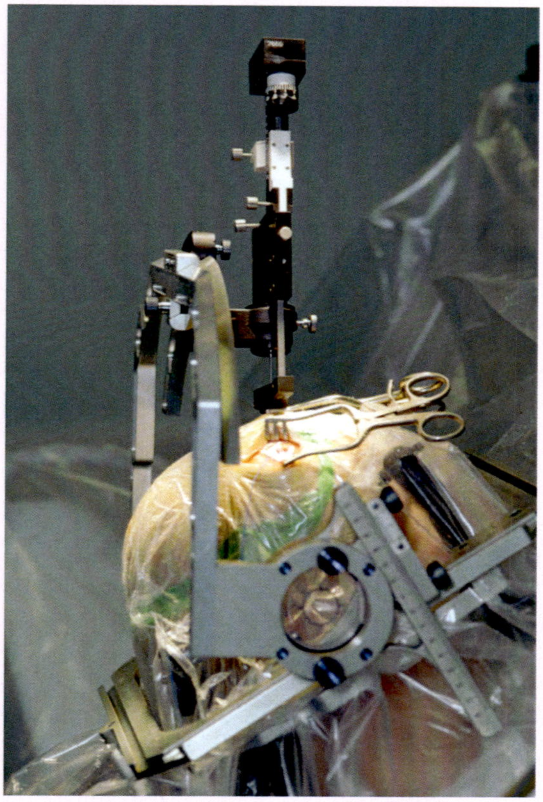

Figure 2.1. *Parkinson's disease diagnosis and treatment.*

Source: CC BY-SA 3.0, https://commons.wikimedia.org/w/index.php?curid=180597.

- ***New Diagnostic Standards for Parkinson's:*** The U.S. developed the gold-standard diagnostic checklist. The Brain Bank of the Parkinson's Disease Society. Doctors used a checklist to assess whether the symptoms they observed were consistent with the illness. However, that's now regarded as antiquated. The International Parkinson and Movement Disorder Society has recently adopted new criteria. The information on this list represents the state of knowledge as of right now. It enables medical professionals to make a more precise diagnosis, enabling patients to start treatment earlier.
- ***What Doctors Look for When Diagnosing Parkinson's:*** A patient will typically decide to visit a doctor in response to specific physical signs and symptoms that they or their loved ones have noticed.

These are the symptoms most often noticed by patients or their families:

- Shaking or tremor: Called resting tremor, a trembling of a hand or foot that happens when the patient is at rest and typically stops when he or she is active or moving
- Bradykinesia: Slowness of movement in the limbs, face, walking or overall body
- Rigidity: Stiffness in the arms, legs or trunk
- Posture instability: Trouble with balance and possible falls

Once the patient is at the doctor's office, the physician:

- Takes a medical history and does a physical examination.
- Asks about current and past medications. Some medications may cause symptoms that mimic Parkinson's disease.
- Performs a neurological examination, testing agility, muscle tone, gait and balance.

2.1.2. Symptoms and Causes of Parkinson's Disease

Parkinson's disease is a progressive neurological disorder that affects the nervous system and the body's nerve-controlled regions. Symptoms develop gradually. An almost imperceptible tremor in one hand may be the initial symptom. In addition to tremors, the disorder can also cause stiffness or slower movements.

In the early stages of Parkinson's disease, you may have a reduced facial expression. Your arms may not swing freely as you walk, and you may begin to speak more slowly or with a slur. As Parkinson's disease progresses, so do its symptoms. While there is currently no known cure for Parkinson's disease, medication can significantly reduce symptoms. In some cases, a medical professional may recommend surgery to target specific brain regions and alleviate symptoms.

- **Symptoms:** Each person may experience Parkinson's disease symptoms differently. Early signs might not be noticeable or be mild. Even after symptoms start to affect the limbs on both sides, they typically start on one side of the body and tend to stay worse there.

Parkinson's symptoms may include:

- ***Tremor:*** Rhythmic shaking, called tremor, usually begins in a limb, often your hand or fingers. You may rub your thumb and forefinger back and forth. This is known as a pill-rolling tremor. Your hand may tremble when it's at rest. The shaking may decrease when you are performing tasks.
- ***Slowed Movement, Known as Bradykinesia:*** Over time, Parkinson's disease may slow your movement, making simple tasks difficult and time-consuming. Your steps may become shorter when you walk. It may be difficult to get out of a chair. You may drag or shuffle your feet as you try to walk.
- ***Rigid Muscles:*** Muscle stiffness may occur in any part of your body. The stiff muscles can be painful and limit your range of motion.
- ***Impaired Posture and Balance:*** Your posture may become stooped. Or you may fall or have balance problems as a result of Parkinson's disease.
- ***Loss of Automatic Movements:*** You may have a decreased ability to perform unconscious movements, including blinking, smiling or swinging your arms when you walk.
- ***Speech Changes:*** You may speak softly or quickly, slur, or hesitate before talking. Your speech may be more of a monotone rather than have the usual speech patterns.
- ***Writing Changes:*** It may become hard to write, and your writing may appear small.
- **Causes:** Parkinson's disease is characterized by the progressive degeneration or death of specific brain cells known as neurons. The loss of neurons in the brain that generate the chemical messenger dopamine is the cause of many Parkinson's symptoms. Reduced dopamine levels lead to erratic brain activity, which exacerbates movement disorders and other Parkinson's disease symptoms.

The cause of Parkinson's disease is unknown, but several factors appear to play a role, including:

- ***Genes:*** Researchers have identified specific genetic changes that can cause Parkinson's disease. But these are uncommon except in rare cases with many family members affected by Parkinson's disease.

However, certain gene variations appear to increase the risk of Parkinson's disease but with a relatively small risk of Parkinson's disease for each of these genetic markers.

- ***Environmental Triggers:*** Exposure to certain toxins or environmental factors may increase the risk of later Parkinson's disease, but the risk is small.

Researchers also have noted that many changes occur in the brains of people with Parkinson's disease, although it's not clear why these changes occur. These changes include:

- ***The presence of Lewy Bodies:*** Clumps of specific substances within brain cells are microscopic markers of Parkinson's disease. These are called Lewy bodies, and researchers believe these Lewy bodies hold an important clue to the cause of Parkinson's disease.
- ***Alpha-Synuclein is Found Within Lewy Bodies:*** Although many substances are found within Lewy bodies, scientists believe that an important one is the natural and widespread protein called alpha-synuclein, also called a-synuclein. It's found in all Lewy bodies in a clumped form that cells can't break down. This is currently an important focus among Parkinson's disease researchers. Researchers have found the clumped alpha-synuclein protein in the spinal fluid of people who later develop Parkinson's disease.

2.1.3. Risk Factors

Risk factors for Parkinson's disease include:

- **Age:** Young adults rarely experience Parkinson's disease. It ordinarily begins in middle or late life, and the risk increases with age. People usually develop the disease around age 60 or older. If a young person does have Parkinson's disease, genetic counseling might help make family planning decisions. Work, social situations and medicine side effects are also different from those of an older person with Parkinson's disease and require special considerations.
- **Heredity:** Having a close relative with Parkinson's disease increases the chances that you'll develop the disease. However, your risks are still small unless you have many relatives in your family with Parkinson's disease.
- **Sex:** Men are more likely to develop Parkinson's disease than women.
- **Exposure to Toxins:** Ongoing exposure to herbicides and pesticides may slightly increase your risk of Parkinson's disease.

1. ***Complications:*** Parkinson's disease is often accompanied by these additional problems, which may be treatable:

- **Thinking Difficulties:** You may experience cognitive problems, such as dementia, and thinking difficulties. These usually occur in the later stages of Parkinson's disease. Such cognitive problems aren't usually helped by medicines.

- **Depression and Emotional Changes:** You may experience depression, sometimes in the very early stages. Receiving treatment for depression can make it easier to handle the other challenges of Parkinson's disease.

You also may experience other emotional changes, such as fear, anxiety or loss of motivation. Your healthcare team may give you medicine to treat these symptoms.

- **Swallowing Problems:** You may develop difficulties with swallowing as your condition progresses. Saliva may accumulate in your mouth due to slowed swallowing, leading to drooling.
- **Chewing and Eating Problems:** Late-stage Parkinson's disease affects the muscles in the mouth, making chewing difficult. This can lead to choking and poor nutrition.
- **Sleep Problems and Sleep Disorders:** People with Parkinson's disease often have sleep problems, including waking up frequently throughout the night, waking up early or falling asleep during the day.

People also may experience rapid eye movement sleep behavior disorder, which involves acting out dreams. Medicines may improve your sleep.

- **Bladder Problems:** Parkinson's disease may cause bladder problems, including being unable to control urine or having difficulty in urinating.
- **Constipation:** Many people with Parkinson's disease develop constipation, mainly due to a slower digestive tract.

You may also experience:

- **Blood Pressure Changes:** You may feel dizzy or lightheaded when you stand due to a sudden drop in blood pressure (orthostatic hypotension).
- **Smell Dysfunction:** You may experience problems with your sense of smell. You may have trouble identifying certain odors or the difference between odors.
- **Fatigue:** Many people with Parkinson's disease lose energy and experience fatigue, especially later in the day. The cause isn't always known.
- **Pain:** Some people with Parkinson's disease experience pain, either in specific areas of their bodies or throughout their bodies.
- **Sexual Dysfunction:** Some people with Parkinson's disease notice a decrease in sexual desire or performance.

2. ***Prevention:*** There is no known cause of Parkinson's disease, therefore there are no effective methods to stop it from happening. Regular aerobic exercise may lower the risk of Parkinson's disease, according to some research. Further studies have revealed that those who drink caffeine, which is present in coffee, tea, and cola, have a lower incidence of Parkinson's disease than non-drinkers. There is also a link between drinking green tea and a lower chance of Parkinson's

disease. It is still unknown, though, whether coffee prevents Parkinson's disease or if it has some other connection. At the moment, there is insufficient data to support the idea that consuming coffee might prevent Parkinson's disease.

2.2. Parkinsonism and Tremor Disorders. a Clinical Approach

Tremor is a prominent feature of a spectrum of neurological conditions known as Parkinsonism and tremor disorders. These conditions are characterized by abnormalities in movement. PD and other atypical Parkinsonism syndromes are examples of Parkinsonism. The condition is characterized by tremor, rigidity, bradykinesia, and postural instability. On the other hand, tremor disorders can manifest as a single tremor without the whole range of Parkinsonian symptoms.

When treating Parkinsonism and tremor disorders clinically, a thorough evaluation is necessary to differentiate between different etiologies and adjust treatment plans accordingly. To rule out secondary causes, this assessment entails a detailed review of the patient's medical history, a thorough physical examination that focuses on motor symptoms and other neurological signs, and occasionally additional investigations like neuroimaging or laboratory testing.

It can be challenging to distinguish idiopathic Parkinson's disease from other Parkinsonism causes, such as vascular Parkinsonism, progressive supranuclear palsy, and multiple system atrophy. According to clinicopathological investigations, 76% of cases of idiopathic Parkinson's disease can be correctly diagnosed clinically. Furthermore, particularly in the early stages of the disease, it may be difficult to distinguish between essential tremor or drug-induced Parkinsonism and tremor-prominent Parkinsonism clinically. Given the distinct clinical progression of these disorders, it is imperative for the clinician to address the concerns of the patient and family regarding prognosis from a solid diagnostic basis.

Subsequently, there have been significant advancements and modifications in our comprehension of the etiology, clinical characteristics, and management of the illness bearing his name. There are no biological markers available to diagnose this condition, so the diagnosis is still based on clinical presentation. The majority of patients have an easy time being diagnosed with idiopathic Parkinson's disease. However, a lot of patients, especially in the early stages of the disease, have diagnostic challenges related to Parkinsonism and tremor disorders. Clinico-pathological investigations have revealed that 24% of patients who receive a clinical diagnosis of idiopathic Parkinson's disease (from a geriatrician or neurologist) actually have a different diagnosis because they do not meet the pathological criteria. The primary pathological diagnoses in such cases are vascular disease, multiple system atrophy, and progressive supranuclar palsy. When compared to a clinical setting, the pathological studies introduce bias because they do not include essential tremor or drug-induced Parkinsonism.

First, there are differences in clinical progress and survival from the more benign essential tremor through idiopathic Parkinson's disease to multiple system atrophy or progressive supranuclar palsy. This is why it is important to differentiate between idiopathic Parkinson's disease and other causes of Parkinsonism and tremor disorders, especially in the early stages. As a result, the clinician should respond to the patient's and family's concerns regarding the prognosis and offer precise prognostic information. Second, the initiation and modification of medication therapy are customized based on the state and advancement of the patient, e.g., Levodopa withdrawal is an option for patients with a revised diagnosis of essential tremor who were previously suspected of having idiopathic Parkinson's disease. Ultimately, a precise diagnosis would define a patient cohort for clinical research studies and aid in understanding the etiology and pathophysiology of various causes of Parkinsonism and tremor disorders.

2.2.1. Definition and Classification of Parkinsonism

Bradykinesia, or slowness of movement, hypokinesia, or reduced movement, akinesia, or loss of movement, rigidity, or increased resistance to passive extension and flexion, and tremor, or mainly occurring during rest, are the clinical symptoms of Parkinsonism.

Parkinsonism may be classified as:

1. Idiopathic Parkinson's disease, of unknown etiology.
2. Parkinsonism as part of other neurodegenerative disorders, such as MSA, and PSP.
3. Parkinsonism with identifiable causes, such as VP and DIP.

Idiopathic PD: Parkinsonism in PD patients is pathologically marked by a loss of neurons in the substantia nigra along with Lewy bodies. Lewy bodies have also been found in other conditions, including MSA, PSP, and Lewy body dementia. Lewy bodies may also be discovered by chance in older patients who do not exhibit any clinical symptoms of Parkinson's disease; these cases likely indicate pre-clinical or early stages of the disease.

Idiopathic Parkinson's disease is the common cause of Parkinsonism, with an annual incidence of 20.5 per 100,000 of the population and a prevalence of 164 per 100,000. The prevalence of the disease increases with age from 47 per 100,000 for ages 40–49 years, to 832 per 100,000 for 70–79 years. The mean age at the onset of PD is between 55–65 years, with a slight male predominance of 60%, and the mean age of death is 75.5 years.

Most Parkinson's Disease patients do not have a family history of Parkinsonism. However, some patients, particularly those with early-onset disease, may have the familial form of Parkinsonism if they have a positive family history. Numerous genetic variations have been discovered, including the autosomal recessive and dominant forms of the parkin gene. Lewy bodies are absent in some of these cases. In the ensuing years, our knowledge of Parkinsonism's genetics would change our perception of the disease's etiology.

Typically, patients arrive with nonspecific aches and pains, stiffness, handwriting abnormalities, or a general slowing down. Examination typically reveals reduced voice volume, loss of facial expression, loss of arm swing, tendency to drag a leg, trouble moving the hands, lead-pipe rigidity or cog-wheel rigidity if tremor is superimposed, and tremor that is mostly at rest.

Asymmetric onset is present in 72% of the patients. 70% of patients have tremor as their presenting feature; 42% have tremor only, without bradykinesia or rigidity; and 11% have tremor dominant disease, or Benign Tremulous Parkinson's disease, as it is known.

Tremor dominant disease has a better prognosis than akinetic rigid presentation. Patients experience swallowing and speech problems in the later stages of Parkinson's disease. Additionally, up to 40% of late features include dementia, autonomic dysfunction, falls, and gait issues. Levodopa therapy works for almost all PD patients.

2.2.2. Multiple System Atrophy (MSA)

MSA is a neurodegenerative disease with a sporadic adult onset. It's a clinicopathological entity that can manifest as any combination of autonomic dysfunction, Parkinsonism, and cerebellar and/or pyramidal signs. In many brain structures, including the substantia nigra, striatum, locus coeruleus, pontine nuclei, cerebellar Purkinje cells, inferior olives, and Onuf's nucleus in the spinal cord, it is pathologically characterized by cell loss, gliosis, and α-synuclein positive oligodendroglial cytoplasmic inclusions.

The following subtypes of MSA have been defined in a clinicopathological study:

1. Shy-Drager syndrome, in which autonomic failure predominates.
2. Striatonigral degeneration, in which Parkinsonism predominates.
3. Olivopontocerebellar atrophy, in which cerebellar features predominate.

However, Oertel and Quinn argue against using the term Shy-Drager syndrome because autonomic dysfunction is almost universal in MSA.

They define MSA subtypes as follows:

1. Striatonigral degeneration (MSA-Parkinsonian type or MSA-P).
2. Sporadic olivopontocerebellar atrophy (MSA cerebellar type or MSA-C).

Although exact incidence statistics for this disorder are unknown, it has been hypothesized that MSA accounts for 3–6% to 22% of incident cases of Parkinsonism. Two to four times as many people have MSA-P as MSA-C. With a mean age of onset of 54 years, a mean age at death of 60 years, and a mean illness duration of 6–9 years, MSA is slightly more common in male patients.

Nearly all patients typically have autonomic dysfunction, with impotence being the most prevalent symptom in men. Other symptoms include urinary incontinence, urinary retention, and postural faintness.

Pyramidal signs are evident in 50% of MSA patients, and cerebellar signs, primarily gait ataxia, are present in half of the cases. Most patients have Parkinsonism; akinesia is the most common symptom, rest tremor occurs in less than half of cases, and classical pill-rolling tremor is observed in only 10% of patients. Stridor and spasms in the muscles were additional symptoms, although MSA rarely causes dementia. Levodopa only produces a response in about one-third of patients, and this is typically not long-lasting.

- ***Progressive Supranuclear Palsy (PSP) or Steele-Richardson-Olszewski Syndrome:*** Progressive supranuclear palsy was the term given by Steele, Richardson, and Olszewski in 1964 to describe the clinical and pathological characteristics of nine patients with a progressive disorder of vertical gaze, axial rigidity, dysarthria, pseudobulbar palsy, and mild dementia. Neurofibrillary tangles, neuropil threads, and tufted astrocytes are pathological features of PSP that are found in the pallidum, subthalamic nucleus, substantia nigra, midbrain, and pontine reticular formation. The atypical histopathological inclusions consist of tau phosphoprotein aggregates that are insoluble. The pathological characteristic of PSP is tau-positive glial inclusions.

It typically manifests in the seventh decade and is slightly more common in males. More than half of the patients present with postural instability and falling, while one-third have dysarthria. About 15% of patients initially experience visual disturbances such as diplopia, blurred vision, burning eyes, and light sensitivity. Changes in cognition or behavior typically ensue. Additional clinical features include dysphagia, neck dystonia, frontal lobe symptoms, bilateral bradykinesia, axial rigidity, dysphonic, palilalia, ataxic, and incoherent speech, and personality changes. The primary clinical characteristic of PSP that is most significant is vertical downward palsy. Even though upward gaze and convergence are affected, other disorders of the basal ganglia and aging also cause this. The disorder is supranuclear because the oculocephalic maneuver is preserved (except very advanced stages). Additional ocular symptoms include blepharospasm, apraxia of opening or closing the eyes, diminished pupillary light reflexes, lid retraction, a significantly lower blink rate, supranuclear ophthalmoplegia, and the absence of Bell's phenomenon. The patient's expression becomes stunned, fixed, and staring as a result of these changes. A few pathologically proven cases of PSP have been reported, although down-gaze palsy is a necessary finding to secure the diagnosis. These cases do not exhibit this abnormality during life.

- ***Vascular Parkinsonism (VP):*** When Critchley (1929) outlined five distinct clinical presentation types of what was then known as arteriosclerotic Parkinsonism, the concept of VP was born. The primary clinical signs were short-stepping gait, rigidity, and fixed faces. Additional features included pseudo-bulbar, dementia, incontinence, and pyramidal or cerebellar signs. Critchley renamed the illness arteriosclerotic pseudo-Parkinsonism in 1981 after multiple clinical investigations in the 1960s and 1970s revealed no connection between arteriosclerosis and Parkinson's disease. The idea of VP was resurrected with the advent of CT and MRI, however, there are currently no widely recognized clinical standards for diagnosing this illness.

Several clinical characteristics link brain vascular lesions to Parkinsonism. a gradual onset of Parkinsonism that can occasionally be mistaken for PD, including a levodopa reaction. Conversely, vascular lesions in the basal ganglia caused two patients to present with acute onset Parkinsonism; however, recovery without anti-Parkinsonian medication had been documented. Another term for patients with VP is lower body Parkinsonism (LBP), which refers to a subset of patients—likely hypertensive—who typically have absent tremor, symmetrical rigidity, difficulty with gait, and no or minimal response to levodopa therapy.

Two studies examined the relationship between vascular risk factors and ischemic stroke; in one, PD patients had a lower incidence of ischemic stroke than controls, but in the other, an association was discovered. Therefore, PD and cerebrovascular disease may coexist, but due to the distinct risk factors associated with each condition, there may be a decreased likelihood of a coincidental relationship. There is clear evidence from post-mortem studies that patients with Parkinsonism may have cerebrovascular disease but no pathological features of Parkinson's disease, and that patients with PD may also have this condition. LBP provides the most lucid clinical description of Parkinsonism in relation to cerebrovascular disease. Nonetheless, patients with less than pure lower body features may have vascular etiology, and upper body signs and symptoms are not ruled out in these cases.

- ***Essential Tremor (ET):*** The most prevalent movement disorder is essential tremor, which is estimated to affect 4 to 39 people per 1000 people worldwide. There are roughly 23 cases per 100,000 people each year. Men and women are equally affected by a bimodal distribution with peaks in the second and fifth decades, according to some studies, but familial cases tend to start earlier and typically occur around 45 years of age. In a study of 20 kindreds, there was no indication that the disease skipped a generation, indicating autosomal dominant inheritance. Penetrance is typically complete by the age of 65. But as of yet, no single gene has been found to be responsible.

The tremor usually affects the hands and forearms, is postural (occurs when one voluntarily maintains one's position against gravity), rarely goes away, and is usually exacerbated by emotion. It begins sporadically and eventually becomes permanent. There may then be tremors in the legs, voice, head, and tongue. Unlike Parkinsonian tremor, which primarily affects muscles that are fully supported against gravity while at rest, ET occurs in these muscles during activity. Even though this description suggests that the tremor types are clearly separated, there is frequently some overlap, which makes ET one of the conditions that is most frequently misdiagnosed as PD, especially by less experienced doctors. "No single type of tremor can be pathognomonic of a particular disorder" is an important reminder to keep in mind. The literature contains contradictory information regarding the relationship between ET and PD; some studies find no evidence of a relationship, while other studies provide evidence in support of the opposite conclusion. ET does not have any particular pathological characteristics.

A review of all service-based and community-based published studies of familial aggregation in ET revealed that a range of 17–100% of patients reported affected relatives, clearly suggesting variation in data collection techniques. It is commonly stated that 30–50% of ET patients have an affected relative. Furthermore, even though ET is benign and has no effect on life expectancy, it can cause social embarrassment and impair bodily functions like eating, drinking, and writing. Due to the disability brought on by the tremor, up to 15% of patients retire early. After drinking alcohol, up to 50–66% of ET patients report that their tremor has improved. This was also noted for Parkinsonian tremor in one study, but it wasn't repeated in another.

- ***Drug-Induced Parkinsonism (DIP):*** The most common adverse effect of neuroleptics is DIP. o10-15% of psychotic patients receiving these medications may develop Parkinsonism as a result of either phenothiazines or non-phenothiazines. Parkinsonism can be brought on by anti-emetic medications like metoclopramide and prochlorperazine. DIP has also been associated with other medications, including tetrabenazine, sodium valproate, and calcium channel blockers like cinnarizine. It can be challenging to distinguish DIP-unmasked Parkinson's disease from pure DIP, particularly since DIP can take months or even years to reverse after the offending drug is stopped. The best course of treatment for DIP is obviously to stop the offending drug, but this can be challenging, particularly when using neuroleptic medications. Amantadine, pyridoxine, and anticholinergic drugs may be able to lessen Parkinsonian symptoms in DIP patients.

2.3. Diagnosis and Treatment of Tremor in Parkinson's Disease Using Mechanical Devices

The degeneration of dopamine neurons in the substantia nigra is the main characteristic of PD, a progressive degenerative disorder. Tremor, stiffness, bradykinesia, akinesia, and postural instability are some of its primary symptoms. One of Parkinson's disease's most prevalent motor symptoms is tremor. Patients with predominant akinesia/rigidity, or akinetic-rigid type (ART), and those with a tremor-dominant type (TDT) are the two subtypes of PD. Compared to TDT-PD, PD-ART shows more cognitive impairment and advances more quickly. Given their importance in identifying the illness and its symptoms, it is necessary to comprehend the status of tremors. Normal individuals can exhibit mild physiological tremors that are not pathological. Over 0.4% of people have pathological tremor, and as people age, both the incidence and prevalence of the condition rise significantly.

The precise underlying mechanism of tremor is unknown, and it can be caused by a wide range of conditions. Of these, PD patients are more likely to experience incidental tremors, such as essential tremor (ET), which is a major differential diagnosis. The sole bilateral upper limb movement tremor that has been present for at least three years without the presence of any other neurologic symptoms is the hallmark of ET, according to the 2018 Movement Disorders Consensus Criteria. Tremor in patients with ET and PD can occasionally be confusing. PD is a complicated neurodegenerative illness that is typically accompanied by tremor, postural instability, muscular rigidity, and asymmetrical onset bradykinesia. Except in the early stages, patients with PD exhibit resting tremor in addition to other symptoms. Walking and carrying out activities like calculating can frequently make resting tremors worse. On the other hand, kinetic tasks tend to exacerbate tremor severity in ET patients. Medical interviews, physical examinations, and blood tests should rule out other common causes of action tremors, such as hyperthyroidism or the side effects of specific medications, even in the absence of a test to confirm the diagnosis.

A neurologist's physical examination serves as the basis for tremor assessment. Current movement disorder scales, such as the Fahn–Tolosa–Marin scale, the Unified Parkinson's disease Rating Scale (UPDRS), and the essential tremor rating assessment scale, are primarily used to help with the phenomenological demonstration of tremor. Accurately diagnosing the various tremor types is crucial for treatment, which may vary depending on the unique etiology of each type. However, 20–30% of cases may result in a misdiagnosis of tremor due to confusion between PD and ET. For this reason, technological solutions may enhance diagnosis quality and enable the measurement of disease stage.

Researchers have looked closely at wearable technology in the past few years to determine the difference between patients with PD and healthy people, as well as between these patients and people with ET. The accuracy of these diagnostic methods has increased significantly with the application of cutting-edge technologies like machine learning. Even for experts, diagnosing PD can be challenging at times. The aforementioned methods help. Researchers are also looking into wearable sensor-based technologies for tremor assessment and monitoring. Unlike assessments conducted at clinics and other facilities, which consist of a time-limited snapshot, monitoring reflects routine symptoms.

These assessments are now feasible and simpler to manage thanks to well-known gadgets like smartphones and smartwatches.

Given that tremor is merely one PD symptom (e.g., motor, and non-motor symptoms), it is important to assess each symptom to determine the patient's overall health. The main treatment for PD in terms of tremors is medication. Another useful treatment for medically refractory tremors is deep brain stimulation (DBS). About 30% of tremor patients either do not respond to pharmaceutical intervention or have intolerable side effects. The detection of tremors using local field potential (LFP) is a potentially noteworthy upcoming technique in DBS. This tremor detection technique will be available in adaptive DBS (aDBS), which functions on the principle of closed-loop interaction. Electrical muscle stimulation (EMS) has the potential to be a safer alternative to deep brain stimulation (DBS) for treating symptoms while minimizing side effects. One approach to tremor suppression with EMS involves the use of orthoses. Another common technique involves estimating the tremor and applying a reverse cancellation signal. EMS also includes a closed-loop system that detects tremors and stimulates them accordingly, effectively suppressing tremors (Fujikawa, 2023) (Figure 2.2).

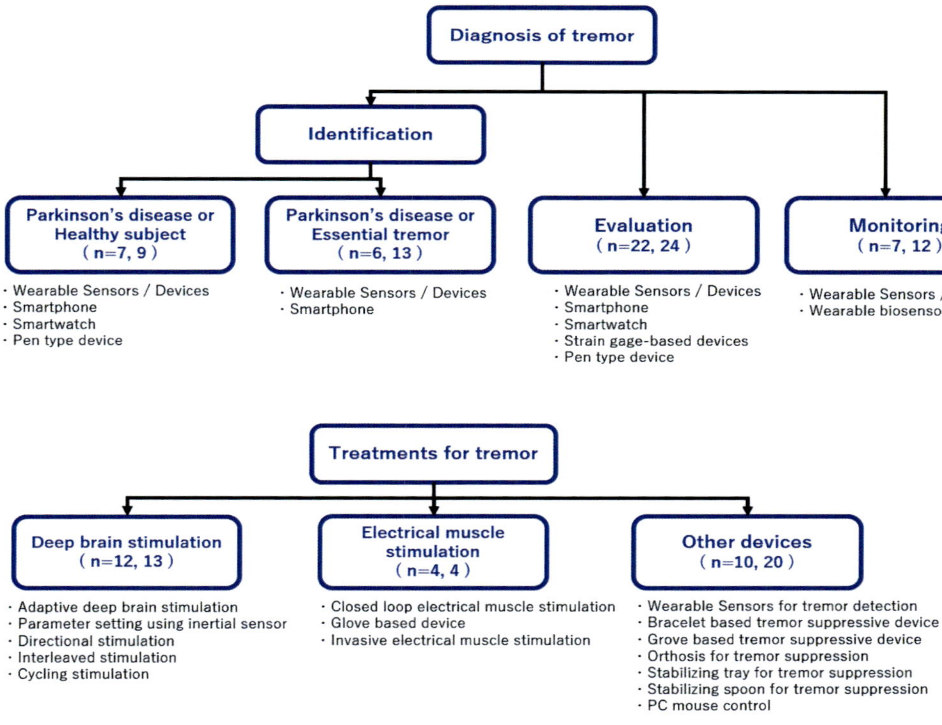

Figure 2.2. *An overview of the diagnostic and treatment devices for tremor.*

Source: Fujikawa J, Morigaki R, Yamamoto N, Nakanishi H, Oda T, Izumi Y, Takagi Y. Diagnosis and Treatment of Tremor in Parkinson's disease Using Mechanical Devices. Life. 2023; 13(1):78. https://doi.org/10.3390/life13010078.

2.3.1. Essential Tremor

A movement disorder called essential tremor makes certain parts of your body tremble. You are powerless over this type of shaking, and you cannot stop yourself from doing it. Although it can also affect your head, voice, and other body parts, essential tremor typically affects your hands and arms. When this illness reaches a severe stage, it can seriously interfere with even the most basic activities and aspects of daily life, like eating, drinking, and getting dressed. Many people also experience anxiety or embarrassment when they think about the symptoms of this illness.

A tremor is an uncontrollably twitchy or oscillating movement of one or more body parts caused by a mildly rhythmic muscle contraction and relaxation. Of all the involuntary movements, it is the most prevalent and can affect the hands, arms, eyes, face, head, vocal folds, trunk, and legs. Hands are where most tremors originate. A tremor may be a sign of another neurological condition in certain individuals. A common neurological symptom seen in clinical practice is tremor, which is an oscillatory movement of one or more body parts that is rhythmic and involuntary. It may show up as the main ailment or as a secondary symptom of many different mental, metabolic, or neurological conditions. The clinical features of tremor, such as the body part affected, frequency, amplitude, and conditions under which it occurs, are usually used to classify it.

Based on its activation state, tremors can be classified into three main categories: resting tremor, postural tremor, and action or kinetic tremor. Resting tremor, which frequently manifests as a pill-rolling motion of the hands in Parkinson's disease, happens when the affected body part is fully supported against gravity and at rest. Postural tremor is a common symptom of essential tremor, the most common movement disorder. It occurs when sustaining a position against gravity, such as holding the arms extended. Action tremor is a tremor that arises from the voluntary contraction of muscles. It can be further classified into two types: kinetic tremor, which happens during movement, and intention tremor, which gets worse as the limb gets closer to a target.

The frequency and amplitude of a tremor can also be used to describe it. High-frequency tremors, exceeding 8–10 Hz, are more frequently observed in essential tremor, while low-frequency tremors, usually below 4-5 Hz, are frequently linked to Parkinson's disease. The degree of movement, from mild to sharp oscillations, is referred to as the tremor's amplitude.

Measuring the frequency and amplitude of tremors helps to focus the differential diagnosis and direct treatment choices. Moreover, the laterality and distribution of tremor can offer important diagnostic hints. Tremor can be unilateral or bilateral, affecting the hands, arms, legs, head, or voice, among other body parts. Some tremor syndromes have distinctive involvement patterns; examples include the vocal tremor in spasmodic dysphonia and the head tremor in cervical dystonia.

Effective management of tremor requires knowledge of its underlying pathophysiology in addition to its clinical features. Tremor is thought to result from aberrant oscillations within the central nervous system, involving intricate interactions between neuronal circuits, neurotransmitters, and oscillatory networks, though the precise mechanisms underlying this phenomenon are still unclear. Essential tremor is associated with dysfunction in the cerebello-thalamo-cortical pathway, while Parkinson's disease tremor is caused by abnormalities in the basal ganglia-thalamo-cortical circuitry.

Tremor treatment strategies, which are frequently adapted to the particular tremor subtype and underlying etiology, are to reduce symptoms and enhance quality of life. In some circumstances, pharmacotherapy—which includes beta-blockers, anticonvulsants, and dopaminergic agents—may be able to relieve symptoms. For refractory tremor, surgical procedures like deep brain stimulation (DBS) that target the thalamus or globus pallidus may be taken into consideration. Occupational therapy, physical therapy, assistive devices, and other non-pharmacological strategies can also help manage symptoms.

A complex and heterogeneous neurological symptom, tremor has a wide range of clinical manifestations and etiologies. For precise diagnosis and individualized treatment, a methodical approach to tremor assessment that includes clinical evaluation, classification, and knowledge of the underlying pathophysiology is necessary. Through the treatment of the underlying cause and symptomatic relief, clinicians can effectively reduce disability associated with tremors and enhance the general quality of life for affected individuals.

2.3.2. Tremor Diagnosis Using Devices

Accelerometers, gyroscopes, and electromyo graphy (EMG) to monitor, classify, and identify tremors and distinguish between tremors resulting from PD, tremors from other causes (like ET), and tremors in healthy individuals. Furthermore, gyroscope and accelerometer features on modern smartphones and smartwatches make them useful monitoring instruments.

- **Distinguishing Between Patients with PD and Healthy Individuals, Using Devices:** It can be difficult to differentiate between PD and ET when diagnosing tremors. As a result, scientists are working hard to find methods that will enable objective evaluation of devices in differential diagnosis. The initial stage of diagnosis involves differentiating between a sick person and a healthy one. Giulia and team employed wearable inertial sensors to distinguish between PD patients and healthy participants. 36 PD patients and 29 healthy controls used the inertial sensors to complete seven motor tasks from the MDS-UPDRS III, which is sponsored by the Movement Disorder Society: resting tremor, postural tremor, fast alternating hand movement, foot tapping, heel-to-toe tapping, timed up and go test (TUG), and a pull test. SVM was used to perform these endpoints using highly relevant items, such as tremor, bradycardia, pull test, and TUG, and it achieved a high accuracy of 97% in differentiating between PD patients and healthy controls. The A-WEAR wristband as well, which employed 3D acceleration and gyroscopes to diagnose PD with a precision of 91.7% based on K-nearest neighbors. These studies have been conducted on smartwatches and smartphones. They created a smartphone app to measure the upper limb tremor of patients. By using machine learning, the app accurately identified 82% of patients and 90% of healthy individuals, respectively, using information from the accelerometer and gyroscope on the smartphone. Smartwatches have also been used in the development of prototypes.

This system was trained on a sample of 192, 75, and 51 patients with Parkinson's disease, other movement disorders, and healthy individuals, respectively. It was tested using artificial neural networks, random forests, and SVM. Artificial neural networks performed the best, with precision and recall of 0.94 (SD 0.03) and 0.92 (SD 0.04) respectively, in differentiating healthy participants from others, including those with PD and other movement disorders. Furthermore, SVM showed the best performance with precision and recall of 0.81 (SD 0.01) and 0.89 (SD 0.04), respectively, in differentiating patients with PD from those with other motor disabilities and healthy participants. Furthermore, there have been additional validations of diagnostics using commercially available smartwatches. For example, a study that employed the widely distributed Apple Watch series 3 and 4 assessed the accuracy of the devices by contrasting them with a Nanometrics seismometer. With a maximum error of, series 3 and 4 were both found to be accurate<0.01 Hz from the seismograph. The patient performed a test designed by a disability specialist to obtain acceleration data while wearing the smartwatch. Machine learning was used to discriminate between patients with PD, healthy participants, and those with motor impairments other than PD (ET, Parkinsonism, etc.). The machine learning classifiers used were as follows: SVM, CatBoost, multilayer perceptron, and simple deep learning architecture. SVM, CatBoost, and multilayer perceptron displayed a balanced accuracy of > 80%, and recall and precision rates exceeding 90% for both healthy individuals and PD patients.

The multilayer perceptron showed balanced accuracy, precision, and recall of 74.1%, 86.5%, and 90.5%, respectively, in an advanced task that differentiates between motor impairment caused by PD and non-PD. Thus, even with consumer goods, significant identification accuracy can be attained. Another study assessed plate-to-mouth (PtM) in seven healthy participants and 21 patients with PD using inertial data from a commercially available smartwatch. The study also looked into eating behavior and the reduction of motor symptoms in PD. PtM is a metric used to describe how long it typically takes for hands to move food from a plate to the mouth during eating. PtM values were higher in PD patients than in healthy individuals. In addition, a PtM-based patient classification model with scores of 0.882, 0.714, and 0.789 for precision, recall, and F1 (harmonic mean of fit and recall) was found. However, because they call for specific knowledge of system operation and maintenance, a few of the previously mentioned techniques are challenging to use. Researchers created a tool that can be used in conjunction with a standard pen to provide a more straightforward and easy way to diagnose PD. The tool uses a basic diadochokinetic paper test to identify PD patients from healthy individuals, which helps identify the disease in its early stages. An accelerometer and gyroscope were built into the device, and naive Bayes, logistic regression, linear discriminant analysis, regression trees, K-nearest neighbors, and SVM were used to classify the collected data. The outcomes demonstrated that, for multiple classifiers, the overall accuracy was close to 100%.

- **Distinguishing Between PD and ET Using Devices:** Iodine-123-labeled N-omega-(flu-oropropyl)-2beta-carbomethoxy-3beta-(4-iodophenyl) tropane and iodine-123-labeled 2β-carbomethoxy-3β-(4-iodophenyl) tropane dopamine transporter imaging with single-photon emission computed tomography using nuclear imaging techniques are the classic method of distinguishing PD tremor from ET. Nevertheless, its precision might be inferior to that of a clinical diagnosis made by experts in movement disorders. Moreover, nuclear imaging methods are not widely accessible due to their high cost and time requirements, as well as their use of radiopharmaceuticals. This justifies taking into account how PD and ET can be identified using widely accessible, reasonably priced wearable technology. The frequency ranges where PD and ET tremors overlap, but the accelerometer power spectrum analysis signals can discriminate between the two.

The researchers attached six-axis inertial sensors to the participants' index fingers and asked them to complete three tasks: kinetic, postural, and resting. They then proposed a novel method for extracting temporal features based on variations in the frequency of tremors with state. It took 10 seconds to finish each task. For individuals with PD and ET, there were significant differences in the elliptical regions of their two-dimensional representations of the resting task (p. < 0.05). They developed a small, low-cost, wearable device with an inertial sensor. The device was worn on the wrist, and four standardized tasks were performed to acquire data and build a classification model, which achieved an average accuracy of > 90%. The acceleration from a smartwatch has also been utilized by researchers to identify PD and ET. By using the mean harmonic peak power obtained from the accelerometer, a receiver operating characteristic (ROC) analysis could make it easier to calculate the optimal discrimination threshold (sensitivity 90%, 95% confidence interval 58.7–99.8%; specificity 100%, 95% confidence interval 76.8–100%; and Cohen's kappa = 0.91, SE = 0.08). Additionally, an analog accelerometer was used to assess the smartwatch's accuracy and produce reliable estimates of the peak frequency and proportional harmonic power. Research has also been done with smartphones: This application classifies data using SVM and discrete wavelet transforms while the user holds the smartphone in their hand to obtain acceleration information. It reported an accuracy rate of more than 96%.

Smartphones were also utilized to identify PD and ET patients. Patients whose diagnosis was unclear were included in the assessment and reassessed a year later. Smartphones were positioned on the dorsal side of the hands for the experiment, and recordings were made for 30 s of rest and 30 s of arm stretching. To determine a threshold to distinguish between participants who trembled and those who did not, they computed the ROC of the total spectral power. The findings showed that 27 out of 32 patients had an accurate PD or ET diagnosis (84.38% discrimination accuracy). Two out of four ET cases and all PD cases were correctly classified out of the patients with undecided diagnoses. Additionally, machine learning classification was carried out using the linear acceleration of tremor recorded by the smartphone's built-in accelerometer, and results ranged from 90 to 100 points of sensitivity and 80 to 100% specificity. Moon and team evaluated the effectiveness of many machine-learning techniques, such as gradient boosting, neural networks, SVM, K-nearest neighbor algorithms, decision trees, and random forests. They employed six inertial sensors—on the wrist, back of the foot, sternum, and hip—to assess gait characteristics and balance to differentiate between PD and ET.

The F1 score (harmonic mean of fit and recall), which is the most commonly used performance metric in machine learning, was 0.61, 0.59, 0.56, 0.55, 0.53, and 0.49 for neural networks, gradient boosting, random forest, SVM, decision tree, and K-nearest neighbors, respectively. It was superior to conventional logistic regression, thus confirming the usefulness of machine learning for diagnosis. Most studies were diagnostic, based on data obtained from inertial sensors, although some studies were conducted using EMG. A study investigating the EEG characteristics of resting tremor in patients with ET and PD confirmed that the parameter that best differentiated the two disorders was the pattern of muscle activation, developed a μEMG device worn on the wrist to record resting tremor Comparison with common EMG recordings confirmed a good correlation between tremor frequency (r = 0.93, $p < 0.001$) and phase difference (r = 0.92, $p < 0.001$). Thus, wearable devices have been used to classify PD and ET with high accuracy. Further validation may provide more efficient diagnostic and prognostic tools that can assist clinicians in decision-making processes.

2.3.3. Tremor Evaluation Using Devices

Apart from the identification process, it's critical to measure the level of tremor quantitatively. In clinical practice, the UPDRS tremor scores are frequently utilized for tremor evaluation. Additionally, wearable device evaluation systems are frequently made to correlate sensor readings with the UPDRS.

- **Tremor Evaluation Using Wearable Sensors:** Researchers utilized EEG and EMG data to analyze tremors in patients with PD. Surface electromyography (sEMG) is commonly used to characterize and monitor tremors in PD patients. A study compared 30 PD patients with a control group by attaching bipolar sEMG to the biceps brachii muscle and evaluating muscle activity. The PD group had significantly higher recurrence and determinism rates, which were correlated with UPDRS scores. Inertial sensors have become popular in recent years, with a study showing their superior accuracy compared to EMG motion tracking. Data-processing methods vary among different studies.

The acceleration resulting from pure translational motion was measured using a gradient descent algorithm, and the tremor severity was successfully estimated based on features extracted from a hidden Markov model and acceleration obtained using accelerometers attached to body segments. The features gleaned from these accelerations and angular velocities were used to build a multiple regression model of UPDRS. The model's performance was $r^2 = 0.95$ for resting tremor and $r^2 = 0.93$ for postural tremor. They created SNUMAP, a wrist-mounted assessment tool featuring a gyroscope and three-axis accelerometer. They trained a convolutional neural network (CNN) on recordings from 92 PD patients to produce an estimated UPDRS model. The findings showed a linearly weighted kappa of 0.85 and an average accuracy of 85%. CNNs may outperform straightforward machine learning techniques like SVM or regression in terms of accuracy. These machine learning-based techniques have gained popularity recently, and a lot of research has been done on them. They tested several machine learning techniques, and extracted characteristic values from acceleration signals in the time, frequency, and spectral domains. The study used data from an accelerometer-based wearable device attached to the patient's upper extremity. The results showed that the neural network model was more accurate than the SVM, random forest, and multivariate linear regression models. Another method using CNNs is to learn a convolved 2D image of the frequency response of the tremor signal.

The results revealed an average accuracy rate of 91% and a linearly weighted kappa of

0.91. Researchers have proposed using fuzzy inference instead of machine learning to estimate UPDRS. Fuzzy theory suggests that truth values are not strictly binary, but rather encompass a range of intermediate values, accounting for uncertainty. This approach is easily adjustable and scalable, mirroring the human inference process.

- **Tremor Evaluation Using Smartphones and Smartwatches:** In recent times, smartphones have emerged as the most widely used gadgets. Research has been done on the assessment of tremors with these devices. They have rapidly increased their computing power, which is partially to blame for this. A standard smartphone to assess the frequency of tremors in PD patients. Showed that accelerometer data acquired through smartphone applications and a clinically acquired EMG had good consistency (Pearson > 0.8, p). < 0.001) In one study, 22 patients with diagnoses of PD, ET, and Holmes' tremor were tested, and three apps were evaluated. The smartphone detected data on hand tremors, and the UPDRS hand tremor scores revealed a good correlation (r > 0.7 and p < 0.01) The majority of these studies have been carried out in controlled settings, like laboratories; nonetheless, some have also been carried out in unconfined spaces. To handle noisy data, researchers have developed an algorithm for classifying tremors that uses a multiple-instance learning technique based on smartphone acceleration. The amplitude at peak frequency varied among the sensors, suggesting that distal worn sensors tended to measure higher amplitudes relative to proximal ones. The study compared accelerometers made in laboratories with those found in consumer products. In addition to having significantly lower barriers to use, tremors can be detected and evaluated with high precision without the need for specialized sensors, suggesting that sensor placement may be crucial in determining tremor amplitude.

In addition to smartphones, some models of smartwatches have gained popularity in recent years. Because smartwatches are worn on the wrists, they might be appropriate for tremor assessment. Several studies used wrist-mounted sensors to assess tremors. They measured the tremor intensity parameters of resting tremors by taking the root mean square of the angular velocity, which they obtained from a smartwatch. In addition, they statistically analyzed the quantified data in conjunction with the UPDRS-III score, and the results showed a strong correlation with a Spearman's correlation coefficient (ρ) of 0.81 (p < 0.001). Furthermore, there was a high level of satisfaction with the device. Researchers have found that a multitasking CNN that accepts both raw signals and spectral data representations as inputs can achieve high tremor detection performance.

Tremors can also be classified using machine learning based on triaxial acceleration data from commercially available smartwatches. Researchers are investigating the features of data measurement required for the precise identification of Parkinson's disease symptoms. After comparing and contrasting smartwatches that are sold commercially and multifunctional measurement sensors, it was found that tremors could be accurately detected using only the accelerometer data from the smartwatch.

Acceleration was needed to detect tremors at a sampling rate of at least 30 Hz. They also looked into the effects on the accuracy of the machine learning features (time, frequency, entropy, correlation, and derivative). It was found that entropy was crucial for tremor detection. Battery consumption and real-time performance are impacted by entropy, which is computationally costly. When combined, smartwatch-based tremor detection has become feasible and is anticipated to be used. For routine care and assessment of patients with PD, the most practical and least taxing method is to use wearable technology at an affordable price.

2.3.4. Tremor Monitoring

While many innovative devices are being developed to evaluate tremors at particular intervals, several studies have focused on continuous monitoring. Clinic and other setting assessments are time-limited and might not capture common symptoms. This calls for an assessment and ongoing surveillance to precisely determine the state of the disease. Such monitoring is also anticipated to serve as screening for the use of cutting-edge treatments, like DBS. Several tests were taken daily in early studies of this kind, but more recently, a continuous monitoring system has also been implemented. Assessments of 13 patients with PD showed that the ratings by ROC curves were consistent with the clinician's UPDRS-III ratings of the video recordings (ROC area > 0.8). The data was collected for six daily activities, including eating and brushing teeth. Researchers have proposed wearable sensors attached to the wrist and chest combined with questionnaire-based assessment for continuous monitoring of PD symptoms in daily life. Overlapping frequency components can make it difficult to distinguish between daily activities and tremors; nonetheless, a method has been proposed for detecting tremors using a two-step algorithm. Another device that can detect PD hand tremors from daily movements is the PD-Watch. This device enables detection by checking for movement frequency and supination–pronation characteristics. Results from 24 patients with PD showed a maximum correlation of 0.96 in gradient tree boosting (Heldman, 2016).

It was shown that there was a correlation between the UPDRS score and the index that was computed using the 24-hour data from the device. Additionally, a CNN and other techniques from a wearable accelerometer system worn on the wrist were proposed as a machine learning approach to detect tremors in daily life data. This technology allowed the quantification of the number of tremors in daily life. The biosensor patch NIMBLE (MC10, Inc.) was created by researchers as a more comprehensive and user-friendly sensor, Lexington, MA, USA) equipped with a myoelectric mechanism and accelerometer. It can stick to the skin like stickers. Furthermore, the measurements can be wirelessly sent to a cloud server and a smartphone or tablet. Based on the obtained data, prediction scores with a probability of 91% fell within the range of ±1. Additionally, their safety and adherence were assessed. By evaluating tremors at higher frequencies during routine activities, these techniques might enable more effective treatment.

2.3.5. Treatments for Tremor

- ***DBS:*** The accepted standard of care for individuals with movement disorders, including PD, ET, and dystonia, is deep brain stimulation (DBS). For these patients, DBS is a popular and successful treatment, and most of them have positive post-operative clinical outcomes. In addition, DBS is a less risky treatment than stereotactic thalamotomy, with a lower rate of complications. It also improves bradykinesia, gait freezing in Parkinson's disease, camptocormia, and tremor. The most frequently targeted areas for PD stimulation are the internal globus pallidus (GPi) and the subthalamic nucleus (STN). A meta-analysis comparing the effects of DBS on tremor suppression found a significant standardized difference mean effect (effect size = 0.36; 95% CI = 0.316–0.395; p < 0.0001). The measure was the sum of UPDRS III, items 20 and 21. These findings suggest a moderate level of effectiveness. There was no discernible difference in the effect size between GPi and STN (p = 0.56). The results of this study also demonstrated that the extent of tremor control by DBS for STN and GPi was equivalent; however, it may take longer to achieve the same tremor control effect when targeting GPi. A 12-month follow-up study also confirmed its effectiveness in reducing action/postural tremor and resting tremor. Additionally, it has been discovered that the frequency of stimulation affects the therapeutic effect. Meta-analyses have demonstrated that tremor is more affected by stimulation than 100 Hz STN. The method of electrode placement is also important. Diffusion tensor imaging and tractography guided lead placement have been shown to provide more stable placement and better tremor control compared to conventional methods of lead placement Other targets include the ventral intermediate nucleus of the thalamus (VIM), caudal zona incerta, and posterior subthalamic area, which have a striking effect in improving tremors. Therefore, if tremor is the main problem, rather than bradykinesia for patients with PD, these targets are warranted to be considered as first choice. A study of 98 patients with PD and ET showed sustained improvement in tremor scores (UPDRS III, items 20 and 21; Fahn–Tolosa–Marin Tremor Rating Scale) with VIM stimulation (mean improvement, 70% and 66% at 1 year and 63% and 48% at >10 years, respectively, $p <$ 0.05) There was no significant loss of a stimulation effect over time ($p > 0.05$). Thus, the effects of DBS are long-lasting. Tremor can be controlled by maintaining the activities of daily living, and there was high patient satisfaction during the 10-year follow-up However, DBS is not effective in all patients, and patients need to determine whether they are appropriate candidates (Wong et al., 2020).

a. ***aDBS:*** New research and development, as well as continuous advancements in DBS technology, are underway. Among the most cutting-edge methods is aDBS. Based on the closed-loop interaction principle, an aDBS device can detect the effect of stimulation and modify it based on the observed effect. To create a closed loop in aDBS, LFPs are employed as biomarkers. One benefit of aDBS with LFPs is that it can be accomplished without the need for extra measurement channels through the online analysis of deep brain recordings. PD patients are currently being treated with it because it works well (Hirschmann et al., 2013).

An aDBS device has not been used clinically for tremor suppression. Reducing battery consumption by using DBS only after symptoms appear. Power consumption matters because changing a battery needs surgery. Tremors from the LFP must be detected for aDBS to function. The deployment of aDBS requires accurate symptom identification. There is activity related to tremors throughout the entire motor network. It comprises the thalamus, cerebellum, primary motor cortex, and basal ganglia, which coherently respond to tremor frequencies of 3–7 Hz upon presentation. Additional findings include alterations in high-frequency fluctuations in the subthalamic nucleus and an increase in low gamma power (31–45 Hz). Complex features such as these require the use of advanced techniques, like machine learning. Hirschmann and team, they extracted the LFP from the STN of ten PD patients and classified the tremors using a hidden Markov model. Four frequency domains were used to evaluate the LFP: power at the individual tremor frequency ± 1 Hz, beta power, low gamma power, and high-frequency oscillations power ratio. A mean area under the ROC curve of 0.82 and a standard deviation of 0.15 were shown by the results. Additionally, it demonstrated good accuracy for individual patients even in the absence of training. The feature that is most helpful in detecting tremors is the high-frequency domain. Camara and team created a system that recorded both electromyographic activity in the forearm and LFP in the subthalamic nucleus at the same time. The system used fuzzy inference to identify tremors based on the relationship between the signals, and it was able to detect tremors in four out of ten PD patients with 100% accuracy and >98.7% accuracy in seven patients. By extending this work to synchronization between the thalamic LFP and other brain signals, a full system can be built within the DBS hardware. Shah and team developed a logistic regression-based classifier-based tremor detection system. The system was trained by removing different features from the frequency and time domains of LFPs. The results of the classification performance showed that the power between 31 Hz and 45 Hz was the most discriminating feature, with an AUC ranging from 0.67 to 0.93. As a machine learning-based method, a multi-feature neural network-based tremor detector was presented. In four out of eight patients, it achieved an accuracy of >86%. Accurate treatment of an aDBS system will be made possible by these technologies.

2.3.6. The Optimization of Stimulation Parameters

For DBS to be used effectively, stimulation parameter optimization is crucial. Determining the general DBS parameters frequently depends on subjective assessment, which might not produce the best results. Furthermore, it is imperative to adjust various parameters, including frequency, pulse width, and amplitude, while adhering to time constraints. Therefore, employing wearable sensors as objective markers for establishing stimulation parameters, researchers suggested next-generation techniques to quantify tremors. An algorithm that involved attaching motion sensors to the fingers, such as gyroscopes and accelerometers, to collect motion data. This motion data was then used to set the DBS parameters. The algorithm consisted of two parts: an algorithm to maximize the treatment effect and another to optimize battery life. In comparison to the standard setting method, the algorithm that optimized the treatment effect resulted in a 13% reduction in motor symptoms.

However, it also caused an increase in stimulus amplitude. On the other hand, the battery life optimization algorithm was able to preserve the therapeutic effect level while achieving an average 50% reduction in stimulus amplitude. At the moment, the intraoperative parameter setting is done arbitrarily. To help awake patients undergoing DBS implantation surgery with electrode placement and test stimulus settings, a system was developed. The system enabled the quantitative real-time visualization of motor symptoms, including tremors, captured by an inertial measurement unit during surgery, created a glove-like device that measures the immediate effects of DBS through assessments of stiffness, bradykinesia, and tremors using an inertial measurement unit and force-sensitive resistor.

Summary

- Clinical diagnosis of Parkinsonism and tremor disorders relies on a meticulous approach integrating medical history, physical examination, and sometimes additional investigations.
- Parkinsonism refers to a group of neurological disorders characterized by a combination of movement abnormalities such as tremors, rigidity, bradykinesia (slowness of movement), and postural instability.
- Parkinson's disease is a progressive disorder that affects the nervous system and the parts of the body controlled by the nerves.
- The cause of Parkinson's is unknown, there are no proven ways to prevent the disease. Some research has shown that regular aerobic exercise might reduce the risk of Parkinson's disease.
- Parkinsonism and tremor disorders encompass a spectrum of neurological conditions characterized by movement abnormalities, with tremor being a prominent feature.
- MSA is a sporadic, adult-onset, neurodegenerative disease. It is a clinicopathological entity, which can present with any combination of Parkinsonism, cerebellar and/or pyramidal signs and autonomic dysfunction.
- PD is a progressive degenerative disorder primarily characterized by the degeneration of dopamine neurons in the substantia nigra. Its main symptoms include tremor, rigidity, bradykinesia, akinesia, and postural instability.
- A tremor is an involuntary, somewhat rhythmic, muscle contraction and relaxation involving oscillations or twitching movements of one or more body parts.
- The optimization of stimulation parameters is important for the efficient use of DBS. Setting general DBS parameters often relies on subjective evaluation, which may not yield optimal effects.

References

1. Barrantes, S., Sanchez Egea, A. J., Gonzalez Rojas, H. A., Marti, M. J., Compta, Y., Valldeoriola, F., Simo Mezquita, E., Tolosa, E., & Valls-Sole, J. (2017). Differential diagnosis between Parkinson's disease and essential tremor using the smartphone's accelerometer. *PLoS ONE, 12*, e0183843.
2. Bhatia, K. P., Bain, P., Bajaj, N., Elble, R. J., Hallett, M., Louis, E. D., Raethjen, J., Stamelou, M., Testa, C. M., Deuschl, G., et al. (2018). Consensus statement on the classification of tremors. From the task force on tremor of the international Parkinson and movement disorder society. *Movement Disorders, 33*, 75–87.
3. Boroojerdi, B., Ghaffari, R., Mahadevan, N., Markowitz, M., Melton, K., Morey, B., Otoul, C., Patel, S., Phillips, J., Sen-Gupta, E., et al. (2019). Clinical feasibility of a wearable, conformable sensor patch to monitor motor symptoms in Parkinson's disease. *Parkinsonism & Related Disorders, 61*, 70–76.
4. Buki, E., Katz, R., Zacksenhouse, M., & Schlesinger, I. (2018). Vib-bracelet: A passive absorber for attenuating forearm tremor. *Medical & Biological Engineering & Computing, 56*, 923–930.

5. Daneault, J. F., Carignan, B., Codere, C. E., Sadikot, A. F., & Duval, C. (2012). Using a smart phone as a standalone platform for detection and monitoring of pathological tremors. *Frontiers in Human Neuroscience, 6*, 357.

6. de la Fuente-Fernandez, R. (2012). Role of datscan and clinical diagnosis in Parkinson's Disease. *Neurology, 78*, 696–701.

7. Deuschl, G., Raethjen, J., Lindemann, M., & Krack, P. (2001). The pathophysiology of tremor. *Muscle & Nerve, 24*, 716–735.

8. Di Lazzaro, G., Ricci, M., Al-Wardat, M., Schirinzi, T., Scalise, S., Giannini, F., Mercuri, N. B., Saggio, G., & Pisani, A. (2020). Technology-based objective measures detect subclinical axial signs in untreated, de novo Parkinson's disease. *Journal of Parkinson's Disease, 10*, 113–122.

9. Elble, R., Comella, C., Fahn, S., Hallett, M., Jankovic, J., Juncos, J. L., Lewitt, P., Lyons, K., Ondo, W., Pahwa, R., et al. (2012). Reliability of a new scale for essential tremor. *Movement Disorders, 27*, 1567–1569.

10. Faizan, M. S., & Muzammil, M. (2020). Hand tremor suppression device for patients suffering from Parkinson's disease. *Journal of Medical Engineering & Technology, 44*, 190–197.

11. Fujikawa, J., Morigaki, R., Yamamoto, N., Nakanishi, H., Oda, T., Izumi, Y., & Takagi, Y. (2023). Diagnosis and treatment of tremor in Parkinson's disease using mechanical devices. *Life, 13*(1), 78. https://doi.org/10.3390/life13010078.

12. Fujikawa, J., Morigaki, R., Yamamoto, N., Oda, T., Nakanishu, H., Izumi, Y., & Takaga, Y. (2022). Therapeutic devices for motor symptoms in Parkinson's disease: Current progress and a systematic review of recent randomized controlled trials. *Frontiers in Aging Neuroscience, 14*, 1–25.

13. Heida, T., Wentink, E. C., & Marani, E. (2013). Power spectral density analysis of physiological, rest and action tremor in Parkinson's disease patients treated with deep brain stimulation. *Journal of NeuroEngineering and Rehabilitation, 10*, 70.

14. Heldman, D. A., Giuffrida, J. P., & Cubo, E. (2016). Wearable sensors for advanced therapy referral in Parkinson's disease. *Journal of Parkinson's Disease, 6*, 631–638.

15. Hirschmann, J., Hartmann, C. J., Butz, M., Hoogenboom, N., Ozkurt, T. E., Elben, S., Vesper, J., Wojtecki, L., & Schnitzler, A. (2013). A direct relationship between oscillatory subthalamic nucleus-cortex coupling and rest tremor in Parkinson's disease. *Brain, 136*, 3659–3670.

16. Hirschmann, J., Schoffelen, J. M., Schnitzler, A., & van Gerven, M. A. J. (2017). Parkinsonian rest tremor can be detected accurately based on neuronal oscillations recorded from the subthalamic nucleus. *Clinical Neurophysiology, 128*, 2029–2036.

17. Hossen, A., Muthuraman, M., Al-Hakim, Z., Raethjen, J., Deuschl, G., & Heute, U. (2013). Discrimination of parkinsonian tremor from essential tremor using statistical signal characterization of the spectrum of accelerometer signal. *Biomedical Materials and Engineering, 23*, 513–531.

18. Ibrahim, A., Zhou, Y., Jenkins, M. E., Luisa Trejos, A., & Naish, M. D. (2020). The design of a Parkinson's tremor predictor and estimator using a hybrid convolutional-multilayer perceptron neural network. In *Proceedings of the 2020 42nd Annual International Conference of the IEEE Engineering in Medicine & Biology Society (EMBC)*, Montreal, QC, Canada, 20–24 July 2020; pp. 5996–6000.

19. Ibrahim, A., Zhou, Y., Jenkins, M. E., Trejos, A. L., & Naish, M. D. (2021). Real-time voluntary motion prediction and Parkinson's tremor reduction using deep neural networks. *IEEE Transactions on Neural Systems and Rehabilitation Engineering, 29*, 1413–1423.
20. Jain, S., Lo, S. E., & Louis, E. D. (2006). Common misdiagnosis of a common neurological disorder: How are we misdiagnosing essential tremor? *Archives of Neurology, 63*, 1100–1104.
21. Jitkritsadakul, O., Thanawattano, C., Anan, C., & Bhidayasiri, R. (2017). Tremor's glove-an innovative electrical muscle stimulation therapy for intractable tremor in Parkinson's disease: A randomized sham-controlled trial. *Journal of the Neurological Sciences, 381*, 331–340.
22. Junior, E. P., Delmiro, I. L. D., Magaia, N., Maia, F. M., Hassan, M. M., Albuquerque, V. H. C., & Fortino, G. (2020). Intelligent sensory pen for aiding in the diagnosis of Parkinson's disease from dynamic handwriting analysis. *Sensors, 20*, 5840.
23. Kang, G. A., Bronstein, J. M., Masterman, D. L., Redelings, M., Crum, J. A., & Ritz, B. (2005). Clinical characteristics in early Parkinson's disease in a central California population-based study. *Movement Disorders, 20*, 1133–1142.
24. Koller, W. C., & Vetere-Overfield, B. (1989). Acute and chronic effects of propranolol and primidone in essential tremor. *Neurology, 39*, 1587–1588.
25. Kostikis, N., Hristu-Varsakelis, D., Arnaoutoglou, M., & Kotsavasiloglou, C. (2015). A smartphone-based tool for assessing parkinsonian hand tremor. *IEEE Journal of Biomedical and Health Informatics, 19*, 1835–1842.
26. Kostikis, N., Hristu-Varsakelis, D., Arnaoutoglou, M., & Kotsavasiloglou, C. (2014). Smartphone-based evaluation of parkinsonian hand tremor: Quantitative measurements vs clinical assessment scores. In *Proceedings of the 2014 36th Annual International Conference of the IEEE Engineering in Medicine and Biology Society*, Chicago, IL, USA, 26–30 August 2014; pp. 906–909.
27. Kyritsis, K., Fagerberg, P., Ioakimidis, I., Klingelhoefer, L., Reichmann, H., & Delopoulos, A. (2020). Using IMU sensors to assess motor degradation of PD patients by modeling in-meal plate-to-mouth movement elongation. In *Proceedings of the 2020 42nd Annual International Conference of the IEEE Engineering in Medicine & Biology Society (EMBC)*, Montreal, QC, Canada, 20–24 July 2020; pp. 494–497.
28. Louis, E. D., & McCreary, M. (2021). How common is essential tremor? Update on the worldwide prevalence of essential tremor. *Tremor and Other Hyperkinetic Movements, 11*, 28.
29. Low, H. L., Ismail, M., Taqvi, A., Deeb, J., Fuller, C., & Misbahuddin, A. (2019). Comparison of posterior subthalamic area deep brain stimulation for tremor using conventional landmarks versus directly targeting the dentatorubrothalamic tract with tractography. *Clinical Neurology and Neurosurgery, 185*, 105466.
30. Meigal, A. I., Rissanen, S., Tarvainen, M. P., Karjalainen, P. A., Iudina-Vassel, I. A., Airaksinen, O., & Kankaanpaa, M. (2009). Novel parameters of surface EMG in patients with Parkinson's disease and healthy young and old controls. *Journal of Electromyography and Kinesiology, 19*, e206–e213.
31. Meigal, A. Y., Rissanen, S. M., Tarvainen, M. P., Georgiadis, S. D., Karjalainen, P. A., Airaksinen, O., & Kankaanpaa, M. (2012). Linear and nonlinear tremor acceleration characteristics in patients with Parkinson's disease. *Physiological Measurement, 33*, 395–412.

32. Moon, S., Song, H. J., Sharma, V. D., Lyons, K. E., Pahwa, R., Akinwuntan, A. E., & Devos, H. (2020). Classification of Parkinson's disease and essential tremor based on balance and gait characteristics from wearable motion sensors via machine learning techniques: A data-driven approach. *Journal of NeuroEngineering and Rehabilitation, 17*, 125.

33. Muceli, S., Poppendieck, W., Hoffmann, K. P., Dosen, S., Benito-Leon, J., Barroso, F. O., Pons, J. L., & Farina, D. (2019). A thin-film multichannel electrode for muscle recording and stimulation in neuroprosthetics applications. *Journal of Neural Engineering, 16*, 026035.

34. Papadopoulos, A., Kyritsis, K., Klingelhoefer, L., Bostanjopoulou, S., Chaudhuri, K. R., & Delopoulos, A. (2020). Detecting parkinsonian tremor from IMU data collected in-the-wild using deep multiple-instance learning. *IEEE Journal of Biomedical and Health Informatics, 24*, 2559–2569.

35. Parkinson Study Group. (2001). A multicenter assessment of dopamine transporter imaging with dopascan/SPECT in parkinsonism. *Neurology, 57*, S52–S59.

36. Rissanen, S. M., Kankaanpaa, M., Meigal, A., Tarvainen, M. P., Nuutinen, J., Tarkka, I. M., Airaksinen, O., & Karjalainen, P. A. (2008). Surface EMG and acceleration signals in Parkinson's disease: Feature extraction and cluster analysis. *Medical & Biological Engineering & Computing, 46*, 849–858.

37. Rissanen, S., Kankaanpaa, M., Tarvainen, M. P., Nuutinen, J., Tarkka, I. M., Airaksinen, O., & Karjalainen, P. A. (2007). Analysis of surface EMG signal morphology in Parkinson's disease. *Physiological Measurement, 28*, 1507–1521.

38. Salarian, A., Russmann, H., Wider, C., Burkhard, P. R., Vingerhoets, F. J., & Aminian, K. (2007). Quantification of tremor and bradykinesia in Parkinson's disease using a novel ambulatory monitoring system. *IEEE Transactions on Biomedical Engineering, 54*, 313–322.

39. San-Segundo, R., Zhang, A., Cebulla, A., Panev, S., Tabor, G., Stebbins, K., Massa, R. E., Whitford, A., de la Torre, F., & Hodgins, J. (2020). Parkinson's disease tremor detection in the wild using wearable accelerometers. *Sensors, 20*, 5817.

40. Shah, S. A., Tinkhauser, G., Chen, C. C., Little, S., & Brown, P. (2018). Parkinsonian tremor detection from subthalamic nucleus local field potentials for closed-loop deep brain stimulation. In *Proceedings of the 2018 40th Annual International Conference of the IEEE Engineering in Medicine and Biology Society (EMBC)*, Honolulu, HI, USA, 18–21 July 2018; pp. 2320–2324.

41. Shawen, N., O'Brien, M. K., Venkatesan, S., Lonini, L., Simuni, T., Hamilton, J. L., Ghaffari, R., Rogers, J. A., & Jayaraman, A. (2020). Role of data measurement characteristics in the accurate detection of Parkinson's disease symptoms using wearable sensors. *Journal of NeuroEngineering and Rehabilitation, 17*, 52.

42. Sigcha, L., Pavon, I., Costa, N., Costa, S., Gago, M., Arezes, P., Lopez, J. M., & Arcas, G. (2021). Automatic resting tremor assessment in Parkinson's disease using smartwatches and multitask convolutional neural networks. *Sensors, 21*, 291.

43. Sturman, M. M., Vaillancourt, D. E., & Corcos, D. M. (2005). Effects of aging on the regularity of physiological tremor. *Journal of Neurophysiology, 93*, 3064–3074.

44. Thanawattano, C., Pongthornseri, R., Anan, C., Dumnin, S., & Bhidayasiri, R. (2015). Temporal fluctuations of tremor signals from inertial sensor: A preliminary study in differentiating Parkinson's disease from essential tremor. *Biomedical Engineering Online, 14*, 101.

45. Thenganatt, M. A., & Louis, E. D. (2012). Distinguishing essential tremor from Parkinson's disease: Bedside tests and laboratory evaluations. *Expert Review of Neurotherapeutics, 12*, 687–696.

46. Varghese, J., Alen, C. M. V., Fujarski, M., Schlake, G. S., Sucker, J., Warnecke, T., & Thomas, C. (2021). Sensor validation and diagnostic potential of smartwatches in movement disorders. *Sensors, 21*, 3139.

47. Varghese, J., Fujarski, M., Hahn, T., Dugas, M., & Warnecke, T. (2020). The smart device system for movement disorders: Preliminary evaluation of diagnostic accuracy in a prospective study. *Studies in Health Technology and Informatics, 270*, 889–893.

48. Wenning, G. K., Kiechl, S., Seppi, K., Muller, J., Hogl, B., Saletu, M., Rungger, G., Gasperi, A., Willeit, J., & Poewe, W. (2005). Prevalence of movement disorders in men and women aged 50–89 years (Bruneck study cohort): A population-based study. *Lancet Neurology, 4*, 815–820.

49. Wile, D. J., Ranawaya, R., & Kiss, Z. H. (2014). Smart watch accelerometry for analysis and diagnosis of tremor. *Journal of Neuroscience Methods, 230*, 1–4.

50. Wong, J. K., Viswanathan, V. T., Nozile-Firth, K. S., Eisinger, R. S., Leone, E. L., Desai, A. M., Foote, K. D., Ramirez-Zamora, A., Okun, M. S., & Wagle Shukla, A. (2020). STN versus GPI deep brain stimulation for action and rest tremor in Parkinson's disease. *Frontiers in Human Neuroscience, 14*, 578615.

51. Xu, C., Zhuang, P., Hallett, M., Zhang, Y., Li, J., & Li, Y. (2018). Parkinson's disease motor subtypes show different responses to long-term subthalamic nucleus stimulation. *Frontiers in Human Neuroscience, 12*, 365.

Chapter

DIAGNOSTIC TESTING AND NEUROIMAGING

3

Contents

Introduction

PD presents a complex diagnostic challenge due to its heterogeneous clinical presentation and overlapping features with other Parkinsonian syndromes. Diagnostic testing and neuroimaging play pivotal roles in elucidating the underlying pathology, confirming the diagnosis, and differentiating PD from similar conditions. These modalities not only aid clinicians in early detection but also guide treatment decisions and provide valuable insights into disease progression.

Neurological examination forms the cornerstone of PD diagnosis, focusing on cardinal motor symptoms such as bradykinesia, resting tremor, rigidity, and postural instability. However, the clinical assessment alone may not always suffice, particularly in early or atypical cases. Therefore, adjunctive diagnostic testing becomes indispensable in corroborating clinical findings and refining diagnostic certainty.

Neuroimaging techniques, including magnetic resonance imaging (MRI), positron emission tomography (PET), and single-photon emission computed tomography (SPECT), offer invaluable insights into the neuroanatomical and functional alterations underlying PD. These modalities can visualize structural changes in the brain, such as atrophy in the substantia nigra and basal ganglia, as well as dopaminergic dysfunction in the nigrostriatal pathway. For instance, DaTscan imaging, utilizing radiotracers targeting dopamine transporters, can assess presynaptic dopaminergic degeneration, providing objective evidence to support the diagnosis of PD and distinguish it from other Parkinsonian syndromes.

Ancillary investigations complement clinical and imaging assessments, offering additional diagnostic clues in PD evaluation. Neuropsychological testing evaluates cognitive function, identifying associated deficits that may aid in differentiating PD from dementia with Lewy bodies or other cognitive disorders. Cerebrospinal fluid (CSF) analysis and genetic testing, though not routinely performed in clinical practice, may be considered in specific cases to elucidate underlying pathology or assess genetic risk factors associated with PD.

Orientation and Directional Terms

Term	Definition	Illustration
Magnetic Resonance Imaging (MRI)	It is a noninvasive medical imaging test that produces detailed images of almost every internal structure in the human body, including the organs, bones, muscles and blood vessels.	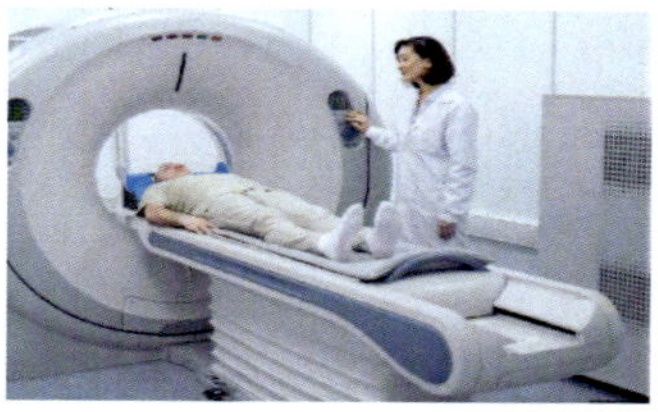
Positron Emission Tomography (PET)	Positron emission tomography (PET) scan is a type of imaging test. It uses a radioactive substance called a tracer to look for disease in the body. A PET scan shows how organs and tissues are working. This is different than MRI and CT scans.	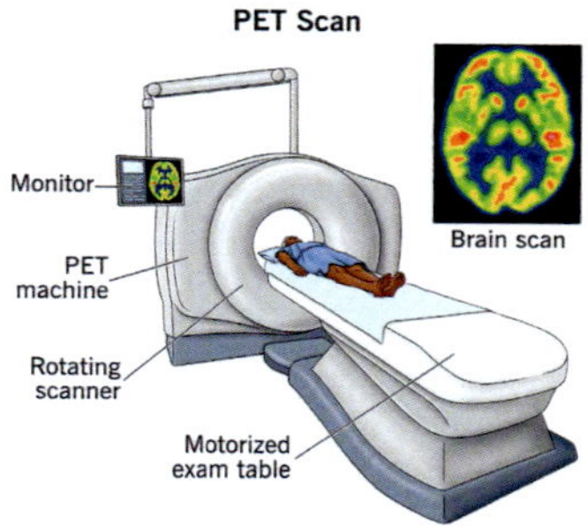
Cerebrospinal Fluid (CSF)	Cerebrospinal fluid (CSF, shown in blue) is made by tissue that lines the ventricles (hollow spaces) in the brain. It flows in and around the brain and spinal cord to help cushion them from injury and provide nutrients.	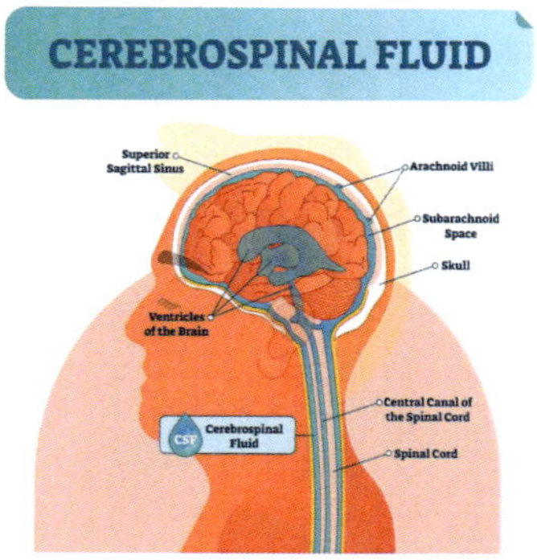
Single Photon Emission Computed Tomography (SPECT)	It is a medical imaging technique that is based on conventional nuclear medicine imaging and tomographic reconstruction methods. The images reflect functional information about patients similar to that obtained with positron emission tomography (PET).	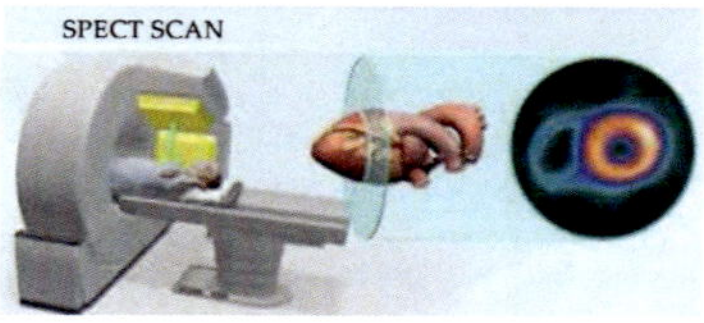
Functional magnetic resonance imaging (fMRI)	Functional magnetic resonance imaging (fMRI) measures the small changes in blood flow that occur with brain activity. It may be used to examine which parts of the brain are handling critical functions, evaluate the effects of stroke or other disease, or to guide brain treatment.	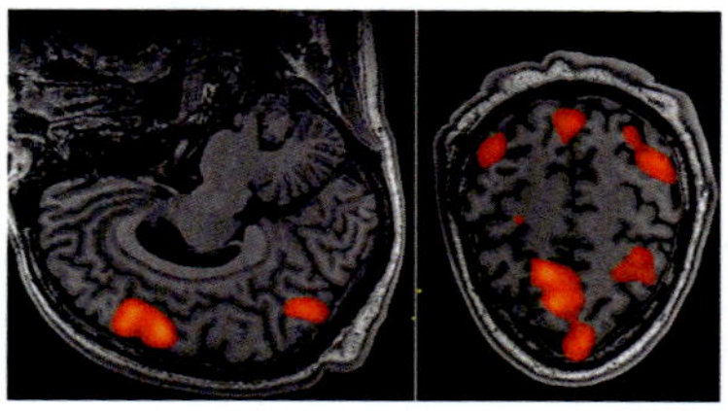

3.1. Clinical Tests

3.1.1. Motor Tests

Clinical tests are widely used to diagnose PD; overview of three test classes: motor tests, pharmacologic challenges, and olfactory tests. In many ways, motor tests are just another form of clinical examination. A variety of motor tasks, such as speech, eye movements, wrist flexion/extension, and visuomotor coordination, have been assessed by researchers. The ability to measure deficiencies and track how well medical and surgical interventions are working has been the main advantage. Motor examinations have failed to distinguish PD from other Parkinsonian syndromes. Combining motor testing with an extensive battery of other tests has demonstrated some capacity to differentiate asymptomatic first-degree relatives of PD patients from healthy controls. These studies show potential in identifying a group of people who are highly susceptible to Parkinson's disease (Stewart & William, 2008) (Table 3.1).

Table 3.1. *Changes in Protein Biomarkers in Brains and Bodily Fluids of PD Patients*

Protein		**Brain**				**Body Fluid**		
	Method	**Change**	**Sample**	**Phase**	**Method**	**Change**	**Sample**	**Phase**
NF-L	IHC	*	SN	Advanced Early	SIMOA, ECLIA	↑	Serum	Advanced Prodromic
					ECLIA	↑	Plasma	Advanced
SP	RIA	↓	SN	Advanced	ELISA	↑	Serum	Advanced
	RIA	↓	Putamen	Advanced	ELISA	↓	Sputum	Early Advanced
	RIA	↓	Caudate	Advanced				
	RIA	↓	GP	Advanced				
P11	qPCR	↓	SN	Advanced	Flow cytometry	↑	Plasma	Advanced
NT	HPLCRIA	↑ ↓	SN Hyp.	Advanced	RIA	↑	Plasma	Early Advanced
ChA	IHC	*	SN cerebellum cerebrum	Advanced	ELISA	↑	Serum	Early Intermediate Advanced
VGF	ELISA	↓	Cortex	Advanced	ELISA	↓	Plasma	Early Advanced
					LC-MS/MS	↓	Urine	with or without LRRK2 G2019S mutation
GFAP	IHC	↑	SN	Advanced	SIMOA	↑	Plasma	Advanced
					ELISA	↑	Serum	Advanced

Source: *Cocco C, Manai AL, Manca E, Noli B. Brain-Biomarker Changes in Body Fluids of Patients with Parkinson's Disease. International Journal of Molecular Sciences. 2023; 24(13):10932. https://doi.org/10.3390/ijms241310932.*

PD = Parkinson's disease; NFL = neurofilament light chain; IHC = immunochemistry; * = abnormal aggregation; SN = substantia nigra; SIMOA = single-molecule array; ECLIA = electrochemiluminescence immunoassay; SP = substance P; RIA = radioimmunoassay; ELISA = enzyme-linked immunosorbent assay; GP = globus pallidus; P11 = S100A10 (S100 calcium-binding protein A10); qPCR = quantitative polymerase chain reaction; NT = neurotensin; HPLCRIA = high-performance liquid chromatography with radioimmunoassay; ChA = chromogranin A; SgII = secretogranin II; VGF = non-acronym; Ct = C-terminus; LC/MS/MS = liquid chromatography/mass spectrometry/mass spectrometry; LRRK2 = leucine-rich repeat kinase2; G2019S = Glycine2019Serine mutation; GFAP = glial fibrillary acidic protein. Hyp: hypothalamus. ↑ = increased concentration; ↓ = decreased concentration.

- ***Pharmacologic Challenges:*** Dopaminergic treatments have been used to identify PD patients in whom there was diagnostic uncertainty because PD responds to these treatments. Researchers have looked into how levodopa and the dopamine agonist apomorphine work therapeutically.

In one study, 250/25 mg of levodopa/carbidopa was administered to 82 patients with Parkinsonian syndrome who did not have a specific diagnosis. When it came to predicting the diagnosis of PD on clinical follow-up two years later, a positive response—defined as more than 30% improvement on the Unified Parkinson's Disease Rating Scale (UPDRS)—had a 71% sensitivity and an 81% specificity. In a practice parameter, the American Academy of Neurology concluded that "levodopa and apormphine challenge tests are probably useful in distinguishing PD from other Parkinsonian syndromes" based on this study and others.

- ***Olfaction:*** The loss of olfactory perception, recognition, or discrimination may occur in Parkinson's disease patients before the onset of motor impairment. The olfactory bulb's neurodegeneration could be the cause of this loss. It has been successfully tested whether olfactory loss can distinguish idiopathic PD from other Parkinsonian syndromes.

The ability to distinguish PD from other Parkinsonian syndromes was discovered through olfactory function in a large study involving 118 patients with PD—29 with multiple system atrophy, 15 with progressive supranuclear palsy, 7 with corticobasal degeneration—and 123 healthy controls. The $27 commercially available University of Pennsylvania Smell Identification test (UPSIT) was utilized to measure olfactory function. Progressive supranuclear palsy and corticobasal degeneration were typical outcomes of multiple system atrophy in people with PD, but marked impairment was observed on the UPSIT in comparison to mild impairment. A sensitivity of 77% and a specificity of 85% were linked to distinguishing PD from other Parkinsonian syndromes when 25 odorants out of a possible 40 were identified on the UPSIT. More generally, severe olfactory deficits in odor identification, recognition, and detection have been consistently found in PD and Alzheimer's disease (ADLD); however, it is more challenging to distinguish between these two neurodegenerative disorders based solely on olfactory function.

A study assessed the effectiveness of combining olfactory testing and imaging with [^{123}I] β-CIT radiotracer and single photon emission computed tomography (SPECT) to identify individuals at risk for PD before symptoms appear.

Ponsen and colleagues screened 361 asymptomatic first-degree relatives of PD patients with an olfactory test followed by SPECT scans. Those who scored in the bottom 10% on the smell test received imaging. Among the 39 individuals with hyposmia, 7 showed significantly reduced [^{123}I] -CIT binding ratios, and 4 of them developed PD after 2 years. No other relatives in the cohort developed PD according to clinical assessment or questionnaire. This study suggests that olfactory testing, combined with other biomarkers, may help identify individuals at high risk for PD.

3.1.2. Blood and Cerebrospinal Fluid Tests

Cerebrospinal fluid (CSF), particularly blood, contains biomarkers that show promise for improving our understanding of PD; as a diagnostic or therapeutic metric, they haven't had much of an impact up to this point. Serum and CSF biomarkers have received a lot of attention, primarily because they are thought to be important in the pathophysiology of PD. In the substantia nigra, mitochondrial complex I levels are lowered.

Researchers have looked at the levels of mitochondrial complex I in platelets and 8-hydroxy-2'-deoxyguanosine as indicators of oxidative stress in an effort to find a peripheral marker. Nevertheless, in one study, there was no difference in complex I levels among platelets, and in another, the elevated levels of 8-hydroxy-2'-deoxyguanosine were not consistent enough to be used as a biomarker in clinical settings.

Low platelet mitochondrial complex I and II/III activities were discovered by other researchers; these findings seem to be connected to the PD etiology. By using electron microscopy, a different study has demonstrated variations in platelet morphology; however, it is unclear what this finding means (Kikuchi, 2002) (Table 3.2).

Table 3.2. *Select PD Biomarkers in the Blood and Cerebrospinal Fluid*

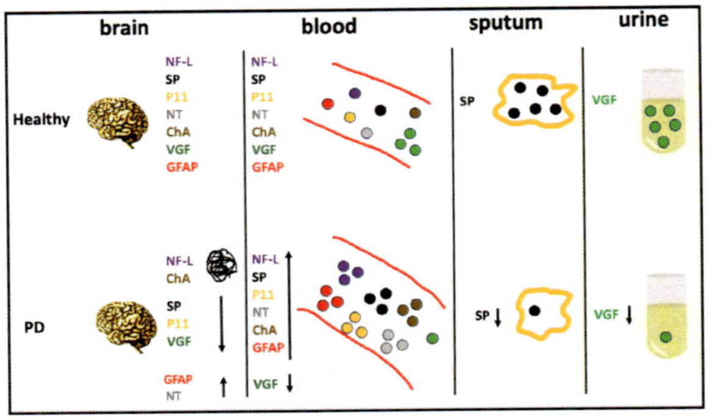

Source: Cocco C, Manai AL, Manca E, Noli B. Brain-Biomarker Changes in Body Fluids of Patients with Parkinson's Disease. International Journal of Molecular Sciences. 2023; 24(13):10932. https://doi.org/10.3390/ijms241310932.

The pathophysiology of PD was investigated by the researchers using oxidative stress as well as other proteins and processes. The pathologic hallmarks of Parkinson's disease, Lewy bodies and Lewy neurites, are made up of insoluble fibrils of α-synuclein. Comparing PD patients to controls, researchers discovered that PD patients had noticeably higher levels of soluble aggregates of the protein α-synuclein. Proteasome activity in peripheral blood lymphocytes is lower in PD patients compared to healthy controls, and defects in the ubiquitin-proteasome system, which breaks down polyubiquinated proteins, may play a role in the pathogenesis of Parkinson's disease. One study has shown the potential of a platelet biomarker to respond to treatment. The increased monoamine oxidase B activity seen in platelets of individuals with PD can be reversed with the addition of selegiline, an inhibitor of monoamine oxidase B.

3.1.3. Genetic Testing

Genes may be thought of as PD biomarkers since they are markers of pathogenic processes. Genetic factors do not appear to be a significant factor for most people with Parkinson's disease. On the other hand, identical twins of PD patients whose onset occurs before age 50 have a higher incidence of PD, and those with a family history of the disease are about two to four times more likely to develop PD. In 1997, Polymeropoulos discovered that PD in a sizable Italian family was caused by a mutation in the α-synuclein gene. Since then, numerous genes linked to Parkinson's disease have been discovered by researchers (Table 3.3). The genes are inherited in different ways: autosomal dominant (e.g., PARK1) to recessive autosomal (e.g., PARK7/DJ-1) to bestow genetic vulnerability (e.g., PARK10). Given that many patients with PD owing to genetic causes have a different clinical course than those with sporadic PD, genetics plays a useful role in diagnosis and patient education for cases of early onset with a family history (see Table 3.3). While progress in using genetic markers is unclear in sporadic PD occurring in adults over 50, it is still being made. In populations descended from Europe, sporadic PD is caused by a mutation in LRRK2, which is present in 1–8% of cases. Higher proportions of certain subpopulations have also been found to carry this mutation (Forman, 2004; Pankratz, 2005).

Table 3.3. *Genes Linked to Parkinson's Disease*

Locus	Gene/Protein	Inheritance Pattern	Clinical Phenotype
PARK1	SNCA/α-synuclein	Autosomal dominant	Mid-age onset (45-60 years old) with typical PD +/− dementia
PARK2	PARK2/parkin	Autosomal recessive	Juvenile (<20) onset with atypical features
PARK3	Unknown	Autosomal dominant	Typical PD
PARK5	UCH-L1	Autosomal dominant	Mid-age onset with typical PD
PARK6	PINK1	Autosomal recessive	Early onset (20-45) PD with slow progression
PARK7	PARK7/DJ-1	Autosomal recessive	Early onset PD with slow progression
PARK8	LRRK2/dardarin	Autosomal dominant	Mid-age onset with typical PD +/− dementia & amyotrophy
PARK10	Unknown	Genetic susceptibility	Typical PD
PARK11	Unknown	Genetic susceptibility	Typical PD
FTDP-17	MAPT/tau	Autosomal dominant	Parkinsonism associated with frontotemporal dementia
SCA2	ATXN2/ataxin-2	Autosomal dominant	Typical PD
SCA3	ATXN3/ataxin-3	Autosomal dominant	Typical PD
Nurr1	NR4A2/NURR1	Likely autosomal dominant	Typical PD
Synphilin-1	SNCAIP/synphilin-1	Likely autosomal dominant	Typical PD
Mitochondria	NADH complex I	Mitochondrial	Typical PD

Source: Stewart a. factor, William j. weiner, Parkinson's Disease Diagnosis and Clinical Management, ISBN-13: 978-1-933864-00-6.

3.2. Functional Neuroimaging in Parkinson's Disease

In order to clarify disease mechanisms, facilitate diagnosis, and evaluate possible novel therapeutic approaches, structural and functional neuroimaging has long been employed in the study of neurological disorders. Over the past ten years, functional neuroimaging has become increasingly useful in clinical and research settings for treating PD and other Parkinsonian disorders. This has led to the development of new therapeutic approaches as well as innovative diagnostic techniques.

This paper examines the use of this type of imaging in Parkinson's disease research.

The progressive loss of nigrostriatal dopaminergic function, which causes downstream alterations in basal ganglia circuitry, is the pathologic hallmark of PD. There has been a lot of interest in learning about the functional effects of dopaminergic pathology, even though direct imaging of the dopaminergic system using positron emission tomography (PET) or single-photon emission computed tomography (SPECT) can be useful for assessing PD. Furthermore, PD symptoms include nonmotor symptoms in addition to the classic characteristics of rigidity, bradykinesia, and tremor. These disease symptoms are caused by widespread functional abnormalities involving multiple neuronal circuits rather than a simple dysfunction of the basal ganglia. Instead of concentrating on individual neurotransmitter systems, functional imaging with MRI (fMRI), PET, and SPECT has become more widely used to evaluate neuronal connectivity. Furthermore, functional imaging can be used to track the advancement of PD symptoms and identify subclinical and early disease in addition to studying the mechanisms underlying the symptoms.

3.2.1. An Overview of Functional Imaging Techniques

- **Radiotracer Imaging***:* Several radiotracers are used in PET and SPECT imaging to evaluate normal and abnormal brain function *in vivo*. The dopamine system in Parkinsonian disorders has been extensively studied using these methods, but other neurochemical systems (e.g., Serotonergic, cholinergic, and other systems) can also be studied. Water or glucose that has been radiolabeled can be used to map cerebral blood flow and glucose utilization.

SPECT imaging is typically more accessible and less costly than PET imaging. Most nuclear medicine departments can perform routine SPECT, and since many radiopharmaceuticals are available commercially, there is no need for an on-site cyclotron. Nonetheless, PET outperforms SPECT in terms of sensitivity and spatial resolution. The resolution in SPECT restricts the caudate and putamen's separation in Parkinsonian disorders. PET's increased sensitivity makes it possible to image patients faster and with fewer motion artifacts. Finally, it is possible to conduct several studies on the same subject in a single day due to the short half-lives of the radiotracers used in PET imaging.

Abnormalities in the striatal storage and release of dopamine in Parkinsonian disorders result from cell loss and dysfunction in the substantia nigra. Therefore, dopaminergic imaging may be useful in determining the severity of a disease. It is possible to comprehend the mechanisms underlying the actions of these tracers by looking at the dopamine production, release, and reuptake pathways.

Tyrosine is first converted to l-3,4-dihydroxyphenylalanine (l-dopa) in nigrostriatal neurons, where it is then further processed by aromatic amino acid decarboxylase (AADC) to produce dopamine (DA). Before levodopa is converted to dopamine, it is actively absorbed when it is administered exogenously as part of dopaminergic therapy. The vesicular monoamine transporter type 2 (VMAT2) then packages dopamine into synaptic vesicles. Following its release into the synaptic cleft, dopamine (DA) interacts with both presynaptic and postsynaptic dopamine receptors. The membrane dopamine transporter (DAT) then either recycles or metabolizes the DA and returns it to the presynaptic terminal. Numerous radiotracers that assess dopaminergic function either pre- or postsynaptically have been developed. The dopaminergic system's radioligand imaging has been the most extensively researched in PD due to the prevalent nigrostriatal pathology. PET and SPECT can also be used to image many other neurochemical systems, including cholinergic, adrenergic, and serotonergic systems.

[^{18}F]-fluorodeoxyglucose (FDG) PET provides a means for imaging cerebral glucose metabolism, reflecting regional synaptic activity. In Parkinsonian disorders, spatial covariance methods have allowed for the detection of symptom-specific or disease-specific patterns that can be used to evaluate disease progression, diagnosis, or treatment effects. Because regional blood flow and cerebral metabolism tend to be largely linked in many neurodegenerative disorders, such pattern analysis can be applied to PET and SPECT imaging of cerebral perfusion as well (e.g., [^{15}O]-water PET or [^{99m}Tc]-technetium-ethylene cysteinate dimer SPECT).

Although applications in Parkinsonian disorders have been limited thus far, radioligand imaging also holds the potential to directly visualize pathology in neurodegenerative disorders. To be more precise, α-synuclein ligands like 2-(1-[6-[(2-[^{18}F]fluoroethyl)(methyl) amino]-2-naphthyl] ethylidene) malononitrile (FDDNP) or [^{18}F]-BF22 can be used to image Lewy bodies *in vivo*. Both of these ligands are not specific to α-synuclein, though. Additionally, they bind to β-amyloid, which means that separate imaging and image subtraction using β-amyloid-specific ligands (e.g., [^{11}C] benzothiazole-aniline, or Pittsburgh Compound B, PIB) are required.

- **Functional Magnetic Resonance Imaging (fMRI):** Since fMRI is widely accessible and doesn't require the injection of a radiotracer, there is no restriction on the total number of scans that can be carried out. For measuring dynamic changes in neural activity, its high spatial and temporal resolution is helpful. Deoxygenated hemoglobin is detectable with fMRI. The proton signal, also known as the blood oxygenation level-dependent (BOLD) contrast, is altered when deoxyhemoglobin interacts with the water molecules that surround blood vessels. Elevated local metabolic demand causes focal blood flow to rise, which in turn causes a relative drop in deoxyhemoglobin and an increase in BOLD signal. Unlike radiotracer imaging, fMRI has a poor signal-to-noise ratio and does not measure an easily understood quantity, even though this is thought to reflect local neuronal activity.

The possibility of using resting-state fMRI to clarify the functional architecture of the brain has surfaced more recently. The BOLD signal sporadic variations are measured using this technique. Then, it is thought that regional correlations in these spontaneous fluctuations represent functional and/or anatomical connectivity throughout those brain regions. In its most basic form, all other brain voxels are correlated with the fluctuations in the BOLD signal from an a priori seed region of interest. Other methods, like independent component analysis (ICA) to examine functional connectivity across brain regions, or hierarchical clustering, which builds a correlation matrix from several seeds, have been developed in response to the limitations imposed by a single seed. Some approaches, like regional homogeneity, measure local activity instead of assuming connectivity. Only a small number of resting-state studies have been methodically applied to PD to date.

3.2.2. Functional Imaging of Motor Symptoms and Motor Physiology

- **Dopaminergic Dysfunction and Motor Symptoms:** The integrity of the nigrostriatal system in PD can be directly studied using dopaminergic imaging. By measuring the activity of AADC, [^{18}F]-6-fluorodopa (FDOPA) PET offers a way to quantify the density of dopaminergic nerve terminals. Striatal FDOPA uptake is correlated with pathological measures and consistently and significantly reduced in patients with PD and other Parkinsonian disorders. The reduction is not consistent throughout the striatum; the putamen exhibits an anterior-posterior gradient and the caudate experiences the least amount of reduction. Furthermore, the reduction is asymmetric, with the more prominent reduction occurring on the hemisphere of the brain opposite the more severe motor signs. Additional radiotracers that measure dopaminergic presynaptic function (e.g., Similar results are shown by DAT and vesicular monoamine transporter [VMAT] ligands), which all decrease as the disease worsens.

The degree of FDOPA reduction appears to be most strongly correlated with bradykinesia and, to a lesser extent, rigidity; however, it does not reflect all motor symptoms equally. Putaminal FDOPA uptake seems to be more closely associated with motor function than caudate FDOPA uptake. Similarly, measurements of stiffness, gait, bradykinesia, and facial expression are correlated with imaging of the dopamine transporter system (DAT). It's interesting to note that there doesn't seem to be a correlation between dopaminergic deficits and tremor, which is not always responsive to dopaminergic therapy. Moreover, dopaminergic loss may not always be directly linked to gait dysfunction. Bohnen and team found that fall risk in PD is correlated with cortical and thalamic cholinergic hypofunction rather than dopaminergic denervation, possibly due to thalamic innervation from the pedunculopontine nucleus (PPN). It has not been established whether there is a correlation between the decline in extrastriatal monoaminergic function as indicated by FDOPA PET and motor or nonmotor symptoms, but at least one study indicates that this decline occurs independently of the nigrostriatal system.

- **Metabolic Networks and the PD-Related Motor Patterns:** FDG PET provides a means for mapping spatially distributed regional changes in cerebral glucose metabolism, and potentially relating these changes to specific diseases and symptoms. Spatial covariance analysis has been extensively used to detect network-level functional abnormalities in a variety of neurodegenerative disorders, including PD), atypical Parkinsonian syndromes such as multiple system atrophy (MSA) and progressive supranuclear palsy (PSP), Huntington's disease, and dementia. The details of this method based on principal component analysis (PCA) have been reviewed elsewhere. Briefly, the scaled subprofile model (SSM), a double-centered log-normalized PCA, is applied to multivoxel metabolic imaging data in a combined sample of scans from healthy subjects and patients. Once a pattern is identified that distinguishes one group from the other, its expression can be prospectively quantified on an individual basis, and the resulting subject scores (i.e., the PCA scalars) can be correlated with clinical and physiological measures of interest.

Using this technique on resting-state FDG PET scans of patients with Parkinson's disease has consistently shown an aberrant spatial covariance pattern associated with the disease involving components of the CSPTC circuitry. The pallido-thalamic and pontine metabolic activity are elevated in this Parkinson's disease-related pattern (PDRP), while the premotor cortex, supplemental motor area, and parietal association regions are relatively reduced. In addition to differentiating between PD patients and healthy individuals, PDRP expression also makes a distinction between PD and atypical Parkinsonian syndromes.

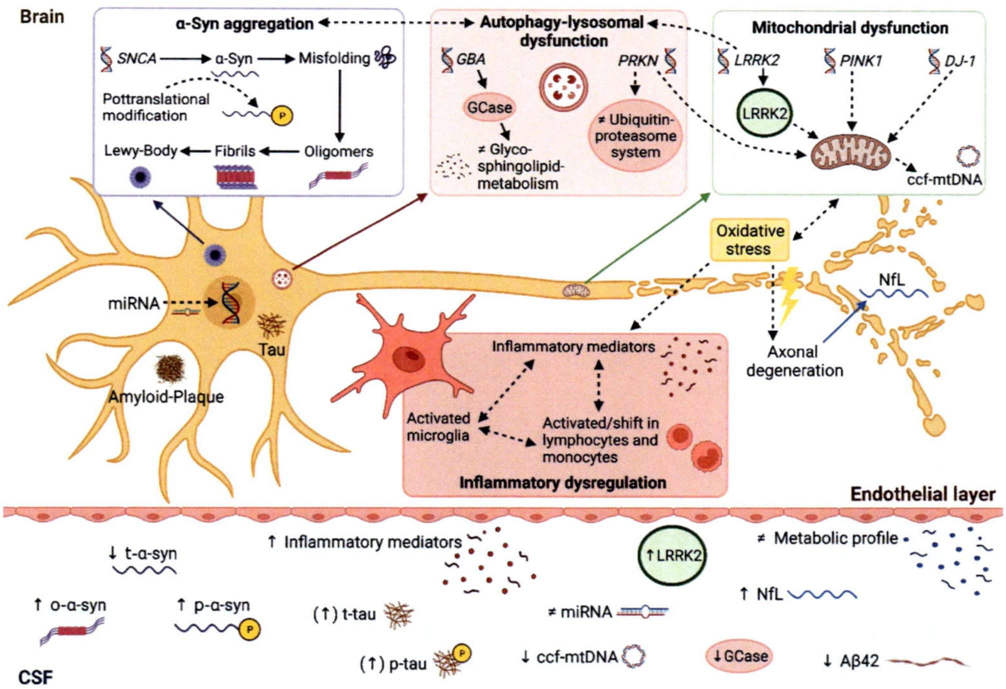

Figure 3.1. *Synopsis of CSF biomarkers under investigation in Parkinson's disease. Pathophysiological links between autophagy-lysosomal disruption, mitochondrial dysfunction and neuroinflammation leading to α-synuclein accumulation. Accordingly, molecular changes can be detected in CSF serving as candidate biomarkers in Parkinson's disease. Solid lines represent direct relations, whereas dotted lines represent multi-step processes. ↑ increased; ↓ decreased; ≠ unaltered; Aβ42, amyloid beta peptide 1-42; α-syn, α-synuclein; ccf-mtDNA, circulating cell-free mitochondrial DNA; miRNA, microRNA; NfL, neurofilament light chain; o-α-syn, oligomeric α-synuclein; p-α-syn, phosphorylated α-synuclein; t-α-syn, total α-synuclein; p-tau, phosphorylated tau; t-tau, total tau protein.*

Source: *Kwon EH, Tennagels S, Gold R, Gerwert K, Beyer L, Tönges L. Update on CSF Biomarkers in Parkinson's Disease. Biomolecules. 2022; 12(2):329. https://doi.org/10.3390/biom12020329.*

It has been possible to identify the PDRP topography in multiple distinct patient populations. Excellent within-subject reproducibility has been observed in subject scores indicating pattern expression in individual patients on test-retest evaluation. PDRP expression can also be measured in scans of resting cerebral perfusion obtained with [^{15}O]H_2O PET, ^{99m}Tc-ethylcysteinate dimer (ECD) SPECT, or with arterial spin labeling MRI methods because metabolism and cerebral blood flow are coupled, at least in the absence of dopaminergic medication (Ma et al.. 2007) (Figure 3.1).

Unified Parkinson's Disease Rating Scale (UPDRS) motor ratings and individual subject PDRP expression values consistently correlate. Similar to dopaminergic imaging, rigidity and bradykinesia rather than tremor are the main correlates of abnormally elevated PDRP subject scores. Furthermore, these findings link the nigrostriatal dopaminergic pathway degeneration to the aberrant PDRP functional topography. Remarkably, a 1-methyl-4-phenyl-1,2,3,6-tetrahydropyridine (MPTP) primate model of Parkinsonian bradykinesia and rigidity has recently been reported to exhibit a similar pattern.

PDRP expression rises steadily over time and is correlated with both putaminal dopaminergic function and motor function decline. Like dopaminergic imaging, PDRP expression is asymmetric, being worse on the side contralateral to the more affected body side. The PDRP can be measured independently in each hemisphere. Both hemispheres exhibit comparable progression over time, maintaining the initial asymmetry. Furthermore, the expression of PDRP in distinct individuals (i.e., the "subject scores") has been found to consistently correlate with UPDRS motor ratings. However, there are only weak correlations (R^2 30–40%) between the longitudinal declines in presynaptic dopaminergic function, clinical deterioration, and increases in PDRP expression with advancing disease, indicating that these progression indices are not equivalent. In fact, experimental models of CSPTC circuitry predict large-scale changes in regional synaptic activity, which is consistent with the spatial topography of PDRP. The connection between PDRP and surgical procedures emphasizes the biological significance of this protein. Subthalamic firing rates recorded during surgery, for instance, have a strong correlation with PDRP expression measurements taken before surgery. PDRP reductions comparable in size to those observed with levodopa treatment are observed with both subthalamic lesioning and deep brain stimulation (DBS).

An independent discrete spatial covariance pattern has been associated with Parkinsonian tremor. Utilizing ordinal trends/cannonical variates analysis (OrT/CVA), a within-subject network mapping algorithm based on supervised (i.e., directed) PCA techniques. FDG PET scans of the ventral-intermediate (Vim) thalamic nucleus were obtained at baseline (tremor present) and during high-frequency stimulation (tremor suppressed) in PD patients with a predominance of tremor. Increased metabolic activity in the caudate and putamen, primary motor cortex, cerebellum, and dorsal pons characterizes this repeatable pattern. The UPDRS tremor subscale ratings and accelerometric tremor measurements are correlated with PDTP expression, whereas the UPDRS akinesia-rigidity subscale ratings are not correlated with it.

- **Resting Studies of Motor Symptoms and Altered Motor Circuit Connectivity:** The study of brain disorders has made greater use of resting-state imaging in recent years. When PD patients were scanned at baseline, it was discovered that there was less functional connectivity in the pathways connecting the inferior parietal cortex and the posterior putamen, but there was no difference in the connectivity between the caudate nucleus and the dorsal prefrontal cortex or the anterior putamen and the pre-MSA. Reduced functional connectivity in PD patients receiving no treatment has not been observed in other studies. Instead, the results showed that dopaminergic treatment normalized baseline increases in cortico-striatal functional connectivity. Apart from the circuits that make up the classical cortico-striato-pallido-thalamocortical (CSPTC) circuit model of motor pathways, the role of the so-called "hyperdirect" pathway between motor cortex and STN in the motor physiology of PD has drawn focus recently. Increased resting-state functional connectivity between cortical motor regions and the STN has been observed in Parkinson's disease patients. The results of the subgroup analysis showed that PD patients with and without tremor differed from one another. Tremor patients had higher STN connectivity with the primary motor cortex and primary sensory cortex when compared to controls, while non-tremor patients also had higher STN connectivity with midline cortical motor areas. Similarly, tremor in Parkinson's disease has been linked to brief increases in functional connectivity between the motor cortex and basal ganglia. The putamen and globus pallidus (GPi and GPe) are momentarily activated at the start of tremor episodes in patients with PD, while activity in the cerebellar pathways cofluctuates with tremor amplitude in these patients. These findings imply that aberrant interactions between the basal ganglia and the cerebellothalamocortical circuit cause tremor in Parkinson's disease.

- **Motor Complications of Therapy—Dyskinesias:** Levodopa is a highly effective treatment for PD, but most patients experience both motor and nonmotor complications after a prolonged course of treatment. Of them, levodopa-induced dyskinesias (LID) affects up to 90% of patients with PD following nine years of therapy. An earlier age of onset, a longer duration of the disease, and the length and dosage of levodopa treatment are all linked to an increased risk of developing LID. The overactivity of the direct striatal pathway is thought to be a key characteristic of LID; however, the pathophysiology of LID is complicated and most likely involves both pre- and postsynaptic changes in the nigrostriatal system. Given that healthy individuals with a functioning presynaptic dopaminergic system do not develop LID, it is assumed that presynaptic dopaminergic denervation is required for the development of LID. Furthermore, the application of levodopa, an exogenous dopamine precursor, and endogenous dopaminergic denervation are likely to interact to cause the development of LID. Indeed, abnormal presynaptic handling of levodopa as well as hyperactive postsynaptic dopamine responses have been linked to LID in rodent and other animal models. In both PD patients and animal models, pulsatile levodopa administration appears to increase the risk of LID. Once established, LID patients are more likely to experience relapses, even after a protracted break from treatment. Functional imaging has provided additional information about this therapy-related complication since levodopa administration can consistently cause peak-dose LID in a large number of patients.

On the presynaptic side, dyskinesia severity is correlated with decreased FDOPA uptake, which is likely indicative of a more severe disease. The availability of postsynaptic dopamine D_2 receptors, as determined by [^{11}C]-raclopride PET, was also implicated in that study. Similarly, patients treated with the agonist had less reduction in putaminal FDOPA uptake and a lower incidence of LID in a longitudinal study comparing levodopa versus ropinirole. However, striatal dopaminergic denervation is insufficient to cause LID to manifest. There was an equal decrease in striatal DAT binding between patients with LID on low-dose levodopa and patients without LID on high-dose levodopa. Dopamine turnover might be involved in this. When estimating synaptic dopamine turnover early in the disease, kinetic modeling of FDOPA time-activity curves (TACs) over extended scanning epochs has shown an increase. Younger patients showed an even more marked relative increase in dopamine turnover in the early stages of the disease, which may have contributed to larger fluctuations in dopamine levels and explained those patients' increased susceptibility to motor complications. Using [^{11}C]-raclopride PET, higher synaptic dopamine levels were also observed in LID patients, and the degree of dyskinesia severity is correlated with the size of the levodopa-mediated change in radioligand binding affinity. Remarkably, a multitracer study of VMAT and DAT binding found that dopamine reuptake was comparatively down-regulated in contrast to nerve terminal loss. This adaptation may alleviate symptoms in the early stages of the disease, but as it advances, it may cause oscillatory synaptic dopamine and related motor complications. Long-term levodopa treatment may increase the number of D_1 receptors, according to animal studies. Nevertheless, PD patients in humans have not been demonstrated to exhibit consistent alterations in striatal D_1 and D_2 neuroreceptor binding.

Studies on animals or postmortem brain tissue have suggested the involvement of other neurotransmitter systems in the development of LID. These include the adenosine, serotonergic, opioid, and α_2 adrenergic systems. It was observed that PD patients with LID had less binding of [^{11}C]diphrenorphine (a nonselective marker of opioid receptors) in the striatum, thalamus, and anterior cingulate compared to those without. The opioid system functions as a modulator of dopamine and a cotransmitter within GABAergic neurons. Reduced putaminal binding was linked to a higher degree of LID severity, which may indicate that endogenous ligands in LID patients are more likely to occupy opioid receptors.

Both levodopa and dopamine agonists cause localized increases in cerebral blood flow. When dopaminergic treatment is administered, functional imaging studies using Xenon-133 have shown comparable increases in PD patients and normal subjects. Adverse reactions to levodopa in Parkinson's disease patients have been linked to increased blood flow in the striatum, globus pallidus, and thalamus, while decreased blood flow has been observed in those who do not experience adverse reactions. In a motor activation study, compared to individuals without LID, patients with LID exhibited a significant overactivation in the SMA and bilateral primary motor cortex measured with Xenon-133. Levodopa-induced alterations in blood flow have also been assessed using $H_2^{15}O$ PET. The alterations in blood flow have generally been ascribed to dopamine's direct effects on the local microvasculature.

Levodopa-induced changes in blood flow are in contrast to changes in local metabolism. Increased glucose metabolism is seen in the putamen, globus pallidus, ventral thalamus, and dorsal pons of untreated Parkinson's disease patients. Changes in local synaptic activity at salient nodes of the PDRP metabolic network have been linked to these regional abnormalities. Strong correlations between regional cerebral metabolic rate (CMR) and blood flow (CBF) have been demonstrated during the resting state, supporting the idea that both measures capture local synaptic activity. As a result, there is a significant correlation between the PDRP expression determined by perfusion-weighted MRI, H_2O PET, and FDG PET scans in the same subjects. Nevertheless, it has been discovered that dopaminergic therapy dissociates, or "uncouples," these effects. Levodopa treatment that works lowers abnormally high metabolic activity while raising basal ganglia CBF. It is true that in PD patients receiving levodopa treatment, PDRP network modulation is dissociated between CBF and CMR, but not during STN stimulation with a similar level of clinical efficacy. The putamen and dorsal pons were the regional sites of the flow-metabolism dissociation phenomenon that was seen at the network level. In these regions, patients with LID show higher increases in rCBF with levodopa treatment, which is consistent with exaggerated microvascular responsiveness to monoamines in these individuals. Levodopa treatment induces angiogenesis and endothelial proliferation in animal models, which could be the basis for this observation.

3.2.3. Functional Imaging of Non-Motor Symptoms

PD is defined and clinically diagnosed based on motor signs and symptoms. Nonmotor symptoms, however, can be more noticeable, appear before motor symptoms, and fall into many categories, including neuropsychiatric, sleep, or autonomic dysfunction. Among the premotor symptoms, idiopathic rapid eye movement (REM) sleep behavior disorder and hyposmia both increase the risk of PD, dopaminergic imaging may be abnormal in these patients.

When it comes to clinical disability and the overall outcome of treatment, cognitive functioning can be significantly compromised in PD. With a significantly higher cumulative prevalence, the point prevalence of dementia in PD may reach up to 31%. Early PD can cause cognitive difficulties even in the absence of dementia; these symptoms are comparable to those experienced by PD patients with dementia (PDD), but they are less severe.

Functional imaging studies have linked several mechanisms, such as dopaminergic depletion, cholinergic dysfunction, protein aggregation, and cortical pathology, to cognitive dysfunction and dementia in PD (i.e., formation of Lewy bodies). Cognitive dysfunction in PD has been studied using functional imaging in the resting state and activation paradigms, just like with motor function.

3.2.4. Resting Metabolism

In PD, FDG PET has reliably revealed cortical hypometabolism. Hypometabolism in the frontal and occipital cortices is seen in patients even in those who do not appear to have cognitive impairment. In PD patients with mild cognitive impairment (MCI), this hypometabolism appears more pervasive and may involve the occipital and medial frontal regions in addition to the prefrontal and lateral parietal cortices. In fact, a comparison of patients with single- and multiple-domain MCI, or between patients with and without MCI, suggests that the extent of cognitive dysfunction is reflected in the degree and topography of hypometabolism.

Early research utilizing network analysis and PET imaging revealed distinct patterns of metabolic dysfunction associated with motor, emotional, and cognitive function. Using FDG PET data from a group of PD patients without dementia and spatial covariance analysis, Huang et al. discovered a noteworthy covariance pattern that showed a correlation between executive functioning in particular and cognitive performance. The frontal and parietal association areas show metabolic reductions, while the cerebellar vermis and dentate nuclei show increases in this pattern, which is known as the PD-related cognitive pattern (PDCP). The level of cognitive impairment increased with the expression of PDCP.

It is not functionally dependent on PD on metabolic patterns. While there is a gradual increase in both PDCP and PDRP expression, only PDRP expression changes are associated with concurrent declines in striatal dopaminergic function. Group analysis shows that, in contrast to PDRP, PDCP expression is not affected by levodopa or DBS treatment of Parkinsonian motor symptoms.

Levodopa-mediated alterations in verbal learning, however, are correlated with baseline PDCP expression, and levodopa does impact cognitive function in certain patients. Furthermore, PDCP expression decreases concurrently with meaningful improvement in levodopa-using patients (Huang et al., 2007) (Figure 3.2).

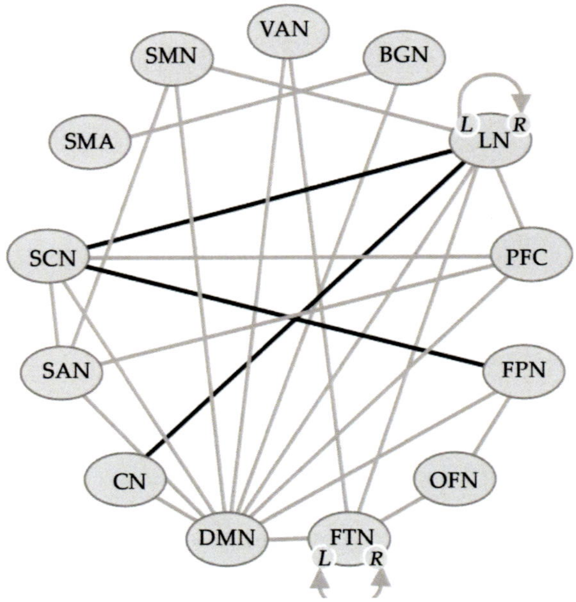

Figure 3.2. *Schematic overview of functional connectivity in some major networks in Parkinson disease with mild cognitive impairment (PD-MCI). gray lines: hypocommunication, black lines: hypercommunication. L, R: left, right hemisphere. network abbreviations: VAN: ventral attention; BGN: basal ganglia; LN: limbic; PFC: prefrontal cortex; FPN: frontoparietal; OFN: orbitofrontal; FTN: frontotemporal; DMN: default mode; CN: cerebellar; SAN: salience; SCN: subcortical; SMA: supplementary motor area; SMN: sensorimotor.*

Source: *Jellinger KA. Pathobiology of Cognitive Impairment in Parkinson Disease: Challenges and Outlooks. International Journal of Molecular Sciences. 2024; 25(1):498. https://doi.org/10.3390/ijms25010498.*

Dopamine levels in various striatal regions (which are influenced by disease severity, genetic factors, and treatment) may have an impact on both the positive and negative effects of Parkinson's disease treatment on cognition. For instance, in a series of studies involving motor sequence learning, GPi and STN stimulation were linked to improved performance, while levodopa was not. Levodopa, however, really helped patients with low baseline performance, while it had the opposite effect on those with high baseline performance. Levodopa specifically inhibited the typical deactivation that takes place during motor sequence learning in the ventromedial prefrontal cortex (vmPFC). Deactivation of the vmPFC was normal in good learners, but levodopa caused abnormal depression. Levodopa-mediated normalization of prefrontal activations has also been observed in other fMRI or H215O PET studies, indicating possible advantageous effects of levodopa on mesocortical pathways (Figure 3.3).

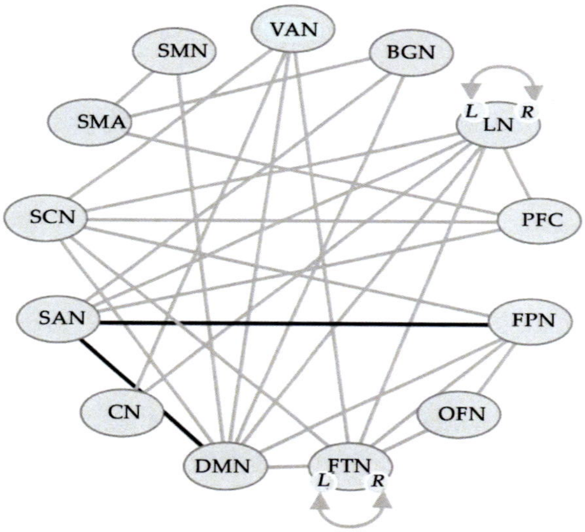

Figure 3.3. *Schematic overview of functional connectivity in some major networks in Parkinson disease dementia (PDD). Gray lines: hypocommunication, black lines: hypercommunication. L, R: left, right hemisphere. network abbreviations: VAN: ventral attention; BGN: basal ganglia; LN: limbic; PFC: prefrontal cortex; FPN: frontoparietal; OFN: orbitofrontal; FTN: frontotemporal; DMN: default mode; CN: cerebellar; SAN: salience; SCN: subcortical; SMA: supplementary motor area; SMN: sensorimotor.*

Source: *Jellinger KA. Pathobiology of Cognitive Impairment in Parkinson Disease: Challenges and Outlooks.International Journal of Molecular Sciences. 2024; 25(1):498. https://doi.org/10.3390/ijms25010498.*

- **The Default Mode Network:** Executive task impairments are a common feature in PD patients. It has been known for the past ten years that deactivating a baseline network may be necessary to accomplish numerous executive or attentional tasks. The medial prefrontal cortex, posterior cingulate cortex, precuneus, and lateral parietal and temporal cortices are part of this network, also known as the default mode network (DMN), which can be detected using fMRI or PET imaging. Patients with dementia or neuropsychiatric disorders, as well as those who are aging normally, may exhibit impaired DMN deactivation. It is not unexpected that deactivation of the DMN would be compromised in PD given that dopamine loss in this condition results in functional impairment of CSPTC pathways and modulation of frontal lobe activity.

Few studies have looked at the DMN in Parkinson's disease thus far Tinaz et al. used fMRI in conjunction with a semantic event sequencing task discovered that during task performance, patients with PD did not exhibit decreased activation of the DMN, in contrast to controls. In a similar vein, PD patients demonstrated reduced activation of the parietal DMN nodes during the control task and less deactivation of the same regions during a Montreal card sorting task. This opposite pattern of activation and deactivation from that observed in healthy aging may point to anomalies unique to PD associated with dopaminergic dysfunction. The degree of DMN deactivation is correlated with task complexity in young, healthy subjects; this relationship may disappear in older, healthy subjects and patients with Parkinson's disease.

Interestingly, apomorphine appears to restore this correlation in both PD patients and healthy controls.

- **Imaging of Specific Neurotransmitters in PD Cognition:** It has been noted that both PD patients with and without cognitive impairment have reduced striatal dopaminergic function. Having said that, PD's cognitive deficits could be influenced by dopaminergic dysfunction in the caudate. Indeed, compared to PD patients without dementia, there is a greater loss of tracer uptake in the caudate in the former group. Jokinen and colleagues observed additional associations with hippocampal and prefrontal atrophy, but they also observed a significant correlation between verbal and visual memory functioning and caudate FDOPA uptake. Numerous other studies have demonstrated connections between decreased frontal lobe, executive, and memory function and decreased caudate dopaminergic tracer uptake. PD patients demonstrated a connection between caudate DAT binding and accurate target acquisition during sequence learning. Furthermore, the dorsolateral and ventral prefrontal cortices' learning-related activation exhibited strong correlations with caudate DAT binding in normal subjects, a relationship that was absent in Parkinson's disease patients. It has been observed that there is a correlation between PDCP expression and caudate, but not putamen DAT binding.

Cognitive function and extrastriatal dopaminergic function may also be related. For instance, drug-naïve patients may have increased dorsolateral frontal cortex uptake of FDOPA, which is linked to poorer performance on sustained attention tests. On the other hand, more FDOPA uptake in the anterior cingulate and medial frontal cortex is linked to better results on tests of suppressed attention. The results may indicate compensatory modifications in dopaminergic transmission in early PD, but they may also indicate increased activity of the AADC in areas related to the noradrenergic and serotonergic neurotransmitter systems.

Evidence of cholinergic dysfunction in the thalamus, striatum, and cortical areas has regularly been found during postmortem examinations of PD patients, and Ruberg et al. reported larger reductions in the frontal cortex of patients with demented Parkinson's disease than did the control group. PD seems to be associated with a loss of cholinergic function in the brain stem, in contrast to Alzheimer's disease (AD). Various radiotracers can be used for *in vivo* imaging of acetylcholinesterase (AChE), nicotinic and muscarinic acetylcholine receptors (nACHR and mAChR), and acetylcholine vesicular transporter (VAChT). AChE function can be evaluated using [^{11}C]-methyl-4-piperidinly proprionate (PMP) or [^{11}C]-methyl-4-piperidyl acetate (MP4A). Diffuse Lewy body disease (DLB), PD, and PDD patients have decreased cortical AChE activity. Compared to their counterparts without dementia (10.2%–12.9%), PD patients with dementia experience a more severe reduction in cognitive function (17% to 29.7%). Furthermore, compared to AD, cortical AChE deficits may be more pronounced in PDD and DLB. This loss of cortical cholinergic function seems to start early in the course of the illness and gets worse when dementia sets in. Tests of attention and cognitive function show a stronger correlation with cholinergic dysfunction than do the length of the disease and the intensity of motor symptoms. PDD patients have relatively lower cortical MP4A binding, but both PD and PDD patients exhibit reductions in striatal FDOPA uptake. However, decreases in striatal FDOPA binding and cortical MP4A are associated with PDD, indicating that a combined decline in the two neurotransmitter systems contributes to the condition in these patients.

Similar cortical reductions, primarily in the parietal and occipital cortices, have been seen in imaging of the VAChT system with [^{123}I]-iodobenzovesamicol (IBVM) in patients with nondemented Parkinson's disease (PDD). These reductions are more extensive and severe in PDD patients. Research on nAChR in PD has consistently reported decreased cortical receptors along with a decrease in subcortical tracer binding.

Even though the majority of these studies involved nondemented PD patients, patients with DLB were assessed for nAChR activity using [^{123}I]-5-I-A-85380 SPECT. They discovered a relative increase in the occipital cortex and decreased tracer binding in the striatum, frontal, temporal, and cingulate areas, which may indicate a connection between cholinergic function and visual hallucinations in that region. Imaging studies of mAChR have revealed elevated frontal and occipital receptor activity in patients with PD and PDD, in contrast to the nicotinic system.

This increase was not seen in demented PSP patients, though, which may indicate that there is no direct correlation between cognitive dysfunction and the muscarinergic system. The visual abnormalities observed in DLB and PDD may be caused by an increase in occipital mAChR activity, similar to an increase in occipital nAChR activity. Cortical cholinergic dysfunction seems to be a common feature of cognitive impairment in PD. These findings are in line with the improvement in cognition that was seen in demented Parkinson's disease patients receiving AchE inhibitors in clinical trials.

- **Protein Aggregation:** As in other neurodegenerative diseases, the pathology of PD is associated with the accumulation of misfolded proteins, namely, Lewy bodies. Lewy bodies, neuronal intracellular inclusions that contain α-synuclein, are more widespread in PDD and DLB. Additionally, β-amyloid deposition, i.e., Alzheimer pathology, is seen in both PDD and DLB, and may be associated with poor clinical outcome. The past few years have seen the development of radioligands for *in vivo* imaging of amyloid deposition. Of these, 2-(1-{6-[(2-[^{18}F] Fluoroethyl) (methyl) amino]-2-naphthy}ethylidene) malononitrile (FDDNP) is relatively nonspecific, labeling senile plaques and neurofibrillary tangles in AD, prion plaques, amyloid deposits, and cortical Lewy bodies *in vitro*. In contrast, [*N*-methyl-C-11]2-(4′ -methylaminophenyl)-6-hydroxybenzothiazole (Pittsburgh Compound B, PIB) binds strongly to amyloid plaques in AD, but not significantly to Lewy bodies. Indeed, limited autopsy studies suggest that in PDD or DLB, *in vivo* PIB imaging does reflect β-amyloid rather than Lewy body pathology. Two of the three had elevated PIB uptake. All three had abundant cortical Lewy bodies, but the two individuals with elevated PIB uptake were also found to have abundant diffuse Aβ plaques.

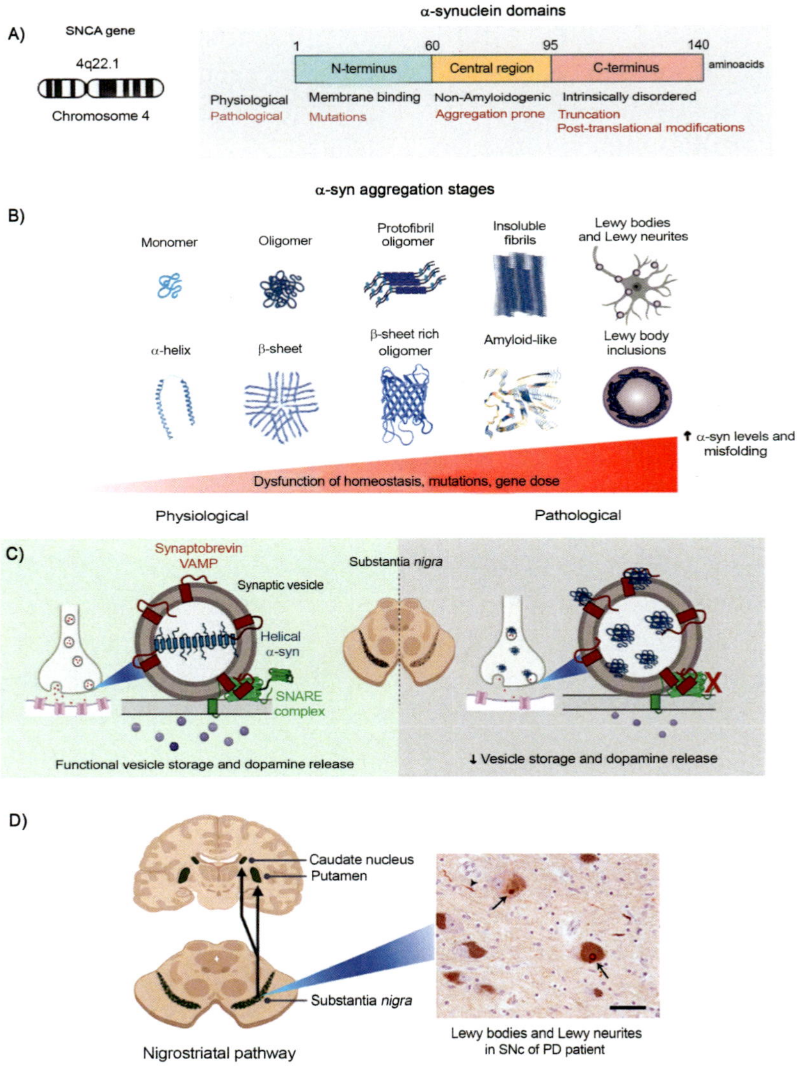

Figure 3.4. *Misfolding and aggregation of α-syn in PD. (**A**) Left: SNCA gene coding for the α-syn on chromosome 4. Right: Structure of α-syn (Protein Data Base, PDB, 1XQ8) highlighting its different domains and its involvement in cell physiology (black) as well as in various alterations that come to affect its function (red). (**B**) Aggregation states of α-syn: structure (above) and three-dimensional composition (PDB 6OSJ) (below) by crystallography. (**C**) α-syn activity under physiological conditions (left), as well as in alterations to its function (right). Image modified from Burré et al. (2010). (**D**) Left: Nigrostriatal pathway, which originates in the SNpc and projects to the dorsal striatum. Right: α-syn inclusions in the form of LBs (arrows) and neurites (arrowheads) from a PD patient (20×).*

Source: Padilla-Godínez FJ, Ramos-Acevedo R, Martínez-Becerril HA, Bernal-Conde LD, Garrido-Figueroa JF, Hiriart M, Hernández-López A, Argüero-Sánchez R, Callea F, Guerra-Crespo M. Protein Misfolding and Aggregation: The Relatedness between Parkinson's Disease and Hepatic Endoplasmic Reticulum Storage Disorders. International Journal of Molecular Sciences. 2021; 22(22):12467. https://doi.org/10.3390/ijms222212467.

PIB has been used in several studies to assess patients with synucleinopathies (PD, PDD, DLB). Patients with PD who are cognitively normal typically do not have elevated PIB binding. On the other hand, DLB patients exhibit aberrantly high cortical PIB binding, at levels similar to those of AD patients. Normal cortical PIB binding is typically linked to PDD, a disorder that may fall under the same umbrella as DLB or be more closely related to PD. In PDD patients, PIB elevation is typically less than in DLB patients (Fig. 3.4(A)), and there might be no correlation between amyloid load and dementia severity indicators. However, occipital PIB binding was higher in the synucleinopathies than in AD patients, and visuospatial impairment was linked to amyloid deposition in the parietal and posterior cingulate regions. While the majority of demented patients did not have elevated PIB binding, another recent study found that amyloid deposition was associated with lower MMSE scores in patients with dementia (DLB and PDD). This suggests that other factors may be involved in the cognitive decline associated with Lewy body disease (Figure 3.4).

3.3. Controversies in Neuroimaging

There are some conjectural claims that, when combined with convincing visuals, could help to explain why functional imaging research on PD is so popular in academic journals and scientific conferences.

The argument goes like this: In PD, symptoms start to appear when 70% of nigrostriatal dopaminergic neurons are lost, according to postmortem data. [18F]Dopamine presynaptic transporter ligand single photon emission computed tomography (DAT-SPECT) and dopa positron emission tomography (dopa-PET) measure the integrity of these dopaminergic neurons in the living human brain. Therefore, these methods can be used to identify asymptomatic individuals with preclinical disease (those with no symptoms but fewer than normal dopaminergic neurons) and confirm the diagnosis in PD patients (those who are symptomatic and have less than 70% dopaminergic neurons). Additionally, the methods enable objective assessment of the disease's dopaminergic pathology's progression. The bulk of dopa-PET and DAT-SPECT studies have demonstrated that the illness has a brief preclinical period and a rapid rate of progression, which contradicts the "long latency" theory. As a result, these indices can be used as biomarkers in neuroprotection studies. Levodopa is toxic in ELLDOPA, a third study, while agonist medications have been shown to have a neuroprotective effect in CALM and REAL, two imaging endpoint studies. These studies also showed that some patients who were recruited and given a clinical diagnosis of PD had normal scan results. These patients are probably misdiagnosed; they have been classified as SWEDDs (symptomatic without evidence of dopaminergic deficit). DAT-SPECT is more likely than dopa-PET to become the indispensable tool for diagnosis and disease monitoring that has long been required due to its lower cost and simpler use. In the end, and with additional funding, the population could be screened to identify those who are at risk of developing PD using dopa-PET and DAT-SPECT. For those who are most vulnerable, neuroprotective treatment may then be started.

Every time this series or any of its component statements have been questioned, controversy has ensued. This chapter examines this collection of claims along with the arguments put forth to support and refute them. It also presents a different perspective on how dopa-PET and DAT-SPECT add to our understanding of Parkinson's disease. The techniques and ligands that are most widely available, have been the subject of the most claims and disputes, and are therefore the only ones covered in this chapter: dopa-PET and DAT-SPECT.

3.3.1. The Controversies and the Evidence

- ***In Parkinson's Disease, Symptoms Begin When 70% of Nigrostriatal Dopaminergic Neurons Have Been Lost:*** This statement has served as supporting evidence for the findings of numerous imaging studies, even though it isn't the subject of a dispute in imaging. Ehringer and Hornykiewicz's groundbreaking research, which identified dopamine's critical role in PD, helped pave the way for the understanding that the nigrostriatal dopamine system is severely damaged at the onset of symptoms 46 years ago. A postmortem study by Bernheimer and colleagues on 69 cases of Parkinsonism and 28 controls was published in 1973. It revealed severe dopamine depletion in the striatum (more than 80%) in PD and a correlation between striatal dopamine and nigral cell count. These data were later interpreted by other authors to suggest that nigral cell loss was at least 50% advanced at the onset of symptoms. Using this and additional data, Calne and Langston conjectured that the development of PD was probably the result of aging normally on top of a prior striatal injury. Fearnley and Lees, on the other hand, predicted an exponentially progressing disease course, a short preclinical period (4.7 years), and symptom onset when the nigral dopaminergic cell count was 69% of normal based on their analysis of postmortem specimens from patients with a wide range of disease severity and duration. All of these postmortem studies have their share of challenges, such as disagreements regarding the best cell counting technique, the impact of the time lapse between death and analysis on biochemistry, and extrapolating results from patients whose illnesses are clinically advanced and whose duration is unavoidably long. A new assessment of the connection between pathology and symptoms has been offered by Braak and team. The nigral melanoneurons are not the first brain structures to develop PD-related lesions, as these authors emphasize, and they postulate a pathologic progression both before and during the progression of symptoms. The most crucial thing to remember about this chapter is that contrary to what Braak's research suggests, either dopamine or massive nigral cell loss is not always present at the onset of symptoms, nor is the loss of dopaminergic nigrostriatal neurons the primary pathologic or biochemical indicator of preclinical Parkinson's disease.
- ***Dopa-PET and DAT-SPECT Measure the Integrity of Nigrostriatal Dopaminergic Neurons:*** Regarding dopaminergic pathology, it is unclear what dopa-PET and DAT-SPECT mean. The important (and often missed) realization is that they offer biochemical measurements instead of pathological or anatomic

ones. A multi-author review found a dearth of evidence supporting their potential as pathology markers. Dopa-PET most likely measures either aromatic acid decarboxylase (AADC) or stored [18F]dopa in the structure that is being studied, but it is unclear how this relates to the real number of cells or terminals. It is true that there has been a correlation between the number of nigral neurons in MPTP monkeys and dopa-PET results; however, the human study that reports this correlation (which is frequently cited in dopa-PET papers) only looked at five subjects, four of whom did not have Parkinson's disease. Presynaptic dopamine reuptake transporter availability can be measured using DAT-SPECT; this transporter's concentration decreases in Parkinson's disease patients, although it is unclear how this decline relates to pathology. The biochemical measurements derived from DAT-SPECT and dopa-PET may be susceptible to up- or down-regulation in response to medication or the course of the disease. They undoubtedly result from intricate biochemical and mathematical analyses, and various tools and techniques produce various outcomes.

We can be certain that the results of dopa-PET and DATSPECT are related to the clinical progression of PD, but we cannot be certain that they measure cell count. Though these methods can be used in theory to detect preclinical illness (i.e., One consistent finding in dopa-PET and DAT-SPECT studies has been a correlation between their indices and clinical severity (i.e., where the result is unrelated to symptom severity). Any aspect of disease severity that is clinically measured and that which is measured by these biochemical tools are probably not perfectly correlated.

It is highly probable that the diverse symptom progression of PD is caused by altered neurochemistry and pathology, rather than a single anatomical and biochemical group of neurons being studied. Clinical measurements, DAT-SPECT, Dopa-PET, and other tests are not error-free, and different medications may have different effects on them depending on the stage of the disease.

The potential benefits of biomarker measurements over clinical measurements have been thoroughly examined. In summary, they provide (theoretically) a single objective, potentially linear, continuous measurement that is unaffected by mood or drug side effects. The cost, radiation exposure, and unavailability stand in opposition to that.

Therefore, the meaning of the results of the DAT-SPECT and dopa-PET tests is that they measure something that deteriorates with clinical progression and is probably connected in some way to the pathologic and biochemical processes that underlie progression. To conclude that they measure the integrity of nigrostriatal dopamine neurons is oversimplified, if not inaccurate.

- ***What Happens to Dopa-PET and DAT-SPECT Results With Normal Aging?*** This is a significant question that hasn't received a satisfactory response despite being thought about. It is reasonable to note that the pathophysiology of the nigrostriatal dopaminergic system in aging appears to be equally ambiguous. While one study found no loss in older subjects, another suggests that pigmented nigral neurons decline with age (5.8% per decade). The answer to this question is critical to understanding imaging results: if pathology changes with aging but biomarkers do not, human biochemistry must be able to compensate to maintain normal dopaminergic function, which in turn presumably results in normal dopa-PET and DAT-SPECT readings. If the pathologists' estimates of the 70% loss before the onset of symptoms are accurate, then upregulation or built-in redundancy is required to allow for the continuation of normal function (up until this point). The question seems appropriate in evaluating the validity of the technique in differentiating PD from normal. If the system does in fact upregulate, how can the techniques be used to measure dopaminergic cell count? Should age be taken into account when adjusting results for the normal population?

An early PET controversy examined how normal aging might alter dopa-PET results. In the first study, ten subjects between the ages of 22 and 80 showed a 53% decline in striatal Ki. In the second published study, which included 26 healthy participants, there was no age-related decrease in putamenal Ki or caudate. This prompted the author, Sawle, to directly and controversially refute Calne and Langston's long-latency theory, arguing that the progression observed in PD and possibly detectable through dopa-PET was not an effect of aging.

Sawle's findings were corroborated by a later study conducted on 19 people by Eidelberg and colleagues. Kumakura and team have, however, returned to the topic and, using a novel analytical technique, discovered a 58% decrease in [18F] dopa storage in the aging human brain. This uncertainty and debate around a population as seemingly simple as the aging normal population highlights numerous issues that frequently arise in functional imaging research, including small sample sizes, disagreements over methodology, and defensive arguing.

Studies of aging using DAT-SPECT seem to be more cohesive. It has been shown in cross-sectional studies that the binding of striatal DAT decreases by 6.6% (n = 126) (33), 5% (n = 13), and 7% (n = 36) per decade.

Unfortunately, it is not possible to conclude that DAT-SPECT is a more accurate marker of neuronal integrity than dopa-PET (assuming that all other factors such as reproducibility, sensitivity, and resistance to confounders are equal) without unity (or at least a firm majority) in pathologic studies.

All DAT-SPECT studies, whether they are diagnostic or tracking progression, need to be modified if these aging studies are accurate in suggesting that dopamine reuptake transporter does not upregulate with age.

- ***Can DAT-SPECT and Dopa-PET Reliably Discriminate Normal From PD at Symptom Onset and Can They Usefully Detect Preclinical PD?*** It is possible to assume that healthy individuals with results outside of the normal range have preclinical disease, while symptomatic individuals with dopa-PET and DAT-SPECT scan results in the normal range (SWEDDs) are misdiagnosed.

Any measurement in a population that is healthy will have a distribution of results around the mean that follows a normal distribution. Numerous factors influence the standard deviation, or amount of spread, around the mean.

Imaging depends on anatomical, physiological, or biochemical variations within the population as well as technique reliability. The outcome of an unreliable technique is results that are dispersed around a mean, regardless of whether the populations are healthy or unhealthy (Table 3.4).

Table 3.4. *Main Comparison of Aggregated Proteins Involved in PD, AATD, and HHHS*

Protein/ Disease	**α-Syn/PD**	**AAT/AATD**	**FG/HHHS**
Native Structure	15 kDa Monomer *N*-terminal alpha-helix region, a central domain or NAC region and A C-terminal acidic tail	52 kDa Monomer Nine alpha-helices, two β-sheets and a reactive center loop	340 kDa triple fibrinogen Aα, Bβ, and γ chains Two lateral globular parts containing the *C*-terminus of Bβ and γ chains, a central nodule, containing the *N*-terminus of all chains
Polymerization steps	Monomer → dimer → oligomer → fibrils	Monomer → Dimer → Oligomer → Inclusion	Monomer → Oligomer → Protofibril → Fibril
Amyloid structure	Amyloid β-sheets in oligomers and fibrils	Amyloid β-sheets in dimers and oligomers	Amyloid fibril protein fibrinogen Aα
Inclusion bodies	LBs with more than 90 protein components	Inclusions with dense material and a clear halo in the periphery	Type I: Polygonal shape Type II: Ground glass appearance Type III: Eosinophilic globules, granular structures in the periphery
Inclusion proteins	α-syn, Tau protein, ubiquitin, neurofilament protein, β amyloid, among others	AAT M-Z and ZZ alleles	Mutated fibrinogen γ-chain
Organelles affected in the cell	α-syn aggregates can be found in all organelles	Only present in the ER	Only present in the ER

Protein/ Disease	α-Syn/PD	AAT/AATD	FG/HHHS
ER Stress response	UPR Chaperone activation PERK-dependent pathway	IL-6 and IL-8 protein production. Possible UPR activation. ER overload pathway	No available data
Organs affected	Across the brain tissue	Liver and lungs	Liver and lungs
Onset of disease	Chronic: Duplication/Triplication of *SNCA*: Symptoms from the age of 40 Idiopathic: From the age of 55	Chronic: Symptoms from early childhood	Chronic: Symptoms from early childhood or adulthood

Source: Padilla-Godínez FJ, Ramos-Acevedo R, Martínez-Becerril HA, Bernal-Conde LD, Garrido-Figueroa JF, Hiriart M, Hernández-López A, Argüero-Sánchez R, Callea F, Guerra-Crespo M. Protein Misfolding and Aggregation: The Relatedness between Parkinson's Disease and Hepatic Endoplasmic Reticulum Storage Disorders. International Journal of Molecular Sciences. 2021; 22(22):12467. https://doi.org/10.3390/ijms222212467.

* PD, and endoplasmic reticulum storage disorders (ERSDs), like alpha-1-antitrypsin deficiency (AATD) and hereditary hypofibrinogenemia with hepatic storage (HHHS)

To estimate the ability of the technique to detect abnormality, either in healthy or unhealthy populations, it is necessary to know or to estimate the threshold for symptom onset. This can be estimated by:

1. Examining either side in patients with a pure hemiParkinsonian syndrome (i.e., one striatum is connected to an asymptomatic side, the other to a symptomatic side, so the threshold lies somewhere between).
2. Correlation in a cross-sectional study. The threshold is assumed to be the value of the imaging marker when the clinical measurement is zero. The flaw in this approach is the assumption of a linear relationship between a multicomponent ordinal scale such as the Unified Parkinson's Disease Rating Scale (UPDRS) and the imaging measurement.
3. Extrapolating back from a longitudinal study, where the imaging measurement at symptom onset can be estimated. An assumption must be made here of either linearity or nonlinearity in index progression over time (Table 3.5).

Table 3.5. *Summary of the Main Characteristics of the Neurotoxin-Induced PD Models*

Neurotoxin	Pathogenesis	PD Symptoms	Advantages	Disadvantages
6-OHDA	Loss of DA innervation	Rotational motor behavior Sensory motor deficits Akinesia (with bilateral administration)	Activation of glial cells Economical Different variants depending on site and dose administered	Needs intracerebral administration Does not mimic the multisystem pathology of PD Does not induce a progressive nigrostriatal degeneration Does not induce LB formation nor synuclein aggregation
MPTP	Dose-dependent loss of DA neurons Reduced DA levels in striatum and midbrain DA neuron loss	Dose-dependent locomotor alterations Sensorimotor deficits	Translatable to human disease Easy to administer	Not toxic in rats Does not induce LBs Does not mimic the multisystem pathology of PD Variability in behavioral and biochemical results High mortality
Rotenone	DA neuron loss in SNpc Nigrostriatal dopaminergic denervation	Motor disturbances Sensory-motor deficits	Easy to administer Induces most motor symptoms of PD	Toxicity in other organs Causes nonspecific cerebral damage High mortality High interindividual variability

Neurotoxin	Pathogenesis	PD Symptoms	Advantages	Disadvantages
Paraquat	Controversy across studies Recent studies describe a reduction in dopaminergic neurons in the SNpc	Decreased locomotor activity and sensory-motor function	Easy to administer Translatable to human disease Increased synuclein immunoreactivity and LB-like structures in DA neurons of the SNpc Increased synuclein immunoreactivity in enteric neurons	Controversial results Important toxic effects, which can difficult the interpretation of behavioral tests High mortality (if using high doses)

Source: Ortega Moreno L, Bagues A, Martínez V, Abalo R. New Pieces for an Old Puzzle: Approaching Parkinson's Disease from Translatable Animal Models, Gut Microbiota Modulation, and Lipidomics. Nutrients. 2023; 15(12):2775. https://doi.org/10.3390/nu15122775.

Abbreviations: 6-OHDA, 6-hydroxydopamine; DA, dopamine; LB, Lewy bodies; MPTP, 1-methyl-4-phenyl-1,2,3,6-tetrahydropyridine; PD, Parkinson's disease; SNpc, substantia nigra pars compacta.

A healthy person could have a result up to 60% (two SDs) below or above the mean in the study with the widest range in the normal population, with an inevitable overlap between the lower limit of normal and the estimated symptom threshold (of 47% to 72). A brief observation is that, despite the desire to designate those below the normal mean as "preclinical," no one has (yet, maybe) described the group above the normal mean as having dopaminergic superiority, or PD resistance. "Those who started at the normal mean would now be at 47% to 72% of normal, but those who started at 160% of the normal mean might still have a result above the normal mean if everyone within that broad but normal population lost enough dopaminergic metabolism to reach their personal threshold for disease." These latter people would be classified as SWEDDs because they had PD but their results were within the normal range. In a similar vein, certain individuals (those who begin 50–60% below the mean) in a population considered healthy will fall into the predicted Parkinsonian range. It is not necessary to suggest or assume pathology in this group of healthy individuals with low PET/SPECT indexes, which may be the result of individual biochemistry, anatomy, or measurement error. In a population as widely dispersed as this, the majority of "preclinical" individuals will be concealed within the normal range.

Calculating the sensitivity and specificity of the method is made possible by understanding the threshold and the distribution around the normal mean. The population at threshold comprises false negatives (i.e., mean = threshold) with a result that is within the normal range (less than two standard deviations from the mean). A subset of the normal population whose results are more than two standard deviations below the normal mean is known as a false positive (Figure 3.5).

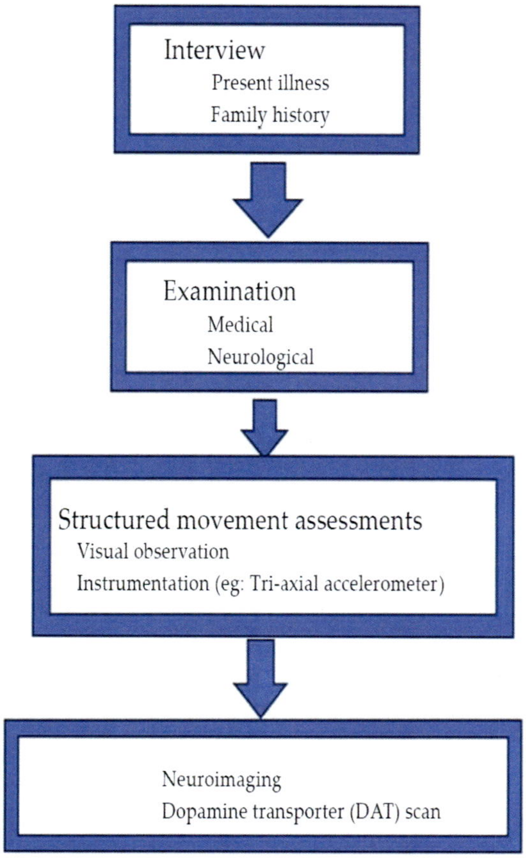

Figure 3.5. *PD diagnosis.*

Source: Elshourbagy T, Brašić JR, Syed AB. Guidelines for the Diagnosis and Treatment of Parkinson's Disease. Biology and Life Sciences Forum. 2021; 9(1):9. https://doi.org/10.3390/ECCM-10859.

Using the Bayes theorem and these estimates of sensitivity and specificity, one can determine the positive and negative predictive values of the methods when applied to populations for which an arbitrary prevalence of abnormality can be assigned. The probability that a person with an abnormal scan will have Parkinsonism or preclinical disease is known as the positive predictive value. Preclinical refers to "abnormal" in this context; however, it does not imply that the person will inevitably develop clinical Parkinson's disease (Figure 3.6).

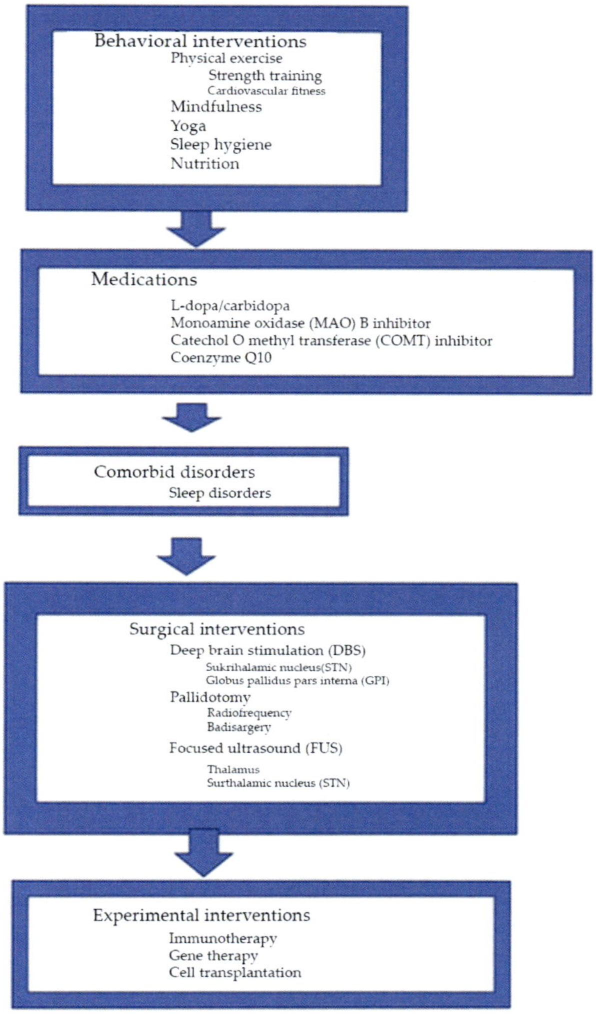

Figure 3.6. *Pathways.*

Source: Elshourbagy T, Brašić JR, Syed AB. Guidelines for the Diagnosis and Treatment of Parkinson's Disease. Biology and Life Sciences Forum. 2021; 9(1):9. https://doi.org/10.3390/ECCM-10859.

Table 3.7's Column 3 displays the probability that an abnormal scan, indicative of an abnormal patient, will occur from a population where 1% is abnormal (e.g., 1% of the presumed-healthy population had preclinical disease). It is evident that only one-third of those identified as such are likely to be "preclinical," even with the smallest SD and lowest threshold. The healthy people who fall on the lower end of the normal range thirds. We are confident that none of the currently available dopa-PET or DAT-SPECT techniques can reliably identify an individual who is truly preclinical (at this prevalence within a population) based on a comparison of these arbitrary SDs and thresholds with the technique's published SDs and thresholds. The situation is different in that half of the healthy individuals may be "preclinical," possibly due to genetic susceptibility. Table 3.5's Column 4 demonstrates that an identified abnormality has a >90% chance of being abnormal or preclinical for each SD and threshold. Consequently, these methods could prove beneficial for studying members of families affected by autosomal dominant Parkinsonism.

- ***What are SWEDDs (Other Than Symptomatic Without Evidence of Dopaminergic Deficit)?*** These computations shed light on a subset of patients, such as those enrolled in the CALM, REAL, and ELLDOPA studies, who have recently developed symptoms. Here, we may predict (based on clinical accuracy knowledge and computation) that 10% of individuals recruited are either healthy or have essential tremor (in which case dopa-PET and DAT-SPECT scans may also be expected to be normal). Following a normal scan, the likelihood of being disease-free is represented by the negative predictive value. The SWEDDs are more likely to have a normal than an aberrant dopaminergic system only if the SD and threshold are as in example 5. Unfortunately, it is unlikely that the 10% of recruits misdiagnosed as SWEDDs in CALM, REAL, and ELLDOPA correspond to the same 10% of identified SWEDDs. Hence, the existence of SWEDDs is not due to inadequate diagnosis, but rather to inadequate technique, which unfortunately combines an excessively broad range of results in the healthy population with an excessively high threshold at symptom onset.

The other consideration, when the technique is used in this way, is reproducibility. The scan-to-scan errors may be sufficient to take any individual's result from unhealthy to healthy and vice versa.

- ***Should Suspected New PD Patients Have a DAT-SPECT or Dopa-PET Scan?*** Positive and negative predictive values can be estimated similarly, using numbers for SD and threshold from studies by Tissingh and Marek using these ligands. Should a clinician, therefore, request a DAT-SPECT scan when unsure whether the diagnosis is PD or ET?93% of patients with abnormal scan results will have Parkinsonism if the patient's chances of being normal (or having ET) or having PD are assumed to be 50/50. This is because an abnormal scan result cannot differentiate idiopathic PD from other akinetic-rigid disorders. Conversely, if the scan results are normal, there is a 57% probability that the patient does not have a positive predictive value (PD). Because it is only slightly more likely that the patient is normal than abnormal, a normal scan will not be helpful in an abnormal patient, but an abnormal scan may be in an abnormal patient. The doctor then needs to inquire as to how much more benefit this technique is likely to have compared to the assessment or opinion of a colleague three months later. Based on the available evidence, the procedures are rarely useful for diagnosis and that the associated costs and radiation exposure are not worth it. The technique's reliability (discussed below) must also be kept in mind by the clinician, as the scan result from today may differ significantly from the one from tomorrow.

- ***What Is the Latency of PD? What Is the Rate of Progression? What Is the Pattern of Progression?*** Since there isn't any proof linking dopa-PET and DAT-SPECT to cell count, conjecture can only address how long the biochemical shift that causes Parkinson's disease takes to occur. The bulk of data gathered using both methods points to a typical biochemical latency of five to twelve years. One must proceed cautiously when evaluating such latency and average rate of progression estimates in Parkinson's disease. Most, though not all, assume linearity, and often a leap from the biochemical data to pathological conjecture is made.

When criticizing the temporal pattern of progression and the latency of PD, commentators may also be committing a logical fallacy by designating a single pattern of progression or latency. We are aware that the rate of progression varies greatly amongst individuals and that dopa-PET and DAT-SPECT provide surrogate measurements of clinical severity. It follows that a broad range in latency and rate of progression, as determined by PET and SPECT, must also exist and that multiple patterns of progression might even exist. Even though the author of the long-latency theory of Parkinson's disease did not intend for it to imply a slow, uniform, linear progression, it seems that many commentators on it do.

- ***Should and Can Dopa-PET and DAT-SPECT Be Used in Longitudinal Studies of Disease Progression and Neuroprotection?*** Here, there are two divisive topics. The first is whether imaging-derived measures are useful in clinical trials because they adequately capture the clinical or pathologic state of the disease. The challenge with assuming that dopa-PET or DATSPECT measure dopaminergic pathology has already been discussed in this chapter and in a previous comment, which also made the point that Parkinsonian deterioration is heterogeneous and far more widespread than striatal dopaminergic function alone. Nonetheless, the majority of studies indicate a correlation between the indices and global clinical scores. They have value in progression studies if they are to be accepted as an index of something that decreases with a decline in clinical function. It would be extremely alluring to have an objective way to measure a single variable that seems to be both continuous and linear, may not be impacted by mood or medication, and correlates with advancement. It is arguable, however, whether grading an illness using a functional imaging index is more useful than grading it using a clinical or quality-of-life scale. There is a crucial point that can be made here that seems to be overlooked in trial design. In a society where personal freedom and democracy are valued, the question of how one wants their illness to be measured is one of personal choice. When designing and recruiting for medical trials, we do not yet ask whose endpoint it is, unlike in clinical practice where we inquire about whose life and whose illness it is. The more objective measurements of a dopa-PET or DATSPECT scan may be preferred by some, while others may place greater significance on the point at which a disability results in job loss, the point at which dyskinesia causes embarrassment, or the point at which a person needs assistance walking to the coffee shop. Evidence from trials using patient-oriented measures and possibly patient-selected endpoints is required for a patient-oriented therapy decision.

If we do assume that dopa-PET and DAT-SPECT provide a useful measurement, the second bone of contention is whether the techniques, at their existing level of development, can perform that role.

A rate of decline in the PET index of 0.78% of the normal mean per year was measured in the first published longitudinal dopa-PET study of PD; a rate ten times that was found in the second study. Since the patients and PET machines were nearly identical, the analysis techniques from the past (Ki in putamen) and the Vancouver study (total striatal ratios) were both applied to a single patient group to explain the discrepancy. This showed that the analysis method determines the measured rate of progression; consequently, some methods may not be sensitive enough or reproducible enough to measure something. To comprehend this, one must adopt a new perspective, moving away from the oversimplified or instinctive notion that the methods measure something as tangible as cell count and toward the idea that method dictates method more so than pathology when determining rate. The key characteristics of any method for measuring progression, whether it be imaging-based or not, are reproducibility and sensitivity to clinical change. Additional characteristics like scale linearity and resistance to confounding are also significant. Numerous cross-sectional studies demonstrate a connection between the clinical state and the DAT-SPECT and dopa-PET index. The concept [and evidence (3)] that some techniques measure a greater change in imaging index than others with a given amount of clinical deterioration appears to be the source of difficulty. If this is not taken into account, there is a risk that a technique or method will be used that is not sensitive enough to measure the tiny variation in striatal dopaminergic biochemistry that goes along with the tiny amount of clinical progression that could be happening, say, in the first year of a progression study. Various dopa-PET indices, for instance, may indicate a clinical change of 10 total UPDRS points, measuring between 3 and 7% of the normal mean. Although some estimates have been made from published data, these have been based on many assumptions and there are no published studies of sensitivity in DAT-SPECT. The technique's usefulness as a measuring tool is limited if it is insensitive to clinical progression and the index changes only slightly.

While sensitivity is important, it is best understood in conjunction with reproducibility; the goal is for the change in imaging index resulting from progression to be substantially larger than the change in index owing to error. Even in the most thorough reviews, reproducibility is often overlooked in PD imaging studies, despite being the most critical factor when assessing medication effect, detecting preclinical disease or PD, or tracking progression. Although studies have addressed the issue, they have rarely done so in a way that is sufficiently critical for the claims being made for the techniques. Would it be too controversial to ask that reproducibility data (in that specific machine with that ligand and method of analysis) be published to accompany every dopa-PET or DAT-SPECT study (Table 3.6).

Table 3.6. *Parkinson's Disease Subtypes*

References	Number of subtypes	Parkinson's disease subtypes	Classification basis
Zetusky et al. (1985) and Jankovic et al. (1990)	3	Tremor-dominant/indeterminate/postural instability and gait difficulty subtypes	Predominant motor symptoms
Schiess et al. (2000), Korchounov et al. (2004), Kang et al. (2005)	3	Tremor-dominant/mixed/akinetic-rigid subtypes	Predominant motor symptoms
Fereshtehnejad et al. (2017)	3	Mild motor-predominant/diffuse malignant/intermediate	Motor symptoms and non-motor symptoms (cognitive decline, RBD, and dysautonomia)
Lawton et al. (2018)	4	Fast motor progression/mild motor and non-motor disease/severe motor disease, poor psychological well-being and poor sleep/slow motor progression	Cognitive impairment, motor and non-motor symptoms
Konno et al. (2018)	4	Tremor-dominant/akinetic-rigid/gait difficulty/mixed subtypes	Predominant motor symptoms
Zhang et al. (2019)	3	Mild Baseline, Moderate Motor Progression/Moderate Baseline, Mild Progression/Severe Baseline, Rapid Progression	Motor and non-motor symptoms, CSF examination, DaTScan

CSF, cerebrospinal fluid; DaTscan, imaging of dopamine transporter using 123^{I}-iofupane single photon emission computed tomography (SPECT); RBD, rapid eye movement (REM) sleep behavior disorder.

Source: Dulski J, Uitti RJ, Ross OA and Wszolek ZK (2022) Genetic architecture of Parkinson's disease subtypes – Review of the literature. Front. Aging Neurosci. 14:1023574. doi: 10.3389/fnagi.2022.1023574.

Techniques that have this much potential for error scanning must be developed to measure something that could change by as little as 1 to 2%, for example, over the course of a year (a figure that is based on both the technique's sensitivity to clinical progression and the actual clinical progression). That could work, but only if the scanned numbers are so large that a positive error always cancels out a negative error. The main challenge for studies on progression is that, regrettably, increased sensitivity to progression seems to only be accompanied by decreased reproducibility; reproducibility is lost and sensitivity is gained through analysis of data obtained from progressively smaller striatal components. The focus of commentary on the data from ELLDOPA and CALM has been on the study of medication and its potential confounding effects. Eliminating a medication's effect should be possible in study design, but studies on medication effects are also susceptible to poor reproducibility, and sample sizes up to this point have likely not been sufficient to allow for definitive results.

There will inevitably be a need for groups that are similar in size to those of studies using clinical indices if PET/SPECT indices are surrogate measures, meaning that the range of rate of progression measured by these techniques is likely to be similar to that seen clinically.

- ***How Do We Interpret the 3 Longitudinal Neuroprotection Imaging Studies?*** There has been a lot of correspondence regarding the CALM, REAL, and ELLDOPA studies, and the discussion surrounding each can be seen as helpful for upcoming imaging trials.

REAL recruited 186 new-onset patients who were treated either with L-dopa or agonist; they were assessed by [18F]dopa PET upon starting medication and again at 2 years. Patients were recruited at 34 sites and scanned twice, on any of 6 different PET machines, with data sent to one central unit for subsequent analysis. Centrally, data were normalized to a standard brain volume; the primary outcome measure was a change in mean putamen Ki between the first and second scans. A nonsignificant trend in favor of the dopamine agonist was reported first, in the abstract. The data were published formally in 2003, achieving significance in favor of the agonist after central analysis and the removal of SWEDDs. Putamen Ki dropped by 13.4 (2.14%) from baseline in the ropinirole group and by 20.3 (2.35%) in the L-dopa group, a rate of progression broadly in keeping with other dopa-PET estimates. The study concluded that either ropinirole was neuroprotective or that L-dopa was neurotoxic. Another possibility (if one accepts the adjustment as legitimate) is that L-dopa has a greater biochemical (rather than pathologic) effect on the outcome measure than ropinirole. The removal of SWEDDs was a belated addition to the trial protocol, and the author's reply to criticism of the study design confirmed that 2 datasets (with and without the removal of SWEDDs) were available at study completion. To formally publish only the results that favored the sponsor's product was ill-judged at best. In the trial's favor were the large number of patients scanned and the fact that such a complicated trial and analysis could be accomplished at all. Its failure and its expense make it unlikely to be repeated.

Over a 4-year period, CALM examined 82 new-onset patients using DATSPECT. In comparison to the L-dopa group, which had a decline in striatal B-CIT uptake of 25.5 (14.1%) at 46 months, the agonist group had shown a decline of 16 (13.3%) from baseline. The patients declined in the "defined off" state by 4.1 (9.9) total UPDRS points in the agonist group and 4.0 (8.7) total UPDRS points in the L-dopa group, both to the same extent. The main objection, effectively made by Ahlskog, is that this study might just be proving a biochemical effect. Another counterargument is that, given that we know the imaging technique is probably going to be relatively insensitive to clinical progression, it is difficult to understand how a technique could demonstrate such large changes in dopaminergic function with such small changes in clinical function (see below). We are left to wonder whether the study measured progression, pharmacologic effect, or error when we add the argument of limited reproducibility.

ELLDOPA sought to establish whether L-dopa was likely to be neurotoxic. Here 142 new-onset patients were scanned twice (with a 1-year interval) off medication at the start and then either off medication or on varying doses of levodopa at the end. Striatal B-CIT uptake decreased by 2.6% of baseline in the placebo group and by between 4% and 7% of baseline in the L-dopa groups in that time. The placebo arm of ELLDOPA provides evidence of a lack of sensitivity of the technique to clinical progression. This untreated group deteriorated (typically for PD) by an average of 7.8 total UPDRS points, yet the SPECT index in the subgroup of 29 who underwent scanning changed by only 2.6% of baseline (or only 1.3% of normal if the baseline is assumed to be 50% normal mean). This suggests that the technique has not adequately detected the deterioration in dopaminergic biochemistry that one might have expected to accompany the clinical progression in this group. The result seems particularly inexplicable compared with CALM (which used a similar technique), where changes of 16% (in the L-dopa group) and 25% (in the agonist group) in the SPECT index (from baseline) were accompanied by a clinical (total UPDRS off medication) change of 4 points in each group. Possibly the UPDRS change was undervalued (if the patients were not assessed truly off medication) in CALM. Possibly the apparent huge changes in the SPECT index (for such a small clinical deterioration) measured in CALM were phamacological, and the greater change in the L-dopa group than in the placebo group in ELLDOPA was also a pharmacologic effect. Possibly instead, the subgroups in each study were too small for negative error to cancel positive error and, because of the poor sensitivity of the technique to progression, the only thing the studies are demonstrating is the balance of error (Stewart and William, 2020).

3.4. Clinical Application of Functional Neuroimaging

3.4.1. fMRI – Physiologic Principle

Eloquent brain regions can be found using functional magnetic resonance imaging (fMRI), which is useful for treatment planning. Its most advanced version uses BOLD contrast, which stands for blood-oxygen-level dependent contrast. BOLD contrast, as opposed to conventional Gadolinium contrast, distinguishes between tissues according to the inherent differences in the magnetic properties of oxy- and deoxyhemoglobin. Due to its diamagnetic nature, oxyhemoglobin is repelled by magnetic fields. Deoxyhemoglobin, on the other hand, is paramagnetic and tends to align itself with the static magnetic field provided by the MRI magnet. A given task causes an increase in neural activity, which in turn causes an increase in cerebral blood flow and oxygen metabolism in the surrounding tissues. Sherrington and colleagues first described this physiological reaction to neural activity that is essential to all functional imaging that depends on cerebral hemodynamics was developed in 1890. Relatively high oxyhemoglobin: deoxyhemoglobin ratio results from an increase in blood flow (and oxyhemoglobin) that is typically greater than the metabolic rate of oxygen utilization by the tissue. An extremely sensitive method for identifying changes in the magnetic field is the T2*-weighted sequence, which can be used to measure changes in this ratio. To evaluate the signal changes that take place over time, a dynamic imaging of the brain is required. Temporal resolution comes at the expense of spatial resolution; however, an incredibly quick sequence like Echo Planar Imaging (EPI) enables a whole brain acquisition in about two seconds.

Resting-state fMRI (rs-fMRI) is a relatively new imaging modality that has great potential for learning about neural networks because it operates on the same physical principles. Unlike task-based fMRI, rs-fMRI depends on identifying low-frequency fluctuations (<0.1 Hz) in the BOLD signal when there are no active tasks. Finding synchronization between various regions that may indicate neuronal connectivity is the goal. Similar temporal patterns of activity across different areas suggest connectivity. Networks in a resting state are typically categorized as task-positive or highly connected during active tasks (i.e., auditory, linguistic, etc.), as well as task-negative networks, which are busier at rest (i.e., the network in default mode).

3.4.2. fMRI – Data Acquisition and Processing

The identification of the eloquent cortex through BOLD fMRI data acquisition is dependent on task-based activation of cortical tissue in experiments known as paradigms. Various paradigms can be applied based on where the lesion is located. These comprise tasks involving the motor skills, expressive and receptive language, hearing, and vision. For the accurate identification of the eloquent cortex, multiple paradigms are frequently needed. The hemodynamic response to the corresponding cortical regions being activated can then be seen, as was previously discussed. We'll talk about a common paradigm that's employed to identify cortical motor tissue.

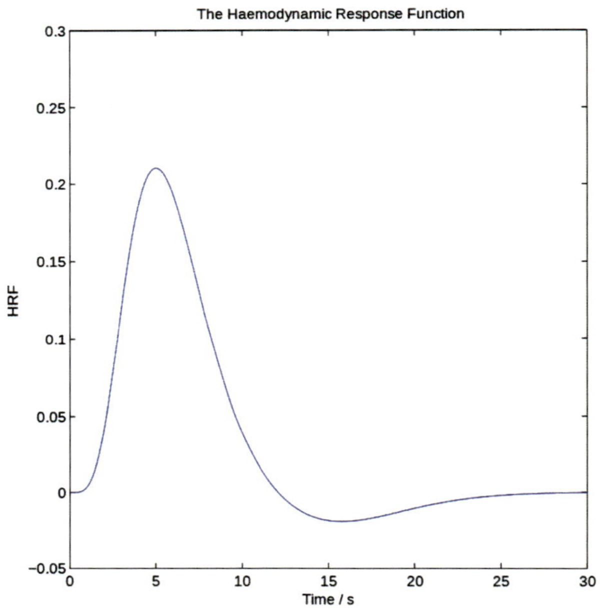

Figure 3.7. *The hemodynamic response curve, shown above, demonstrates the temporal lag of T2* signal (generated by increased Hb/dHb ratio due to increased CBF) relative to neuronal activity.*

Source: By Lionfish0 – Own work, Public Domain, https://commons.wikimedia.org/w/index.php?curid=12683452.

Increases in cerebral blood flow, hemoglobin oxygenation, and relative T2* signal are caused by neuronal activity. The T2* signal (y-axis) is plotted against time (x-axis) in the hemodynamic response curve. A typical HRC is shown in Figure 3.7. The T2* weighted signal and the hemodynamic response follow neural activation in a delayed manner. The corresponding hemodynamic response happens on the order of seconds, whereas neural activation happens on the order of milliseconds. The motor paradigm's temporal organization is determined by the HRC. Robust detection of activated cortical tissue requires many activation and rest trials for a single task since the T2* weighted signal change resulting from oxygenated blood is only approximately 2%.

The most popular design paradigm is the block design paradigm. Typically, a block design has 20 seconds of activation time (i.e., finger tapping) and then taking a 20-second break before repeating the process up to eight times. 160 distinct volumetric brain acquisitions could be made in 320 seconds of study time, after which the T2* weighted signal for every voxel could be plotted over time. The MRI signal displayed by voxels activated by the prescribed task aligns with the hemodynamic response curve's expected shape. The background noise's random fluctuations are visible in the uninvolved areas. The correlation coefficient (CC) is a mathematical measure of the degree of correlation between the fMRI data set and the anticipated hemodynamic response curve. On the fMRI scan, voxels with a high CC are shown as areas of positive activity. It should be mentioned that an fMRI test is a statistical representation of brain activity and that different CC thresholds may be used to display the test results. Post-processing requires some experience because an accurate determination of functional tissue depends on a correlation coefficient threshold that records neuronal activity indicative of task performance. An excessively strict threshold will not elicit enough activations to reliably identify neural activity, while an excessively low threshold will include an excessive amount of background activity. Localizing the activated tissue is then possible by superimposing the post-processed BOLD signal on a volumetric anatomic sequence that was acquired independently, such as post-contrast T1 (Figures 3.8 and 3.9).

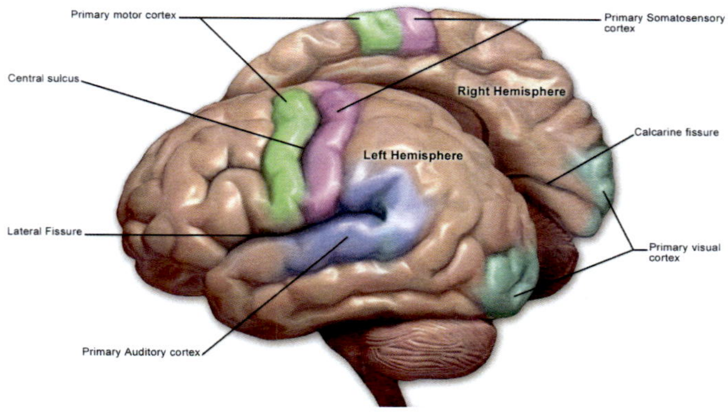

Figure 3.8. *A typical paradigm for identification of the primary motor cortex. Alternating finger tapping is performed for 20 seconds, during which 10 T2* acquisitions are acquired. This is followed by 20 seconds of rest and 10 additional T2* acquisitions. This is repeated as necessary to generate reliable data.*

Source: By BruceBlaus. When using this image in external sources it can be cited as:Blausen.com staff (2014). "Medical gallery of Blausen Medical 2014." WikiJournal of Medicine 1 (2). DOI:10.15347/wjm/2014.010. ISSN 2002-4436. – Own work, CC BY 3.0, https://commons.wikimedia.org/w/index.php?curid=31574257.

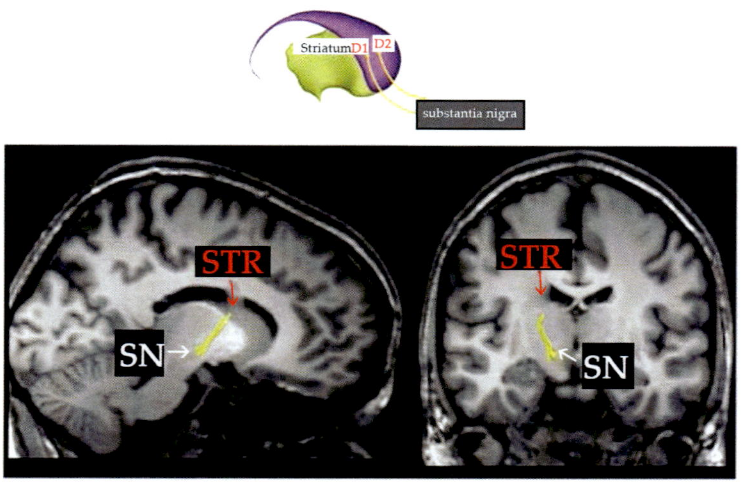

Figure 3.9. *Determining the statistical threshold is an essential part of post-processing. Setting the statistical threshold too high obscures the eloquent cortex, while setting it too low results in excessive background noise and limits specificity.*

Source: Lauretani F, Longobucco Y, Ravazzoni G, Gallini E, Salvi M, Maggio M. Imaging the Functional Neuroanatomy of Parkinson's Disease: Clinical Applications and Future Directions. International Journal of Environmental Research and Public Health. 2021; 18(5):2356. https://doi.org/10.3390/ijerph18052356.

Resting-state fMRI paradigms differ in both data acquisition and analysis. Acquisition is performed in the resting state, without a required stimulus or task, to identify resting state networks. These are networks of related parenchymal tissue that may be involved in either attention-based networks or the default mode network but are active in the absence of performing an active task. The default mode network is an example of a network of neural tissue that functions in the passive state but demonstrates enormous connectivity with different neural systems and is one of the most evolutionarily conserved neural networks in mammals. The default mode network was first identified using fMRI. Multiple methods of analysis can be employed which generally fall into two categories: seed-based (also known as model-based) and data-driven. Seed-based analysis relies on a priori placement of regions of interest (ROIs), or seeds, and comparing data between ROIs. This method offers a practical means to demonstrate functional connectivity to a specific voxel or ROI. The limitation of this method is that the interpretation and power of the study are influenced to a large degree by the placement of the ROIs. It obviously also offers limited utility in the determination of connectivity outside the ROIs. More recently, rs-fMRI has tended towards data-driven analyses. There are numerous methods of data-driven analysis. One of the more popular forms is independent component analysis (ICA). ICA does not require a priori selection of ROIs, rather it relies on a temporal map of the entire brain based on independent components. Temporal patterns of activity are compared between the independent components to assess for correlations that suggest connectivity. Multiple other data-driven forms of analysis allow for parcellation of the brain, including clustering analysis, k-means and edge-finding methods. While increasing in popularity, data-driven analysis of fMRI data presents potential obstacles. Background physiologic activity in the form of respiratory or cardiovascular noise may generate a signal that suggests spurious neuronal connectivity, generating false positive correlations. Specific software packages are often required to mitigate the confounding signal and increase the specificity of temporospatial correlations.

3.4.3. fMRI – Clinical Applications and Limitations

When evaluating patients undergoing neurosurgical treatment, task-based fMRI has proven to be highly valuable in preserving function before surgery. The identification of eloquent cortex, like the primary motor cortex or visual cortex, can be especially useful when pathologic processes cause native anatomy to be distorted, making it more difficult to identify using conventional anatomic landmarks (Figure 3.10). Additionally, fMRI is an effective non-invasive method for precisely localizing the major receptive and expressive language areas, which tend to be quite variable in their anatomic location, as well as for determining hemispheric language dominance, which is crucial for patients undergoing frontal or temporal lobe resections. The surgical approach or the extent of the resection may change depending on the preoperative localization of these regions and their anatomical relationship to the intended surgical target. In the end, its application has improved clinical outcomes and reduced the likelihood of post-operative deficits, though only for a subset of patients. Task-based fMRI preoperative planning requires patient cooperation to complete the tasks within the designated paradigms. The ability to accurately identify the eloquent cortex may be severely limited by changes in mental status, seizure-like activity, patient age, sedation, or limited cognitive function at baseline. This would severely limit the generalizability of fMRI in neurosurgical planning. Recent research indicates that in patients unable to engage in task-based paradigms, rs-fMRI may be helpful in identifying eloquent cortex. In particular, Zhang et al. used a seed-based analysis. proved that the placement of the ROI on the motor cortex that was spared allowed for the accurate identification of the motor cortex that was distorted on the opposite side for the purpose of neurosurgical planning.

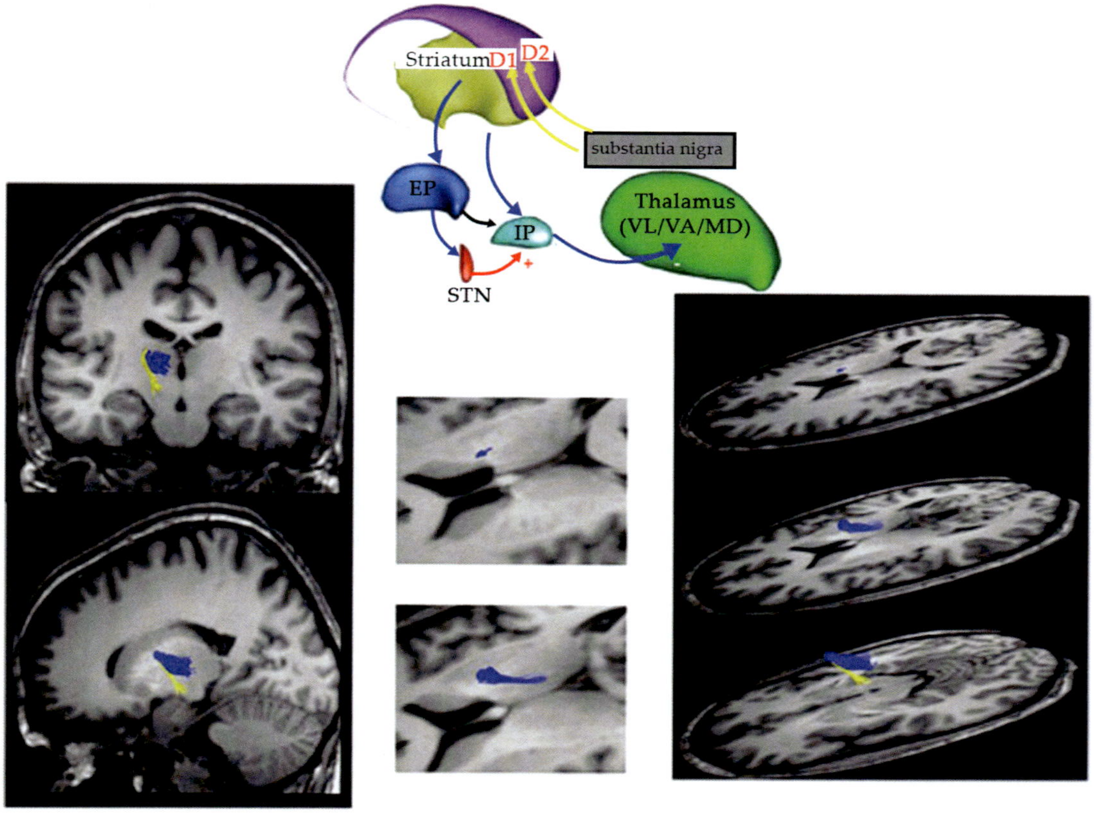

Figure 3.10. *The primary motor cortex may be readily identifiable in normal patients; however, its location can be easily obscured by malignancy and other pathologic processes. Here, a large glioma distorts the right cerebral hemisphere and limits reliable determination of the primary motor cortex. Utilization of a bilateral finger tapping motor allows the identification of the functional motor cortex.*

Source: *Lauretani F, Longobucco Y, Ravazzoni G, Gallini E, Salvi M, Maggio M. Imaging the Functional Neuroanatomy of Parkinson's Disease: Clinical Applications and Future Directions. International Journal of Environmental Research and Public Health. 2021; 18(5):2356. https://doi.org/10.3390/ijerph18052356.*

Recent resting-state fMRI studies show reproducible differences in basal functional connectivity within the temporal lobes in cases of mesial temporal lobe epilepsy. The information points to an overall decline in basal functional connectivity in the epileptogenic temporal lobe and an increase in basal functional connectivity in the contralateral temporal lobe, as well as an asymmetric disruption of specific neuronal networks. With a specificity of up to 91% shown by Bettus et al., indirect localization of the epileptogenic focus through assessment of enhanced basal functional connectivity in the non-epileptogenic temporal lobe seems to be the most accurate measure of localization of the epileptogenic zone. Significantly, in patients without structural insult on MRI, there was a laterality of increased basal functional connectivity within the non-epileptogenic temporal lobe. This suggests that rs-fMRI plays a special role in localizing the epileptogenic zone for pre-surgical planning in cases of drug-resistant epilepsy.

The distinctive patterns of cortical activations and deactivations in various dementia types have been shown in many functional connectivity studies, indicating the diagnostic utility of resting-state fMRI in dementia diagnosis. In particular, even in the early stages of the disease's clinical course, Alzheimer's dementia constantly exhibits decreased default mode network activity during resting states. More thorough functional connectivity studies have also shown that, in comparison to healthy controls, there is increased activity within the salience network—a neural network within the anterior insular cortex and anterior cingulate cortex that monitors external inputs and internal brain activity—and decreased functional connectivity within the medial temporal lobe and posterior cingulate cortex. On the other hand, frontotemporal dementia may show signs of reduced salient network connectivity and increased default network connectivity, which makes a diagnosis more certain in situations where there may be clinical ambiguity.

Since its inception, functional connectivity and resting state network identification have been the main research uses for rs-fMRI. The acceptance of rs-fMRI in clinical settings is still relatively new and has not yet reached the same level of acceptance as task-based fMRI. As was previously mentioned, several recent studies have shown that rs-fMRI has promising diagnostic applications in a range of pathologies. An additional special advantage of resting state fMRI is its ability to examine neural activity in a patient who is comatose or uncooperative. The role of rs-fMRI in the clinical domain is certain to solidify with additional clinically based research and processing tool development.

3.4.4. DTI – Physiologic Principles

Diffusion tensor imaging (DTI) has completely changed the assessment of white matter. Using the same concepts as diffusion-weighted imaging—the Brownian motion of water molecules—DTI enables examination of the brain and visualization of neural tracts. Water molecules diffuse differently across complex cellular membranes; as a result, the diffusion profile reflects the underlying tissue microstructure. Diffusion can be understood directionally by gathering diffusion measurements in at least six non-collinear directions. The resulting data can be shown as a three-dimensional ellipsoid called the "diffusion tensor." Anisotropic diffusion, which is strongly skewed in one direction, causes the resulting tensor to elongate and display a particular orientation. Diffusion perpendicular to the highly organized white matter tracts is typically restricted by cell membranes and myelin sheaths, but diffusion along the tract's axis is comparatively unrestricted within the tracts. There are numerous and extensive clinical uses for DTI in neuroradiology. Tractography, or the capacity to simulate the main white matter tracts found in the brain, is among the most aesthetically pleasing applications.

3.4.5. DTI – Data Acquisition and Processing

DTI measures the three-dimensional diffusion profile of water molecules. Detection of the direction of preferential diffusion depends on applying different diffusion-weighted gradients along the x, y, and z axes and measuring the corresponding diffusion coefficients. Diffusion measurements along a minimum of six non-collinear directions [e.g., (x,y,z) = (1,0,0), (1,1,0), (0,1,0), (0,1,1), (1,0,1), (0,0,1)] are needed to derive the tensor matrix, D, which has six components that represent diffusion coefficient along different directions: D_{xx}, D_{xy}, D_{yy}, D_{yz}, D_{xz}, D_{zz}. The resultant tensor takes the shape of an ellipsoid with its three principle axes aligning with the tensor eigenvectors (v_1, v_2, v_3), each with its own radius or eigenvalue (λ_1, λ_2, λ_3) representing the diffusivity along the three axes (Figure 3.11).

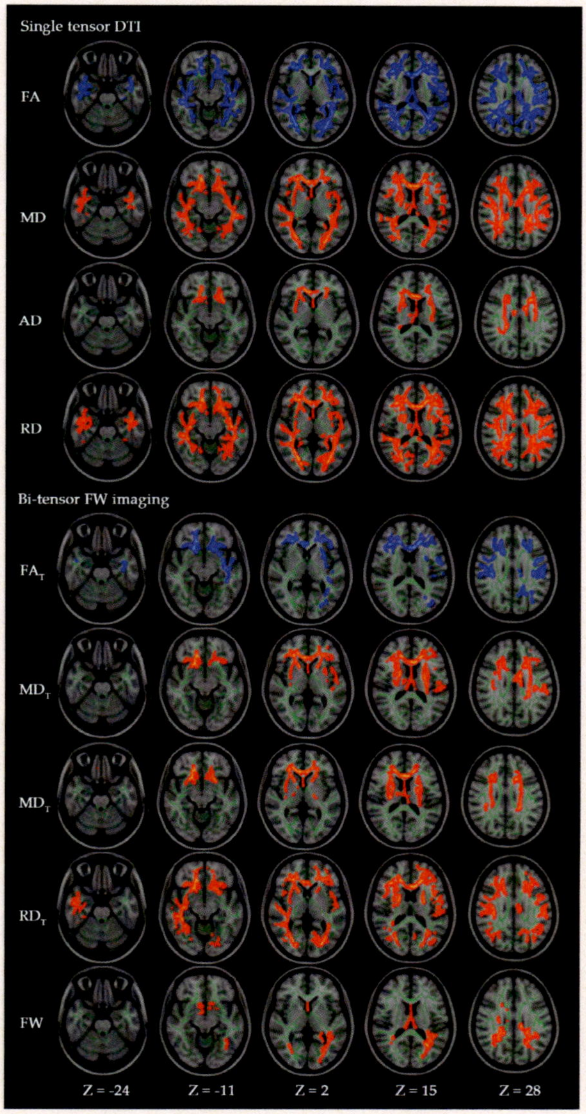

Figure 3.11. *Comparison of DTI (FA, MD, AD, and RD) and FW imaging (FA_T, MD_T, AD_T, RD_T, and FW) indices between healthy controls and patients with PD. TBSS analyses show that patients with PD have significantly ($p < 0.05$, FWE-corrected) lower FA and FA_T (blue/light-blue voxels) and significantly higher MD, MD_T, AD, AD_T, RD, RD_T, and FW (red-yellow voxels) compared with healthy controls. The skeleton is presented in green. To aid visualization, the results are thickened using the fill script implemented in the FMRIB Software Library. AD, axial diffusivity; AD_T, free water-corrected axial diffusivity; DTI: diffusion tensor imaging; FA, fractional anisotropy; FA_T, free water-corrected fractional anisotropy; FW, free water; MD, mean diffusivity; MD_T, free water-corrected mean diffusivity; PD, Parkinson's disease; RD, radial diffusivity; RD_T, free water-corrected radial diffusivity; TBSS, tract-based spatial statistics.*

Source: *Andica C, Kamagata K, Hatano T, Saito A, Uchida W, Ogawa T, Takeshige-Amano H, Zalesky A, Wada A, Suzuki M, et al. Free-Water Imaging in White and Gray Matter in Parkinson's Disease. Cells. 2019; 8(8):839. https://doi.org/10.3390/cells8080839.*

The eigenvalues are typically sorted such that $\lambda_1 > \lambda_2 > \lambda_3$, with the preferential diffusion direction aligning with v_1. As the number of diffusion measurements increases, the accuracy of the tensor data improves. Generally, in the clinical setting, 30-direction measurements uniformly oriented around a sphere are acquired. Fractional anisotropy (FA) is a quantitative scalar measurement indicating the extent to which the diffusivity differs from the expected spheroid distribution (a Gaussian diffusion profile). A FA value of 0 implies a spheroid distribution, whereas 1 implies maximum anisotropy. The FA value does not contain any information regarding the direction of anisotropy. Post-processing software will assign a color for the orientation of the white matter tract, with the intensity of the color signifying the FA value of the voxel (Figure 3.12).

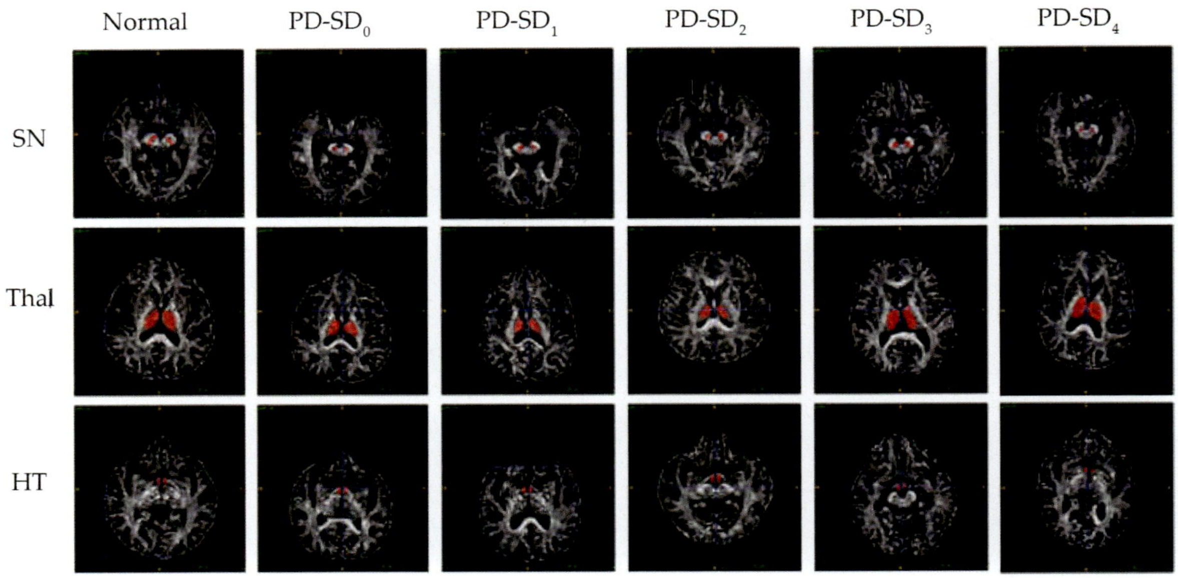

Figure 3.12. *Representative DTI images of SN, Thal and HT in early PD patients with different numbers of SD types. Normal, healthy control; PD-SD_0, PD patients with no SD; PD-SD_1, with one type of SD; PD-SD_2, with two types; PD-SD_3, with three types; PD-SD_4, with four types; SN, substantia nigra; Thal, thalamus; HT, hypothalamus.*

Source: Jiang Y, An H, Xi Q, Yang W, Xie H, Li Y, Huang D. Diffusion Tensor Imaging Reveals Deep Brain Structure Changes in Early Parkinson's Disease Patients with Various Sleep Disorders. Brain Sciences. 2022; 12(4):463. https://doi.org/10.3390/brainsci12040463.

3.4.6. DTI – Clinical Applications and Limitations

DTI has significantly altered how white matter can be examined and seen. On T2 weighted imaging, a variety of pathologic processes, such as inflammation, edema, tumors, gliosis, and demyelination, show elevated signal intensities; on the other hand, DTI can provide quantitative information about the degree of white matter involvement and compromise (via ADC and FA values). One of DTI's clinical applications is in the diagnostic characterization of multiple sclerosis (MS). While T2-weighted/FLAIR MRI is still a vital diagnostic tool, its histopathologic insight into the disease process is limited. Traditionally, this imaging protocol has been used to diagnose and track the progression of MSdot. On MRI, normal-appearing white matter may reveal cellular white matter disease associated with multiple sclerosis. Utilizing sophisticated diffusion metrics during evaluation enables the identification of white matter disease foci that are beneath the soft tissue resolution of magnetic resonance imaging (MRI).

DTI has proven useful in the diagnosis of epilepsy as well. Even though standard MR imaging is an essential part of the diagnostic process for treating epilepsy, some of the more common results on standard MR (i.e., T2 hyperintensity and hippocampus volume loss) might be too subtle for a conclusive diagnosis. The use of DTI in the assessment of epilepsy is based on the cytoarchitecture being distorted due to epileptogenic activity, resulting in decreased anisotropy and increased diffusivity. DTI can identify neoplastic diseases, which also exhibit cytoarchitecture distortion. In this situation, determining the involvement of the white matter tract can be crucial for neurosurgical planning. Tractography, the 3D modeling of white matter tracts based on DTI data, is being used more and more in the clinical setting (Figure 3.13).

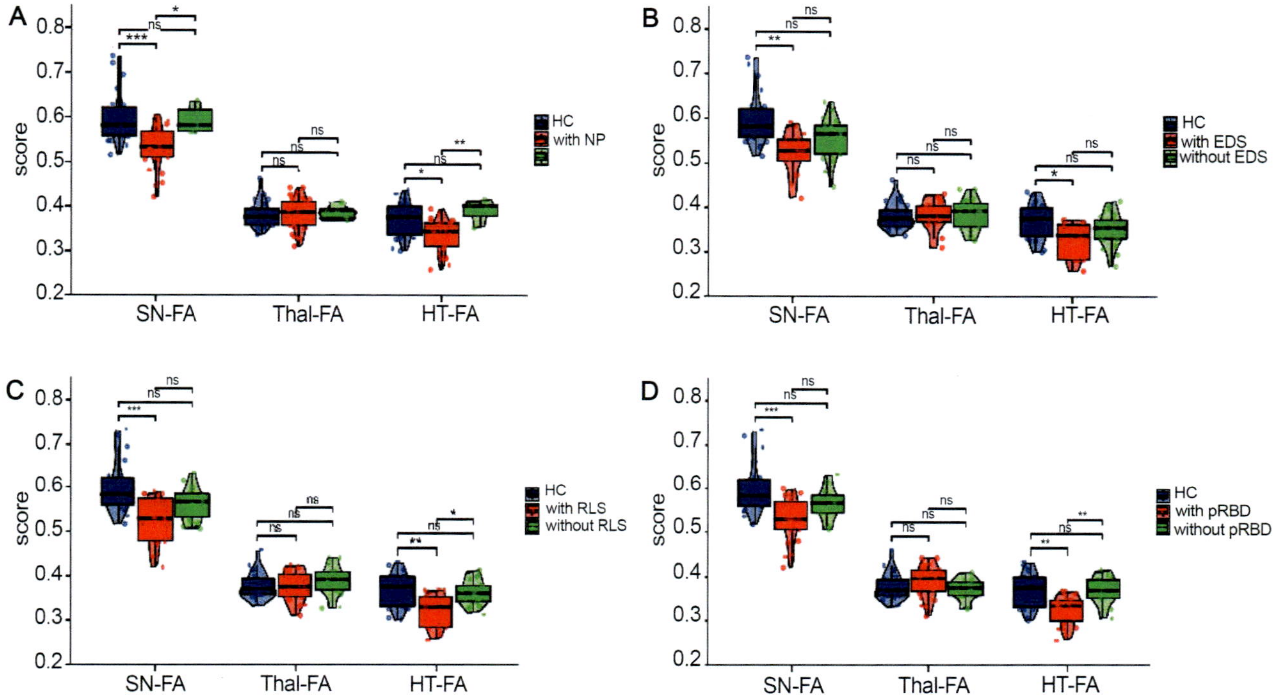

Figure 3.13. *Imaging features of early PD patients with various SDs and healthy controls (A–D). The differences in FA values for SN, Thal and HT among healthy controls, early PD patients with NP (A), EDS (B), RLS (C) or pRBD (D) and those patients without. NP, nighttime problems; EDS, excessive daytime sleepiness; RLS, restless leg syndrome; pRBD, probable REM sleep behavior disorder; ns, no significance; * p < 0.05, **p < 0.01, ***p< 0.001.*

Source: Jiang Y, An H, Xi Q, Yang W, Xie H, Li Y, Huang D. Diffusion Tensor Imaging Reveals Deep Brain Structure Changes in Early Parkinson's Disease Patients with Various Sleep Disorders. Brain Sciences. 2022; 12(4):463. https://doi.org/10.3390/brainsci12040463.

Although DTI has revolutionized white matter visualization, the diffusion metrics employed are predicated on a Gaussian diffusion model, which presupposes that water molecules moving with Brownian motion will exhibit a normal spatial distribution. Numerous experiments have shown that non-Gaussian diffusion characteristics exist within neurologic tissues, so this model of the diffusion profile is not entirely accurate. The resolution is further restricted by the fact that, in a normal DTI analysis, a single diffusion tensor is generated for each voxel, which may measure 2 × 2 × 2 mm. Tens of thousands of axons and glial cells, which probably make up several white matter tracts, can be found at the cellular level in the voxel region. The resulting data are ultimately an average of that voxel's diffusion properties, and they don't provide enough spatial resolution to accurately identify several axonal tracts inside of a single voxel. Furthermore, when assessing white matter appearance on MRI in patients with established white matter pathology (i.e., local aberrations in diffusion metrics in multiple sclerosis) could be so small that they only show up in group analyses, which would restrict diffusion-based white matter interrogation on an individual basis. When it comes to abnormally appearing white matter, DTI is most useful for identifying and characterizing the involved white matter tracts in terms of their spatial configuration when there is anatomic distortion (Stewart William, 2020).

A Closer Look

Epithelium

Neuroimaging has revolutionized our understanding of PD, offering valuable insights into its pathophysiology, diagnosis, and management.

Advanced imaging techniques such as magnetic resonance imaging (MRI), positron emission tomography (PET), and single-photon emission computed tomography (SPECT) provide detailed structural and functional information about the brain, allowing clinicians and researchers to visualize the underlying neurodegenerative changes associated with PD.

In PD, neuroimaging helps detect specific patterns of neuronal loss, particularly in the dopaminergic system, which is central to the disease's pathology. For example, imaging studies using radiotracers targeting dopamine transporters in the nigrostriatal pathway can quantify presynaptic dopaminergic dysfunction, aiding in the differential diagnosis of PD from other Parkinsonian syndromes.

Moreover, neuroimaging modalities such as functional MRI (fMRI) allow researchers to investigate alterations in brain connectivity and network dynamics, shedding light on the neural circuits involved in motor and non-motor symptoms of PD. Resting-state fMRI studies have identified aberrant functional connectivity patterns within the basal ganglia-thalamocortical circuits, providing insights into the pathophysiology of motor fluctuations and dyskinesias in PD patients.

Additionally, neuroimaging plays a crucial role in monitoring disease progression and evaluating treatment responses in PD. Longitudinal imaging studies can track changes in brain structure and function over time, correlating imaging biomarkers with clinical outcomes and disease severity. This facilitates the development of novel therapeutic strategies and personalized treatment approaches tailored to each patient's unique neuroimaging profile.

Overall, neuroimaging serves as a powerful tool in the multidisciplinary management of Parkinson's disease, offering a window into the underlying neurobiology of the disease, and aiding in early diagnosis, differential diagnosis, disease monitoring, and therapeutic interventions. Continued advancements in neuroimaging technology and methodology hold promise for further enhancing our understanding of PD and improving patient outcomes.

Summary

- The development of high-field magnetic resonance imaging (MRI) with three-dimensional (3D) volumetric acquisitions, gray and white matter suppressing inversion recovery sequences and diffusion-weighted imaging (DWI) has led to a more important role for structural imaging in the diagnosis of Parkinsonian disorders.
- Motor tests have not been able to differentiate PD from other Parkinsonian syndromes. Motor tests combined with a battery of other tests have shown some ability to distinguish asymptomatic first-degree relatives of individuals with PD from by normal controls.
- Biomarkers in the cerebrospinal fluid (CSF), especially blood, offer promise for increasing our understanding of PD; to date, however, these have had little impact as a diagnostic tool or therapeutic metric. Much of the focus on serum and CSF biomarkers has been on markers of oxidative stress, which is thought to contribute to the pathophysiology of PD.
- Structural and functional neuroimaging has long been used in the study of neurological disorders to elucidate disease mechanisms, to aid in diagnosis, and to assess potential new therapies. Clinical and research applications of functional neuroimaging to PD and other Parkinsonian disorders have advanced over the past decade, leading to novel diagnostic methods and contributing to the development of new therapies. This article will review how such imaging has been applied to the study of PD.
- PET and SPECT imaging use many radiotracers for *in vivo* assessment of normal and abnormal brain function. These techniques have been extensively used to study the dopamine system in Parkinsonian disorders, but other neurochemical systems (e.g., cholinergic, serotonergic) can also be investigated. Cerebral blood flow and glucose utilization can be mapped with radio-labeled water or glucose.
- fMRI is widely available and does not require the injection of a radiotracer, thus not imposing a limit on the number of scans that can be performed. It has high spatial and temporal resolution, which is useful for measuring dynamic changes in neural activity.
- Functional imaging studies utilizing Xenon-133 have found similar increases in PD patients and normal subjects in response to dopaminergic treatment.
- The clinical diagnosis and definition of PD is based on motor signs and symptoms. Nevertheless, nonmotor symptoms may be prominent, and can precede motor symptoms, and they can encompass a variety of categories, such as neuropsychiatric, sleep, or autonomic dysfunction.

References

1. Benamer, H. T. S., Patterson, J., Wyper, D. J., Grosset, D. G., et al. (2000). Correlation of Parkinson's disease severity and duration with I-123-FP-CIT SPECT striatal uptake. *Movement Disorders, 15*, 692–698.

2. Benamer, T. S., Patterson, J., Grosset, D. G., et al. (2000). Accurate differentiation of parkinsonism and essential tremor using visual assessment of [123I]-FP-CIT imaging: the [123I]-FP-CIT study group. *Movement Disorders, 15*, 503–510.

3. Bernheimer, H., Birkmayer, W., Hornykiewicz, O., et al. (1973). Brain dopamine and the syndromes of Parkinson and Huntington. Clinical, morphological, and neurochemical correlations. *Journal of Neurological Sciences, 20*, 415–455.

4. Braak, H., Tredici, K. D., Rub, U., et al. (2003). Staging of brain pathology related to sporadic Parkinson's disease. *Neurobiology of Aging, 24*, 197–211.

5. Brooks, D. J., Ibañez, V., Sawle, G. V., et al. (1990). Differing patterns of striatal 18F-dopa uptake in Parkinson's disease, multiple system atrophy and progressive supranuclear palsy. *Annals of Neurology, 28*, 547–555.

6. Factor, S. A., & Weiner, W. J. (2008). *Parkinson's Disease: Diagnosis and Clinical Management* (2nd ed.). Demos Medical Publishing.

7. Fearnley, J. M., & Lees, A. J. (1991). Ageing and Parkinson's disease: substantia nigra regional selectivity. *Brain, 114*, 2283–2301.

8. Fischman, A. J., Bonab, A. A., Babich, J. W., et al. (2001). [C-11, I-127] Altropane: a highly selective ligand for PET imaging of dopamine transporter sites. *Synapse, 39*, 332–342.

9. Forman, M. S., Lee, V. M. Y., & Trojanowski, J. Q. (2005). Nosology of Parkinson's disease: Looking for the way out of a quackmire. *Neuron, 47*(4), 479–482.

10. Frost, J. J., Rosier, A. J., Reich, S. G., et al. (1993). Positron emission tomographic imaging of the dopamine transporter with 11C-WIN 35,428 reveals marked declines in mild Parkinson's disease. *Annals of Neurology, 34*, 423–431.

11. Guttman, M., Burkholder, J., Kish, S. J., et al. (1997). [11C] RTI-32 PET studies of the dopamine transporter in early dopa-naive Parkinson's disease: implications for the symptomatic threshold. *Neurology, 48*, 1578–1583.

12. Hu, M. T., White, S. J., Herlihy, A. H., et al. (2001). A comparison of (18)F-dopa PET and inversion recovery MRI in the diagnosis of Parkinson's disease. *Neurology, 56*, 1195–1200.

13. Huang, C., Mattis, P., Tang, C., Perrine, K., Carbon, M., & Eidelberg, D. (2007). Metabolic brain networks associated with cognitive function in Parkinson's disease. *Neuroimage, 34*, 714-723.

14. Hutchinson, M., & Raff, U. (2000). Structural changes of the substantia nigra in Parkinson's disease as revealed by MR imaging. *American Journal of Neuroradiology, 21*, 697–701.

15. Jellinger, K. (1987). The pathology of parkinsonism. In C. D. Marsden & S. Fahn (Eds.), *Movement disorders 2* (pp. 124–165). 1st ed. London: Butterworths.

16. Jellinger, K. A., Seppi, K., Wenning, G. K., & Poewe, W. (2002). Impact of coexistent Alzheimer pathology on the natural history of Parkinson's disease. *Journal of Neural Transmission, 109*, 329–339.

17. Kikuchi, A., Takeda, A., Onodera, H., et al. (2002). Systemic increase of oxidative nucleic acid damage in Parkinson's disease and multiple system atrophy. *Neurobiology of Disease, 9*(2), 244–248.

18. Kish, S. J., Shannak, K., & Hornykiewicz, O. (1988). Uneven pattern of dopamine loss in the striatum of patients with idiopathic Parkinson's disease. *New England Journal of Medicine, 318*, 876–880.

19. Leenders, K. L., Salmon, E. P., Tyrrell, P., et al. (1990). The nigrostriatal dopaminergic system assessed *in vivo* by positron emission tomography in healthy volunteer subjects and patients with Parkinson's disease. *Archives of Neurology, 47*, 1290–1298.

20. Lindvall, O., & Björklund, A. (1979). Dopaminergic innervation of the globus pallidus by collaterals from the nigrostriatal pathway. *Brain Research, 172*, 169–173.

21. Ma, Y., Tang, C., Spetsieris, P. G., Dhawan, V., & Eidelberg, D. (2007). Abnormal metabolic network activity in Parkinson's disease: test-retest reproducibility. *Journal of Cerebral Blood Flow & Metabolism, 27*, 597–605.

22. Marek, K., Seibyl, J. P., Zoghbi, S. S., et al. (1996). [I-123] β-CIT SPECT imaging demonstrates bilateral loss of dopamine transporters in hemi Parkinson's disease. *Neurology, 46*, 231–237.

23. McKeith, I. G., Galasko, D., Kosaka, K., et al. (1996). Consensus guidelines for the clinical and pathologic diagnosis of dementia with Lewy bodies (DLB): report of the consortium on DLB international workshop. *Neurology, 47*, 1113–1124.

24. Morrish, P. K., Sawle, G. V., & Brooks, D. J. (1995). Clinical and [18F]dopa PET findings in early Parkinson's disease. *Journal of Neurology, Neurosurgery & Psychiatry, 59*, 597–600.

25. Pankratz, N., & Foroud, T. (2004). Genetics of Parkinson's disease. *NeuroRx, 1*, 235–242.

26. Rakshi, J. S., Uema, T., Ito, K., et al. (1999). Frontal, striatal, and midbrain dopaminergic function in early and advanced Parkinson's disease: a 3D 18F-dopa PET study. *Brain, 122*, 1637–1650.

27. Rinne, J. O., Bergman, J., Ruottinen, H., et al. (1999). Striatal uptake of a novel PET ligand, [18F] b-CFT, is reduced in early Parkinson's disease. *Synapse, 31*, 119–124.

28. Schrag, A., Good, C. D., Miszkiel, K., et al. (2000). Differentiation of atypical parkinsonian syndromes with routine MRI. *Neurology, 54*, 697–702.

29. Schulz, J. B., Skalej, M., Wedekind, D., et al. (1999). Magnetic resonance imaging-based volumetry differentiates idiopathic Parkinson's syndrome from multiple system atrophy and progressive supranuclear palsy. *Annals of Neurology, 45*, 65–74.

30. Seppi, K., Schocke, M. F., Esterhammer, R., et al. (2003). Diffusion-weighted imaging discriminates progressive supranuclear palsy from PD, but not from the Parkinson variant of multiple system atrophy. *Neurology, 60*, 922–927.

31. Whone, A. L., Moore, R. Y., Piccini, P., & Brooks, D. J. (2003). Plasticity in the nigropallidal pathway in Parkinson's disease: an 18F-dopa PET study. *Annals of Neurology, 53*, 206–213.

32. Forman MS, Lee VMY, Trojanowski JQ. Nosology of Parkinson's disease: Looking for the way out of a quackmire. Neuron 2005; 47(4):479–482.

33. Pankratz N, Foroud T. Genetics of Parkinson disease. NeuroRx 2004; 1:235–242.

Chapter

DRUG TREATMENT OF PARKINSON'S DISEASE

4

Contents

Introduction

A multidisciplinary approach is used to treat PD with the goals of symptom management, quality of life enhancement, and disease progression slowing. Although there isn't a cure for Parkinson's disease, there are a number of medication therapies that can help with both the condition's motor and non-motor symptoms.

The pharmacological management of PD is a cornerstone in alleviating symptoms and improving the quality of life for individuals affected by this neurodegenerative disorder. Characterized by the progressive loss of dopamine-producing neurons in the brain, PD manifests primarily through motor symptoms like bradykinesia, rigidity, tremor, and postural instability. The primary goal of drug treatment is to replenish dopamine levels in the brain, either by directly administering dopamine or by stimulating dopamine receptors. Levodopa, a precursor to dopamine, remains the most effective medication for managing motor symptoms of PD. By crossing the blood-brain barrier and converting into dopamine in the brain, levodopa helps compensate for the deficient dopamine levels. However, long-term use of levodopa can lead to motor fluctuations and dyskinesias, prompting the need for adjunctive therapies. Dopamine agonists, such as pramipexole and ropinirole, mimic the action of dopamine in the brain and can be used as monotherapy in early-stage PD or in combination with levodopa in advanced PD. Additionally, monoamine oxidase-B (MAO-B) inhibitors, such as selegiline and rasagiline, block the enzyme responsible for dopamine breakdown, prolonging its effects. Catechol-O-methyltransferase (COMT) inhibitors, such as entacapone and tolcapone, enhance the efficacy of levodopa by inhibiting its metabolism in peripheral tissues. Anticholinergic drugs and amantadine may also be used to alleviate specific symptoms like tremor and dyskinesias. With a variety of medications targeting different aspects of PD pathology, drug treatment offers a tailored approach to managing symptoms and optimizing patient outcomes. However, balancing efficacy with potential side effects and addressing disease progression remain ongoing challenges in the pharmacological management of PD.

Orientation and Directional Terms

Terms	**Definition**	**Illustration**
Dopamine	Dopamine is a neurotransmitter that helps regulate movement, memory, and motivation in the central nervous system.	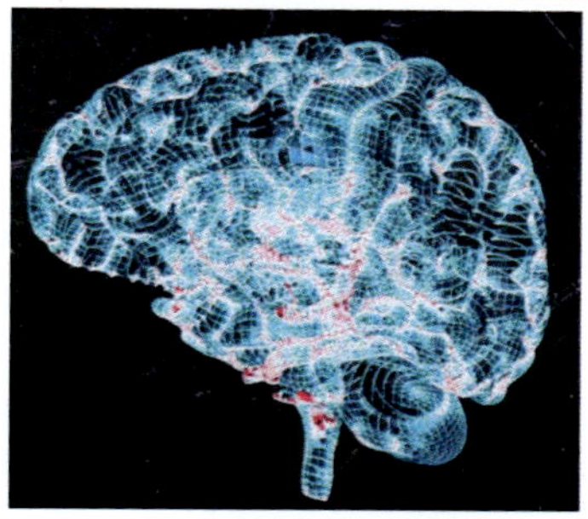
Levodopa	Levodopa is a prodrug of dopamine that is administered to patients with Parkinson's due to its ability to cross the blood-brain barrier.	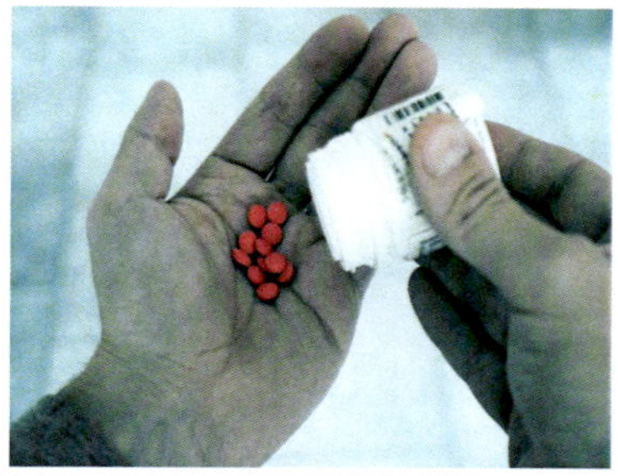
Amantadine	Amantadine is an unbranded form of Parkinson's medication, which comes in the form of capsules and syrup.	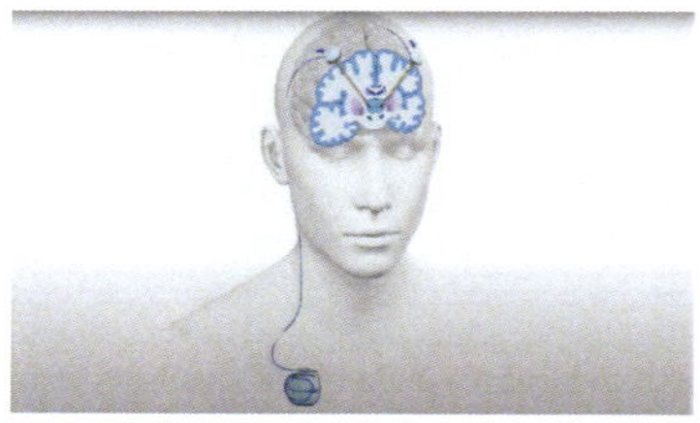
Istradefylline	Istradefylline (Nourianz) is a prescription drug used to treat adults with Parkinson's disease who experience "off" episodes. It's an adenosine A2A receptor antagonist that's used as an add-on treatment to levodopa/carbidopa (L/C).	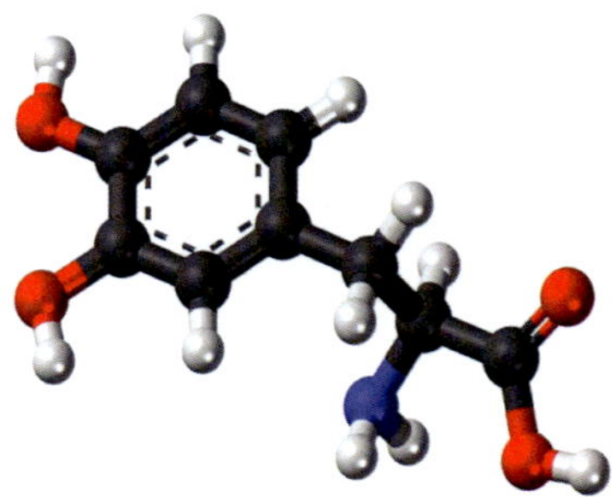
Carbidopa	Carbidopa is a medication used in the management and treatment of PD. It is in the decarboxylase inhibitor class of drugs.	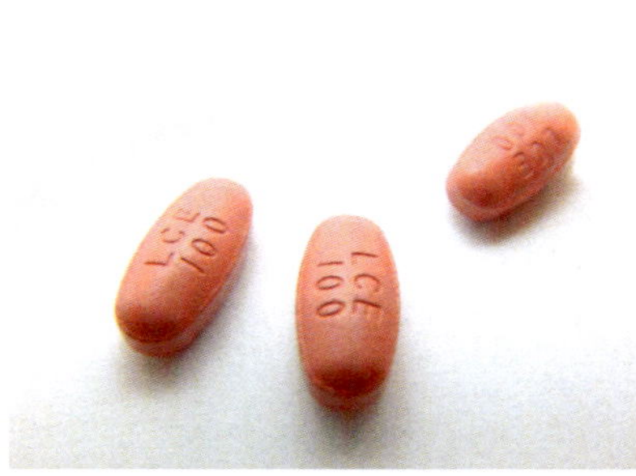

4.1. Parkinson's Disease Treatment

The goal of PD treatment is to enhance quality of life and reduce symptoms. The primary treatment for PD is medication, particularly levodopa, which increases dopamine levels in the brain and is the best medication for managing the disease's symptoms.

Other drugs, such as amantadine or dopamine agonists, may also lessen symptoms. Similar to deep brain stimulation, surgery is typically saved for people who have tried every kind of medication.

4.1.1. Goal of Parkinson's Treatment

The main objective of Parkinson's disease treatment is to lessen symptoms in order to enhance quality of life and everyday functioning.

Parkinson's disease is caused by the degeneration of brain nerve cells that produce dopamine. Because dopamine controls movement, symptoms related to movement such as stiffness, trembling, loss of balance, and slow movements (bradykinesia) result from dopamine depletion.

During the early stages of the disease, Parkinson's disease symptoms are typically mild before gradually getting worse and frequently becoming unpredictable and difficult to control.

4.1.2. Medication for Parkinson's

Parkinson's disease can be managed with a variety of pharmaceutical options. Future medication or surgical options are influenced by the medication a person starts taking early in the disease, as well as by its effectiveness and tolerability. Because of this, it's critical to collaborate closely with a medical professional who has treated Parkinson's disease before.

4.1.3. Dopaminergic Medications

The cornerstone of treating Parkinson's disease is dopaminergic therapy (related to dopamine). There are four primary types of dopaminergic drugs, which are arranged according to decreasing dopamine potency:

- **Levodopa:** For most PD patients, levodopa, also known as L-dopa, is the first medication they take and the most effective medication for reducing symptoms.

Levodopa is typically taken as the tablet combination known as Sinemet (carbidopa-levodopa), which acts by raising dopamine levels in the brain.

By preventing dopamine from being converted outside of the brain, carbidopa reduces side effects and enables levodopa dosages to be lowered while still producing the intended therapeutic effect.

Two possible exceptions to starting PD treatment with levodopa include:

- Levodopa requires frequent daily dosing, so people with mild PD may prefer a once-a-day drug, like a monoamine oxidase type B (MAO B) inhibitor.
- Levodopa is associated with the highest risk of dyskinesia, so people with PD under 50 years may opt to start treatment with a dopamine agonist.

- **Dopamine Agonists:** Drugs known as dopamine agonists activate the brain's dopamine receptors, also known as "docking sites." They can be taken with levodopa or without it.

Dopamine agonists have more side effects than levodopa, including drowsiness, leg swelling, visual hallucinations, and impulse control disorders (e.g., PD). They are also marginally less effective at controlling PD symptoms excessive and uncontrollably gambling or shopping).

Dopamine agonists include:

- Mirapex (pramipexole) is a pill taken once daily (extended-release) or multiple times daily (immediate-release).
- Requip (ropinirole) is a pill taken once daily (extended-release) or multiple times daily (immediate-release).
- Neupro (rotigotine) is a patch applied to the skin once a day.
- Apokyn (apomorphine) is a shot given underneath the skin as needed.

- **MAO-B Inhibitors:** Monoamine oxidase B is inhibited or decreased by MAO-B inhibitors. In the brain, this enzyme degrades dopamine. It has little effect on PD symptoms overall, but it can be taken on its own or in addition to levodopa or other Parkinson's drugs.

MAO-B inhibitors include:

- Azilect (rasagiline) is a pill taken once daily.
- Xadago (safinamide) is a pill taken once daily.
- Eldepryl (selegiline) is a pill usually taken once daily.

- **Amantadine:** Amantadine is an antiviral medication that is thought to function by enhancing the effects of dopamine in the brain. It might also prevent glutamate from docking at brain sites. One brain chemical that affects nerve cell communication in PD is glutamate.

Amantadine has a transient effect and can be taken on its own or in combination with anticholinergic medications or levodopa (see below).

Amantadine is available in three formulations:

- Symmetrel is a pill taken two to three times daily.
- Gocovri is an extended-release pill taken once daily.
- Osmolex is an extended-release pill taken once daily.

4.1.4. Other PD Medications

Catechol-O-methyl transferase (COMT) inhibitors and anticholinergic drugs are two more Parkinson's medications that don't affect dopamine levels:

- **Anticholinergics:** Acetylcholine is a neurotransmitter that helps control movement, and anticholinergic medications block its effects. Anticholinergics should be avoided in older people because of the possibility of side effects, particularly constipation, urine retention, and cognitive/memory impairments.

Anticholinergic drugs used in PD include:

- Cogentin (benztropine) is a pill taken twice daily.
- Artane (trihexyphenidyl) is a pill taken two to three times daily.

- **COMT Inhibitors:** In advanced Parkinson's disease, a COMT inhibitor is a levodopa adjunct therapy used to manage "off" periods. It functions by stopping dopamine from breaking down.

COMT inhibitors include:

    - Ongentys (opicapone) is a pill taken once daily at bedtime.
    - Comtan (entacapone) is taken with each dose of levodopa, up to eight times a day.
    - Tasmar (Tolcapone) is a pill taken three times daily.

- **Istradefylline:** For patients with PD going through "off" periods, the medication Nourianz (istradefylline) is authorized as an adjuvant to levodopa. It is taken once daily and is thought to function by obstructing adenosine receptors on brain nerve cells that produce dopamine.

4.1.5. Surgery for Parkinson's

Levodopa-induced dyskinesia and "off" periods are two motor complications that can arise from long-term Parkinson's disease medication treatment.

In certain cases, surgery can help manage these motor complications and alleviate symptoms when medication is not providing enough relief.

The two main types of Parkinson's surgeries include:

- Device-assisted therapies
- Ablative surgery

1. **Device-Assisted Therapies:** Deep brain stimulation and Duopa therapy (continuous levodopa-carbidopa intestinal gel) are the two main device-assisted therapies. The most popular type of brain surgery used to treat Parkinson's disease is deep brain stimulation, or DBS.

With deep brain stimulation (DBS), a neurosurgeon first inserts an electrode in a region of the brain that controls movement. After that, the electrode is fastened to an implantable pulse generator, which is a device that is positioned beneath the skin close to the collarbone.

Through a wire under the skin, the implantable pulse generator sends electrical signals to the electrode located in the brain.

These electrical signals reduce the motor symptoms associated with PD in a way that is intricate and still poorly understood.

2. **Duopa Therapy**

Levodopa and carbidopa gel known as Duopa is inserted into the intestines continuously (for up to 16 hours per day) using a percutaneous gastrojejunostomy tube, a kind of feeding tube.

The feeding tube is connected to a transportable, battery-operated infusion pump that is worn around the waist or neck in a small bag.

Like levodopa, the goal of duopa therapy is to treat Parkinson's motor symptoms; however, because it has direct access to the intestines, its effects are expected to be more profound. Additionally, "off" periods are decreased by the drug's rapid delivery to the intestines.

4.1.6. Ablative Surgery

With adjunctive surgery, a physician uses advanced imaging methods to target a particular Parkinson's disease-affected brain region.

The surgeon then makes an incision in the skull and uses radiofrequency to kill the surrounding tissue.

A more recent, less invasive technique that uses high-energy ultrasound beams to destroy brain tissue is called magnetic resonance imaging (MRI)-guided focused ultrasound. By using this method, the targeted area can be accessed without requiring a surgical cut to the skull.

4.1.7. Supportive Parkinson's Treatments for Symptom Management

- Healthy lifestyle practices, such as exercise and "brain-healthy" eating habits, may help people better control their symptoms and improve their overall quality of life in addition to medical therapies for Parkinson's disease.
- Furthermore, research indicates that diet and exercise may be able to slow the progression of the illness. Consult your PD care team about visiting a dietitian and a physical therapist for guidance if you have Parkinson's disease.
- The Mediterranean diet, with its abundance of fresh fruits and vegetables, olive oil, fish, nuts, and seeds, may be suggested by a nutritionist. These foods contain antioxidants and anti-inflammatory properties that are beneficial for brain health.
- Similarly, a physical therapist can assist you in creating a customized exercise regimen that meets your needs and goals. Exercises like jogging, dancing, tai chi, and yoga have been shown to help with a number of Parkinson's disease symptoms, such as balance issues and walking difficulties.
- Parkinson's disease management is a lifelong process that calls for careful monitoring with a PD care team and a well-thought-out treatment plan.
- Seek treatment for PD from a neurologist (a physician who specializes in disorders of the nervous system) who has treated cases of the disease. These professionals are also known as movement disorder specialists or Parkinson's specialists.
- The Parkinson's Foundation's Global Care Network is one possible source for locating a Parkinson's expert. This network offers details on Parkinson's disease treatment facilities located in the US and a few other nations.
- In addition to consulting a Parkinson's disease specialist, it makes sense to educate yourself about the illness and make use of resources that could improve your overall health and wellbeing.
- For instance, the American Parkinson's Disease Association (ADPA) is a sizable group committed to assisting people with PD in leading fulfilling lives.
- Numerous free services are provided by the ADPA, such as support groups, instructional webinars, and online classes that include seated exercises, virtual yoga, and tai chi. They also offer details on clinical trials pertaining to Parkinson's disease.

4.2. Levodopa

Dihydroxyphenylalanine, or levodopa, was first used to treat PD, marking a significant advancement in both science and medicine. There are two ways to look at this. Of course, the patients stand to gain greatly first. The second realization is that knowledge of biochemical deficiencies may hint at the successful application of replacement therapy in neurodegenerative illnesses, offering notable symptom relief if not a cure. Efforts to treat AD and other neurodegenerative disorders were greatly influenced by dopa. Unfortunately, dopa did not slow down the neurodegenerative process; rather, its effects were purely symptomatic. This was discovered despite the drug's miraculous effects on patients with both early and advanced PD and the motor benefits it provided. As a result, as the illness worsens, the dosage of dopa needed to control the motor symptoms must be gradually increased. It soon became evident that only the levorotatory stereoisomer, levodopa, of the two dopa isomers had therapeutic benefits, and methods to chemically separate the two isomers were created.

Nowadays, levodopa is the only medication used to treat PD, which has improved safety. It was soon realized that some of the side effects of the medication were caused by the peripheral, as opposed to the central, conversion of levodopa into DA, which has a significant autonomic activity.

Due to its inability to cross the blood-brain barrier (BBB), any DA generated in the peripheral nervous system actually causes serious adverse events, including gastrointestinal and other autonomic disturbances, and does not contribute to the clinical benefits of levodopa. L-amino acid decarboxylase (L-AAD; formerly known as dopa decarboxylase), the enzyme that converts levodopa to dopamine (DA), is a widely distributed enzyme in the body that is concentrated in the liver.

Carbidopa and benserazide are two medications that were created to inhibit it and are still in use today.

At. Currently, levodopa is administered in a fixed-dose combination with one of these inhibitors to almost all patients who need it for treatment. Naturally, the brain must convert levodopa into dopamine (DA), which is why the L-AAD inhibitor must not cross the blood-brain barrier.

An additional, at first overlooked, the effect of inhibiting peripheral L-AAD is that it extends the biological half-life of levodopa, and consequently of dopamine (DA) in the brain. In cases of advanced Parkinson's disease, this effect is significant.

Levodopa has a strikingly positive early-onset Parkinson's disease effect known as the "honeymoon." Levodopa dosages must be increased to make up for the loss of more dopamine-producing neurons as the disease progresses.

First, this is shown as a reduction in the amount of time that individual levodopa doses remain effective; this is known as the "end-of-dose" effect or wearing off. Other symptoms follow, such as dyskinesias associated with the "peak of dose" and unpredictable levodopa responses (also known as "yo-yoing" or "unexpected "on-off" responses). Although the precise mechanism causing this erratic response is still unknown, pharmacokinetic factors like levodopa plasma levels play a role.

Patients' independence is particularly limited by the phenomenon known as wearing off, in which the initial prolonged response to individual levodopa doses is no longer maintained. The inability of the nigrostriatal DA neurons and their terminals to absorb, store, and release DA is likely the cause of wearing off. As more and more terminals degenerate, the issue gets worse. Merely prolonging the drug's biological half-life through blockade of peripheral L-AAD is insufficient to make up for this (Stern, 2001) (Table 4.1).

In PD therapy, levodopa continues to be the "gold standard." It is the strongest anti-Parkinsonian medication on the market. On the other hand, levodopa fails to alleviate or only partially relieves some important Parkinson's disease symptoms.

Table 4.1. *Clinical Definition of Parkinson's Disease and Advanced Parkinson's Disease*

S	Depression
	Dementia
	Anxiety
	Anhedonia
	Apathy
	Psychosis (hallucination and delusion)
	Cognitive dysfunction
	Attention deficit
	Off-period–related panic attacks
	Confusion
Sleep disorders	Insomnia
	Excessive daytime sleepiness
	Nonrapid eye movement sleep-related movement disorders
	Sleep-disordered breathing
	Periodic limb movement disorder
	Rapid eye movement sleep behavior disorder
	Vivid dreaming
	Restless legs syndrome
Autonomic symptoms	Urgency
	Frequency
	Orthostatic hypotension
	Nocturia
	Erectile dysfunction
	Sweating
Gastrointestinal symptoms	Dribbling of saliva
	Ageusia
	Nausea
	Dysphagia
	Reflux and vomiting
	Constipation
	Diarrhea
	Fecal incontinence
	Unsatisfactory voiding of bowel
Sensory symptoms	Primary pain
	Secondary pain
	Fluctuation-related pain
	Paresthesia
	Olfactory disturbance
	Visual dysfunction
Other symptoms	Fatigue
	Ankle swelling
	Non-motor fluctuations
	Blurred vision

Source: Auxiliadora de Paula Vasconcelos, L. (2020). Parkinson's Disease Rehabilitation: Effectiveness Approaches and New Perspectives. IntechOpen. doi: 10.5772/intechopen.89360.

As was previously mentioned, using levodopa for an extended period of time can cause complications later in the disease; the most problematic ones are wearing-off, dyskinesias, freezing episodes, and unpredictable "on-off" fluctuations. Although the exact pathogenesis and pathophysiology of these complications are unknown, it has been proposed that levodopa toxicity or its metabolites may be a factor.

One of the main possible causes could be the pharmacokinetic and pharmacodynamic alterations that occur as the illness worsens. Additionally, there has been conjecture that the toxic effects of levodopa or DA oxidative metabolites could be partially responsible for the complications (Marsden, 1976) (Table 4.2).

Table 4.2. *Recommended Rating Scales for Parkinson's Disease*

MDS-Owned Rating Scales	The European Parkinson's Disease Association (EPDA)
Global assessment scale for Wilson's disease	Unified Parkinson's disease rating scale (UPDRS)
Global dystonia scale	Hoehn and Yahr scale
MDS-unified Parkinson's disease rating scale (MDS-UPDRS)	Schwab and England activities of daily living (ADL) scale
Modified bradykinesia rating scale	PDQ-39
Nonmotor symptoms scale (NMSS)	PD NMS questionnaire
Nonmotor symptoms questionnaire (NMSQ)	NMS survey
PKAN disease rating scale (PKAN-DRS)	Parkinson's disease composite scale
Quality of life essential tremor questionnaire	King's PD pain scale
Rating scale for psychogenic movement disorders	Parkinson's disease sleep scalePDSS-2
Rush dyskinesia rating scale	Lindop Parkinson's assessment scale
Rush video-based tic rating scale	Short-form 36 (SF-36)
UFMG Sydenham's chorea rating scale (USCRS)	Sickness impact profile (SIP)
Unified dyskinesia rating scale (UDysRS)	Mini-mental state examination (MMSE)
Unified dystonia rating scale (UDRS)	Montreal cognitive assessment scale (MoCa)
Unified multiple system atrophy rating scale (UMSARS)	Caregiver strain index (CSI)

Source: Auxiliadora de Paula Vasconcelos, L. (2020). Parkinson's Disease Rehabilitation: Effectiveness Approaches and New Perspectives. IntechOpen. doi: 10.5772/intechopen.89360.

Levodopa reduces the symptoms of the illness, making it difficult to accurately assess the patient's true condition and track the disease's progression. As of right now, stopping levodopa for longer than two weeks is the only way to determine whether something is improving or getting worse. It is obvious that this is not a workable solution, especially when the disease is advanced, and as a result, our capacity to track the rate of disease progression is constrained. There is a continuous search for biological surrogate markers. Techniques like single-photon emission computed tomography (SPECT) and positron emission tomography (PET) are being developed and have demonstrated strong correlations with the overall severity of PD.

Levodopa-based preparations are the cornerstone of today's PD treatment regimen, acting as a dopamine substitute in the striatum. It is not possible to treat PD with dopamine alone because it cannot cross the blood-brain barrier. Levodopa, on the other hand, is a dopamine precursor that can be given as a medication and crosses the blood-brain barrier. DOPA decarboxylase transforms it into the neurotransmitter dopamine after it has been absorbed and passed through the blood-brain barrier. Levodopa is typically started on a low dose for patients, and the dose is gradually increased based on how well the patient responds to treatment and how well the side effects are managed. The majority of patients need multiple daily doses within the range of 150–1000 mg. Growing doses lead to an increased chance of experiencing unfavorable side effects, as will be covered below. Levodopa typically has a rapid clinical effect that can last for several hours, especially in the early stages of the disease. However, the drug's effects usually wear off after shorter periods of time as the disease progresses, necessitating more frequent dosing.

Despite its effectiveness, levodopa has several serious side effects that play a major role in the patient's illness, especially when the disease is advanced. Some of its related side effects are caused by DOPA decarboxylase's peripheral conversion of levodopa to dopamine, which occurs outside of the central nervous system. As will be covered below, administering levodopa in conjunction with peripheral DOPA decarboxylase inhibitors reduces these effects. Extended usage may lead to severe on-off motor fluctuations and major motor complications, such as dyskinesias.

Involuntary twisting hyperkinetic movements, or dyskinesias, typically happen when a drug is at its highest dosage, though they can also happen when the drug is wearing off or even during off-periods. Levodopa dosage reduction may be used to treat problematic dyskinesias. This means that a challenging balance must be struck between maximizing motor symptom control and minimizing side effects. Deep brain stimulation may be taken into consideration for patients who have previously responded well to levodopa but have developed problematic dyskinesias. This may allow for the control of motor symptoms on a lower dosage of levodopa. The term "on-off phenomenon" describes the sudden changes in motor function that patients with advanced Parkinson's disease may encounter. While in the "on" state, levodopa's effects wear off quickly, leaving the patient in the "off" state with severe Parkinsonian motor features. During this time, the patient's motor symptoms are largely under control. These variations can seriously impair function and be especially troublesome. Variable drug absorption and transit across the blood-brain barrier, along with the ensuing oscillations in pre-synaptic and post-synaptic dopamine levels in the nigrostriatal pathway, are likely the root causes of these motor symptoms. Orthostatic hypotension and gastrointestinal disorders like nausea and vomiting are significant additional side effects. Dopamine's "off-target" effects in extranigral brain regions may give rise to neuropsychiatric features such as anxiety and hallucinations.

The lowest effective dose, dose fractionation, and the use of substitute dopaminergic therapies are a few tactics employed to mitigate the side effects of levodopa. Levodopa withdrawals, also known as "levodopa holidays," were once common, but they are no longer advised. Levodopa is given in conjunction with DOPA decarboxylase inhibitors, such as benserazide and carbidopa, to lessen its peripheral side effects. These substances selectively block levodopa from being converted to dopamine in the peripheral nervous system, which lessens the peripheral side effects without breaching the blood-brain barrier. The two combination medications that are most commonly prescribed are benserazide/levodopa (co-beneldopa [trade name Madopar]) and carbidopa/levodopa (co-careldopa [trade names Sinemet, Pharmacopa, Atamet]). These compounds come in a variety of formulations, such as suspensions that may be helpful for patients who have trouble swallowing, and modified release preparations that may help limit symptoms in the morning and control symptoms overnight.

Recently, the continuous intestinal infusion of levodopa gel (Duodopa [AbbVie Limited]), a combination of levodopa with carbidopa, has been found to be more effective in reducing severe motor fluctuations compared to oral levodopa. This is likely due to more consistent absorption of levodopa. However, the high cost of this treatment currently limits its widespread use. Researchers are now concentrating on developing other long-acting oral medications and alternative methods of drug delivery that may improve clinical effectiveness and reduce side effects in the future.

4.3. Catechol-O-Methyltransferase Inhibitors

Levodopa is broken down by the ubiquitous enzyme catechol-O-methyltransferase (COMT) before it can be converted to dopamine (DA). COMT inhibitors often lower the total amount of levodopa required by extending the availability of a single dose without delaying the onset of its effects. The current use of COMT inhibition is as a levodopa adjunctive treatment for patients with advanced Parkinson's disease who have developed wearing-off or "on-off" fluctuations. Nonetheless, by averting or postponing motor complications, COMT therapy in the early stages of Parkinson's disease may also be beneficial. A thorough analysis of COMT inhibition as a novel PD treatment approach has just been published.

Thus far, tolcapone and entacapone have been extensively studied as COMT inhibitors. While tolcapone or entacapone frequently reduces or eliminates motor fluctuations such as "off" periods, peak dose dyskinesias can be enhanced or precipitated, necessitating a reduction in levodopa doses individually. It was shown that both medications enhanced the patients' quality of life. Tolcapone's suspected hepatic toxicity led to its recent removal from the majority of countries' markets. The precise connection to drug exposure is still unclear, though. Some practitioners argue that the drug's withdrawal was premature because of the rarity of these adverse events, and they speculate that the drug may be better than entacapone (though a direct comparison between the two has not been performed).

Entacapone must be taken with each dose of levodopa (or even more frequently) due to its short half-life of about two hours. Levodopa, entacapone, and a decarboxylase inhibitor combined in a single tablet or capsule may be advantageous, particularly for patients receiving concurrent treatment with other medications. Entacapone formulations with sustained release or long-acting derivatives may also be beneficial.

COMT is an additional enzyme implicated in the breakdown of dopamine. Because they lessen the breakdown of endogenous dopamine, inhibitors of COMT also provide a therapeutic way to maintain endogenous dopamine levels. They are primarily used in conjunction with levodopa to extend the latter's duration of action by boosting the latter's half-life and cerebral delivery. Compared to standard levodopa/DOPA decarboxylase inhibitor combinations, this reduces off time and allows for control of motor symptoms in some patients. When levodopa therapy alone is not enough to address end-of-dose "wearing-off," these are frequently prescribed to the patients.

COMT inhibitors are available as tablets and are not typically prescribed as monotherapy because of their limited ability to treat Parkinson's disease symptoms on their own. Entacapone (Comtan), tolcapone (Tasmar), and opicapone (Ongentys) are a few examples of COMT inhibitors. In combination preparations with carbidopa and levodopa, entacapone is frequently used (Stalevo, Sastravi). The two most widely used COMT inhibitors are tolcapone (100 mg three times a day) and entacapone (200 mg four to eight times a day) with each levodopa dosage. It should be highlighted that COMT inhibitors may require a decrease in the levodopa dosage because they can exacerbate levodopa-induced side effects, such as dyskinesias. Since tolcapone carries a rare but potentially dangerous risk of hepatotoxicity, entacapone is typically recommended. Therefore, it is necessary to monitor liver function tests while on tolcapone treatment. Sleepiness, nausea, appetite loss, diarrhea, dizziness, orange urine discoloration, hallucinations, headaches, confusion, dry mouth, and chest pain are other infrequent side effects.

4.4. DA Agonists

For nearly 40 years, DA agonists (DAAs) have been a crucial component of the PD treatment arsenal. First, Calne et al.'s study of DAAs was a turning point in PD treatment. These medications were first prescribed as second- or even third-line treatments when they were first brought to the market, not long after levodopa was discovered. This was due to the fact that they worked well for patients who had grown resistant to levodopa or experienced its negative effects. Their initial application showed that they were effective in reducing tremor and stiffness while also sparing dopa. The potential for lowering the levodopa dosage progressively gained importance as the side effects of long-term levodopa therapy—dyskinesias and motor fluctuations in particular—were identified. These motor disturbances were alleviated when a DAA was used in place of part of the levodopa dose, demonstrating that they are not always an inevitable side effect of long-term Parkinson's disease.

The trend toward using a DAA as early therapy has increased, as delaying the start of levodopa treatment can prevent motor complications. Efforts to use a DAA as monotherapy in advanced cases of Parkinson's disease were abandoned because of its poor efficacy and side effects. Though these studies proved that, some novel DAAs were tested and their utility was clearly demonstrated. Levodopa is more effective than DAAs (apomorphinc being an exception). At first, this might not have much of an impact on Parkinson's disease. But as the illness worsens, more potent DA stimulation is needed, and when higher DAA dosages are impeded by adverse effects, levodopa supplementation is required—albeit once more with the risk of developing motor problems.

While it is undeniable that DAAs can be used initially as monotherapy, it is unclear how many patients can benefit from this treatment for an extended period of time. Based on the information at hand, levodopa will be added in roughly three years. 20% of patients, and 50% of them after five years.

Although the ergot derivatives are unquestionably effective in Parkinson's disease, a number of side effects have complicated their use. Ergots were discovered to be "dirty" medications with the ability to interact with a variety of peripheral and central nervous system receptor types. An essential next step was the creation of the synthetic DAAs pramipexole, ropinirole, and piribedil. These agents did, however, have a lot of side effects in common. Thus, it became evident that the majority of the side effects of these treatments are class effects, even though pleuropulmonary fibrosis might be unique to ergot derivatives. Pergolide has recently been linked to alterations in the heart valves.

Long-term levodopa therapy is associated with motor fluctuations, which are considered (but. not demonstrated) to be connected to the brief plasma half-lives (t1/2=90 min) of individual levodopa dosages. The buffering ability of the remaining DA neurons, which convert levodopa to DA, store it, and then release it in a tonic rather than phasic pattern, explains why the clinical benefit from single doses is longer, at least in the early stages of the disease. A potential benefit is that DAAs are independent of DA neurons, especially in the later stages of the disease when few DA neurons remain viable. This benefit, though, is tied to their longer half-lives, which are usually 4 to 6 hours (and significantly longer for cabergoline). If the development of motor fluctuations is caused by a nonsustained level of DA stimulation, then if cabergoline is to be used in de novo cases, these complications should be significantly delayed.

DAAs may also possess advantageous qualities like antioxidant or antiapoptotic effects, according to a number of studies. It should be noted that because these studies were conducted *in vitro*, they were all quite brief and used doses that weren't entirely relevant to the clinical setting. There is currently no evidence to support the notion that oxidative stress is a key factor in the pathophysiology of PD or that DAAs have any appreciable antioxidant or antiapoptotic effects when used in routine clinical settings in humans. The early inclusion of a DAA stops (or at least postpones) the development of motor issues, however. There is debate as to whether this has a neuroprotective effect. Moreover, it would be exceedingly challenging to demonstrate that DAA can actually halt the progressive loss of DA neurons in the substantia nigra.

Stimulation of presynaptic DA receptors may be a potential mechanism if DAAs slow the progression of Parkinson's disease. Receptors that mediate the synthesis and release of dopamine by negative feedback are likely present in all dopamine (DA) terminals. Reactive oxygen species that are harmful can be produced by the metabolism of endogenous DA. Therefore, it is reasonable to assume that a decrease in the rate of DA synthesis will slow the ongoing harm to DA neurons. The majority of DAAs—possibly all of them—lower the rate of DA of synthesis; however, little is known about how effective each DAA is in this regard. In theory, it is better to use a medication like talipexole that has comparatively high presynaptic stimulation (compared to postsynaptic D2 stimulation). However, it is unclear how this benefit can be shown in patients with Parkinson's disease.

The "ergot-derived" or "ergoline" medications bromocriptine, cabergoline, lisuride, and pergolide are currently in use as DAAs because their chemical structures are derived from the plant alkaloid ergot. Strong promotion is being given to the more recent, "non-ergot" synthetic DAAs, such as piribedil, pramipexole, and ropinirole, which are chemically unrelated to ergot.

Along with levodopa, all DAAs can cause side effects such as nausea, vomiting, dizziness, and orthostatic hypotension. Higher dosages of DAAs have the potential to cause confusion, hallucinations, and psychosis; however, these side effects typically manifest in the later stages of the disease. Other side effects of levodopa and some DAAs include sedation and insomnia, which are most likely unrelated to any particular agonist.

Sleeplessness has recently come to light as a potential side effect of DAAs, including levodopa. Patients receiving DAA treatment have reported experiencing "sleep attacks," or intense urges to sleep. This is a dangerous side effect that could result in auto accidents. This should be taken into account and discussed with the patient, especially if they are engaged in activities where their sleepiness, even if it isn't extreme, could put them or others in danger.

Pleuropulmonary and retroperitoneal fibrosis, as well as digital or coronary vasospasm, are among the adverse effects that have been particularly connected to ergot derivatives. The more recent and secure non-ergot DAAs, ropinirole, pramipexole, and piribedil, are not linked to these.

Currently under development is a transdermal formulation of rotigotine, an experimental D2 selective agonist. In a multicenter phase 2b trial, it was found to lower daily levodopa doses by 30% in patients with mild-to-severe Parkinson's Disease.

As DA itself stimulates both DA D1 and D2 receptors, apomorphine is the most potent DAA and the only one that does so efficiently. Its limited therapeutic range, intricate interindividual pharmaco-kinetics, and pharmacodynamic variability, however, limit its therapeutic effect. However, apomorphine cannot be taken orally. Subcutaneous injections are very beneficial, especially for those who experience protracted periods of not feeling well. Apomorphine can be continuously delivered subcutaneously via a pump, but. is pricey and technically challenging to use. To address these challenges, various endeavors are underway to develop customized controlled delivery methods for apomorphine, such as sublingual and transdermal iontophoresis. This will be especially helpful for controlling fluctuations quickly. A recent study tested an apomorphine powder made of carboxymethyl cellulose as an intranasal sustained-release formulation. Hopefully, these more advanced delivery methods will improve its usage as a life-saving drug in extreme circumstances. DA receptors come in at least five different varieties: D_1, D_2, D_3, D_4, and D_5. It has long been disputed whether D_1 stimulation has a place in the treatment of movement disorders, especially PD. Pergolide is a D_1 agonist and bromocriptine is a D_1 antagonist; ropinirole and pramipexole have no effect on D_1 receptors. The usefulness of D_1 receptors in PD therapy is debatable because all of these DAAs are equally effective in treating PD. But according to recent reports, ABT-431, a particular Drstimulating medication, may also be helpful for Parkinson's disease. Thus, DAA therapy still has a number of unresolved issue (Rascol & Blin, 1999) (Table 4.3).

Table 4.3. *Mechanism of Action and Indications of Dopamine Precursors and Dopaminergic Agonist and Antagonist Drugs*

Drug	**Mechanism of Action**	**Indications**
Precursors		
Levodopa (L-DOPA)	Levodopa mimics the role of endogenous dopamine; crosses the blood–brain barrier through various pathways, and is decarboxylated to form dopamine stimulating the dopamine receptors	Parkinson's disease
L-phenylalanine	Precursor of tyrosine, dopamine, norepinephrine (noradrenaline) and epinephrine (adrenaline)	Antidepressant effects Vitiligo
L-tyrosine	Precursor of dopamine, norepinephrine and epinephrine	Antidepressant
Receptor agonists		
Apomorphine	A nonergoline dopamine agonist with binding affinity to dopamine D2, D3, and D5 receptors	Parkinson's disease

Drug	Mechanism of Action	Indications
Bromocriptine	Ergoline derivative with strong agonist activity on the D2 dopamine receptors	Parkinsonian Syndrome Amenorrhea Galactorrhea Acromegaly Premenstrual syndrome Female infertility
Cabergoline	Ergoline derivative; dopamine agonist (with a high affinity for D2 receptors) and prolactin inhibitor.	Hyperprolactinemic disorders. Parkinsonian Syndrome
DA	Agonist to the D1, D2, D3, D4, D5 dopamine receptors. Interacts on the synaptic terminals, causing neuronal excitation or inhibition at the target neuron	Hemodynamic imbalances Blood pressure Hypotension Poor perfusion of vital organs Low cardiac output
Fenoldopam	Benzazepine derivative; selective dopamine D1 receptor agonist. Decreases peripheral vascular resistance in renal capillary beds	Hypertension
Lisuride	Ergoline derivative, agonist to dopamine D2 receptors. It can be an antagonist to dopamine D1 receptors. Additionally, activates some serotonin receptors	Parkinson's disease
Piribedil	Nonergoline, piperazine derivative, dopamine agonist that acts on D2 and D3 receptors	Parkinson's disease
Pramipexole	Nonergoline, a dopamine agonist showing specificity and strong activity at dopamine D2 receptors	Parkinson's disease Restless legs syndrome
Quinagolide	Nonergoline derivative; it selectively binds to D2 receptors on the surface of lactotroph cells, resulting in reduced adenylyl cyclase activity and inhibition of prolactin secretion from the anterior pituitary	Hyperprolactinemia
Ropinirole	Nonergoline derivative, selectively binds to dopamine D2 receptors, with highest affinity at D3 receptors	Parkinson's disease Restless legs syndrome
Rotigotine	Nonergoline derivative; a nonselective agonist of dopamine receptors with higher affinity at D3 receptors	Parkinson's disease Restless legs syndrome

Drug	Mechanism of Action	Indications
Experimental agonists		
Dihydrexidine (LS-186,899)	Selective full agonist at the dopamine D1 receptors. It has some affinity for the D2 receptor	Scientific research
Pukateine	Aporphine derivative; agonist at the D2 dopamine receptor and antagonist at the α1 adrenergic receptor	Scientific research
Quinpirole	Selective D2 and D3 receptor agonist	Scientific research
SKF 38393	A selective D1-like receptor agonist	Scientific research
Antagonists and receptor blockers		
Typical antipsychotics		
Chlorpromazine	Phenothiazine derivative. It binds strongly to the D2 receptor, blocking its action; this blockade, in the nigrostriatal pathway, is responsible for its extrapyramidal side effects	Schizophrenia, Bipolar disorder Acute psychosis, Nausea and vomiting Relief of apprehension before surgery Persistent singultus (chronic hiccups)
Fluphenazine	Phenothiazine derivative. Blocks postsynaptic mesolimbic dopaminergic D2 receptors in the brain	Management of psychosis in schizophrenia
Haloperidol	It is a first-generation antipsychotic and one of the most frequently used worldwide. It is not selective for the D2 receptor, but, has a strong antagonism to this dopamine receptor in mesolimbic and mesocortical pathways in the brain	Schizophrenia Tourette syndrome Behavioral disorders in children Hyperactivity
Loxapine	Dibenzoazepine tricyclic derivative. Antagonist with high affinity for the D2 receptor, also a serotonin 5-HT2 blocker	Schizophrenia Other psychotic disorders
Molindone	Indole derivative. Antagonizes dopamine D2 receptor sites in the reticular limbic systems in the brain, decreasing dopamine activity	Schizophrenia
Perphenazine	Phenothiazine derivative. It binds to the dopamine D1 and dopamine D2 receptors inhibiting their activity. Its antiemetic effect is mainly due to blockade of D2 receptors in the chemoreceptor trigger zone and the vomiting center	Schizophrenia Other psychotic disorders Nausea and vomiting

Drug	**Mechanism of Action**	**Indications**
Pimozide	Diphenylbutylpiperidine derivative. It binds and inhibits the dopamine D2 receptor	Tourette syndrome Schizophrenia
Thioridazine	Phenothiazine derivative. It blocks postsynaptic mesolimbic dopaminergic D1 and D2 receptors	Schizophrenia Other psychotic disorders Generalized anxiety disorder Depressive disorders
Thiothixene	Thioxanthene derivative. Is a highly potent antagonist of the D1, D2, D3 and D4 dopamine receptors.	Schizophrenia
Atypical antipsychotics		
Amisulpride	Benzamide derivative. It is a selective dopamine D2 and D3 receptor antagonist	Schizophrenia Nausea and vomiting
Clozapine	Dibenzodiazepine derivative. It binds to the D4 dopamine receptors with a higher affinity than D2 receptor. Additionally, it has antagonistic effects at 5-HT2A receptors and is a partial agonist at 5-HT1A receptors	Resistant schizophrenia
Olanzapine	Thienobenzodiazepine derivative. It exerts its action primarily on dopamine D1, D2, D3 and D4 and serotonin 5-HT2A, 5-HT2C, 5-HT3 and 5-HT6 receptors, blocking their action	Schizophrenia, Bipolar disorder
Quetiapine	Thiazepine derivative. Antagonizes to D2 dopamine receptors and to 5-HT2A receptors (it has strong affinity for the latter)	Schizophrenia Bipolar disorder Major depressive disorder
Risperidone	Benzisoxazole derivative. It blocks D2, but more 5-HT2A receptors in the brain.	Schizophrenia, Bipolar mania Autism-associated irritability
Sulpiride	Benzamide derivative. Selective antagonist at dopamine D2, D3 receptors	Schizophrenia
Ziprasidone	Benzothiazolylpiperazine derivative. Binds to 5-HT2A and dopamine D2 receptors with high affinity	Schizophrenia Bipolar mania Acute agitation in schizophrenic patients
Antiemetics		
Domperidone	Benzimidazole derivative. It has strong affinity for the D2 and D3 dopamine receptors, blocking their activity	Peristaltic stimulant, Dyspepsia, Indigestion, Epigastric pain Nausea and vomiting

Drug	Mechanism of Action	Indications
Metoclopramide	Benzamide derivative. Inhibit dopamine D2 and serotonin 5-HT3 receptors	Nausea and vomiting Gastroesophageal reflux disease
Prochlorperazine	Phenothiazine derivative. It mainly blocks the D2 dopamine receptors in the mesolimbic system	Schizophrenia, Schizoaffective Other conditions with psychosis symptoms Nausea and vomiting
Experimental antagonists		
Eticlopride	Antagonizes D2 dopamine receptor	Scientific research
Raclopride	Potent and selective antagonist on D2/D3 dopamine receptors	Trials studying Parkinson's disease
SCH23390	Highly potent and selective of D1 dopamine receptor	Scientific research of drug addiction

Source: Bandala C, Cárdenas-Rodríguez N, Mendoza-Torreblanca JG, Contreras-García IJ, Martínez-López V, Cruz-Hernández TR, Carro-Rodríguez J, Vargas-Hernández MA, Ignacio-Mejía I, Alfaro-Rodriguez A, et al. Therapeutic Potential of Dopamine and Related Drugs as Anti-Inflammatories and Antioxidants in Neuronal and Non-Neuronal Pathologies. Pharmaceutics. 2023; 15(2):693. https://doi.org/10.3390/pharmaceutics15020693.

In 1978, dopamine receptor agonists were introduced to the market to treat Parkinson's disease. Based on receptor specificities, the widely used agonists can be divided into ergot and non-ergot derived groups. All agonists have an ethanolamine moiety. Unlike levodopa, these medications do not require conversion into dopamine in order to activate the dopamine system. Instead, they bind to dopaminergic receptors. For PD patients, especially those who are younger, dopamine agonists are frequently prescribed as an initial treatment. This strategy permits a postponement of levodopa use, potentially mitigating the negative effects of the previously mentioned motor complications. A number of the medications are no longer in clinical use due to notable idiosyncratic side effects. Pergolide, for instance, was taken off the market as a medication in 2007 due to research showing a possible risk of pericardial, retroperitoneal, and pleural fibrosis (Shaunak et al, 1999).

Some of these medications come in tablet, patch, and injection form in controlled or extended-release formulations. For example, rotigotine patches come in handy for patients who are nil-by-mouth during surgery or who are unable to take oral medications. To make sure a patient is receiving enough medication when switching to rotigotine patches in this situation, the levodopa-equivalent dose of their current treatment plan must be calculated. Dopamine agonists can be helpful in patients with mild symptoms, in those who cannot tolerate levodopa, or as an adjunct to levodopa therapy, even though they may be less effective than levodopa in controlling the motor symptoms of PD, with the majority of patients eventually requiring levodopa therapy.

Patients and the kind of agonist prescribed will determine how long a drug will take to take effect and how long its half-life is. When starting dopamine agonists, the dosage is typically increased gradually in accordance with the patient's response and any side effects that may occur. Among the frequently prescribed dopamine agonists, the typical dosage is as follows: up to 31.3 mg of pramipexole, divided into three doses; 9–16 mg (maximum 24 mg) of ropinirole divided into three to four doses; and 4-6 mg of rotigotine taken once daily. Although it is not as commonly used, apomorphine can be helpful when administered as a subcutaneous injection to treat severe "off" episodes or as a subcutaneous infusion to patients who still experience severe motor fluctuations even after other medications have been optimized. Dopamine agonists may have antioxidant qualities and slow the loss of dopaminergic neurons, according to certain preclinical and imaging research, but there isn't enough proof to support the idea that these medications can alter the course of the disease.

Compared to levodopa, treatment with dopamine agonists has been demonstrated to reduce the incidence and severity of dystonia, motor fluctuations, and dyskinesia. They might, however, have additional serious negative effects. Frequent adverse effects include dry mouth, insomnia, peripheral edema, constipation, fainting, hallucinations, nausea, vomiting (caused by stimulation of the area postrema, which is located in the medulla at a site in which the BBB is disrupted), and sleepiness.

Impulse control disorder (ICD), a behavioral disorder characterized by compulsive and impulsive behaviors, is arguably the most significant side effect of dopamine agonists. Hypersexuality, gambling, compulsive buying/shopping, binge eating, punding, and hobbies (such as obsessive Internet use, creative pursuits, and writing) are some possible symptoms. After starting dopamine agonists, it is critical for clinicians to be on the lookout for these issues because they can cause serious financial and social problems for the patient. Interpersonal relationships, caregiver well-being, and overall quality of life can all suffer from ICD. Some behaviors might be more typical in men (e.g., excessive sexuality) or women (e.g., compulsion to shop), and ICD is more prevalent in people who have previously experienced addiction (e.g., to gambling or alcohol). 15 to 20%percent of Parkinson's disease patients who take dopamine agonists experience ICD; levodopa also increases the risk of ICD, but it is significantly lower than that of dopamine agonists. Dopamine agonists' effects on the opiate and serotonin systems, the orbitofrontal cortex, and the mesolimbic dopaminergic pathway have all been suggested as possible mechanisms.

The possibility of developing dopamine agonist withdrawal syndrome (DAWS), which can happen when someone with compulsive or impulsive behavior either quits using dopamine agonists altogether or lowers their dosage, is another crucial factor to take into account. Anxiety, panic attacks, sleeplessness, restlessness, dysphoria, agitation, exhaustion, orthostatic hypotension, diaphoresis, and cravings for drugs are some of the symptoms of withdrawal syndrome. As a result, stopping dopamine agonists gradually and keeping a close eye out for these issues is necessary. Similar to ICD, DAWS can have serious psychosocial repercussions.

4.5. Monoamine Oxidase-B Inhibitors for the Treatment of Parkinson's Disease

A common chronic neurodegenerative disease, PD is characterized by abnormal formation of Lewy neurites and/or Lewy bodies, which are intraneuronal aggregates of proteins (mainly α-synuclein) that spread in an ascending pattern from the medulla oblongata to the pontine tegmentum, midbrain, mesocortex, and neocortex; additionally, there is a decrease in the number of dopaminergic neurons in the substantia nigra (SN), which results in a dopamine deficiency.

There are roughly 10 million PD patients globally, and as people age, the prevalence rises, reaching 1 to 3% in those over 65. Bradykinesia, resting tremor, rigidity, postural instability, and gait disorder are common motor symptoms of PD.

These symptoms are frequently accompanied by a variety of non-motor symptoms, such as sleep disturbance, autonomic dysfunction, depression, and fatigue, which can significantly impair day-to-day functioning.

Therapeutic approaches, such as medication therapy, surgery, and rehabilitation, have been developed despite the fact that the disease cannot be cured. These approaches can reduce symptoms and may even be able to slow the disease's progression.

Nearly all PD patients eventually need levodopa, which is thought to be the most effective symptomatic treatment.

However, levodopa use over an extended period of time can result in dyskinesia and motor fluctuations (also known as "wearing off" or "on-off").

Adjuvants such as dopamine agonists (DAs) or enzyme inhibitors, such as those that inhibit catechol-O-methyl-transferase (COMT) or monoamine oxidase B (MAO-B), are frequently used in conjunction with levodopa to relieve motor complications. While MAO-B inhibitors cross the blood-brain barrier, inhibit central MAO activity in the central nervous system, and thereby decrease dopamine degradation, commonly used COMT inhibitors, such as entacapone and opicapone, inhibit levodopa degradation in the peripheral. Both when used as adjunctive therapy in advanced illness and during the early stages of Parkinson's disease, MAO-B inhibitors have demonstrated excellent efficacy and safety.

Longer periods of exposure to MAO-B inhibitors have been linked to lower levodopa consumption and a slower rate of clinical decline, according to clinical studies.

As of right now, reversible inhibitors like safinamide and irreversible inhibitors like rasagiline and selegiline are approved MAO-B inhibitors. The impact of MAO-B inhibitors on both motor and non-motor symptoms of PD, their mode of action, and potential future developments for these drugs will all be covered in this section.

4.5.1. Mechanism of Action of MAO-B Inhibitors

- **MAO-B Inhibitors Regulate the MAO-B Activity***:* The riboflavin protein monoamine oxidase (MAO) is found on the mitochondria's outer membrane. It is a catalyst for the oxidative deamination of monoamine and tyramine neurotransmitters, including norepinephrine, dopamine, phenethylamine, and 5-hydroxytryptamine. MAO-A and MAO-B are the two isoenzymes that make up MAO. MAO-A is primarily found in the heart, platelets, and gastrointestinal tract. It can speed up the metabolism of food ingredients that contain tyramine, preventing hypertensive crises brought on by tyramine buildup (also known as a "cheese reaction"). Catecholaminergic neurons, including norepinephrine neurons in the locus coeruleus and dopaminergic neurons in the SN, also contain MAO-A. The majority of MAO-B is found in glial cells and platelets, and in the brain, MAO-A makes up about 20% of total MAO activity. MAO-B is mostly found in these cells. Dopamine is one of the amine neurotransmitters that are regulated by both MAO-A and MAO-B. Dopamine released into the synaptic cleft and absorbed by glial cells is metabolized by MAO-B, whereas dopamine metabolized by MAO-A occurs in presynaptic neurons. It has been demonstrated that glial cell density increases with age, and that MAO-B activity naturally rises in neurodegenerative diseases. MAO-B inhibitors selectively raise dopamine levels at synaptic clefts, inhibit MAO-B activity in the brain, block dopamine catabolism, and improve dopamine signaling. Second-generation MAO-B inhibitor rasagiline is 3–15 times more potent than selegiline *in vivo* rat studies, according to preclinical research. Patients with PD can benefit from even low doses of rasagiline (0.5 to 2 mg/day), as opposed to selegiline (10 mg/day). Furthermore, in *in vitro* studies using rat brain, the traditional MAO-B inhibitor selegiline only demonstrates 127 times higher selectivity than safinamide, the most recent generation of MAO-B inhibitor that also possesses sodium and calcium channel blocking activity. Safinamide, on the other hand, shows 5,000 times higher selectivity for MAO-B than MAO-A. Safinamide inhibits glutamate release, voltage-dependently opens sodium channels, and modifies non-dopaminergic systems like calcium channels in addition to preventing dopamine reuptake.

- **MAO-B Inhibitors may have Disease-Modifying Effects:** The ability of a particular agent to prevent, delay, or stop the process of nigral dopaminergic cell death, and thereby prevent clinical deterioration, is known as disease modification for patients with PD. Because the metabolism of dopamine by MAO-B can produce harmful metabolites like dihydroxyacetaldehyde and hydrogen peroxide, MAO-B inhibitors can shield neurons from these harmful processes. In addition to inhibiting MAO-B, selegiline and rasagiline also have neuroprotective effects relating to their propargylamine structures. Selegiline and rasagiline have the ability to play a neuroprotective role by upregulating the expression levels of nerve growth factor, brain-derived neurotrophic factor, glial cell-derived neurotrophic factor, and other nerve growth factors. By either directly or indirectly stimulating anti-apoptotic factors like Bcl-2 and Bcl-xL and suppressing the expression of pro-apoptotic factors like Bax, rasagine can prevent apoptosis. Because rasagline and selegiline have distinct metabolic pathways, rasagline may have a neuroprotective advantage over the latter. For instance, in PC12 cell lines, selegiline and rasagiline can both lessen the cell death brought on by oxygen-glucose deprivation. Nevertheless, oxygen-glucose deprivation-induced cell death was enhanced by 70% by L-methamphetamine, a metabolite of selegiline, rather than aminoindan, the principal metabolite of rasagiline. Rasagiline may also have a neuroprotective effect by stabilizing regional cerebral blood flow perfusion in Parkinson's disease patients, according to brain SPECT scans. Safinamide, in contrast to selegiline and rasagiline, decreases excitotoxicity to dopaminergic neurons, controls glutamate release, and blocks sodium and calcium channels. Safinamide prevents dopaminergic neurons from degenerating and inhibits the activation of microglial cells, according to research on animals.

- **Effects of MAO-B Inhibitors on Mitochondria and Cell Apoptosis:** In PD, mitochondrial dysfunction is typified by elevated production of reactive oxygen species and decreased activity of mitochondrial complex I. Studies conducted *in vitro* have demonstrated that MAO-B inhibitors can enhance the performance of brain mitochondria by blocking nitric oxide synthase activity and lowering hydrogen peroxide production. Furthermore, neurotoxins and oxidative stress can alter the membrane permeability of mitochondria, and MAO-B inhibitors can prevent calcium efflux from occurring in mitochondria. For instance, after crossing the blood-brain barrier, the toxin 1-methyl-4-phenyl-1,2,3,6-tetrahydropyridine (MPTP) is oxidized by MAO-B to form 1-methyl-4-phenylpyridine ion (MPP+). Subsequently, MPP+ impedes the function of mitochondrial complex I, culminating in cellular demise and the discharge of reactive oxygen species, which causes dopaminergic cell death. Studies on animals have demonstrated that selegiline and rasagiline can both considerably lessen MPTP's neurotoxicity.
- **Effects of MAO-B Inhibitors on Alpha-synuclein Aggregation:** Lewy bodies are primarily composed of alpha-synuclein. Studies conducted *in vitro* have demonstrated that MAO-B inhibitors can postpone the alpha-synuclein aggregation nucleation phase, which may slow down the rate at which the disease progresses. Alpha-synuclein is encouraged to form cyclic or dimeric structures by MAO-B inhibitors (Figure 4.1), which also inhibit it from forming the sheet-like and linear structures that are necessary for aggregation. Based on the various pharmacological mechanisms mentioned above, MAO-B inhibitors have shown remarkable efficacy in both early and advanced PD and may have the potential to modify the disease (Kakish et al, 2015).

4.5.2. PD Symptoms Treated by MAO-B Inhibitors

PD-related symptoms treated with MAO-B inhibitors are detailed in Table 4.4:

Table 4.4. *Inhibition of Recombinant Human Monoamine Amine Oxidase-A and B by Propolis Extract, Fractions and Pure Constituents*

Sample Name	Unit	Monoamine Oxidase-A (IC_{50})*	Monoamine Oxidase-B (IC_{50}) *
Propolis Extract (prop-E)	µg/mL	0.60 ± 0.12	6.99 ± 0.09
Fraction 2 (9.0–17.5 min) #	µg/mL	0.33 ± 0.03	0.31 ± 0.02
Fraction 3 (17.5–20 min) #	µg/mL	0.16 ± 0.11	0.23 ± 0.09
Fraction 4 (20–30 min) #	µg/mL	5.36 ± 0.22	0.98 ± 0.08
Fraction 5 (30–35 min) #	µg/mL	26.16 ± 0.29	22.19 ± 3.34
Galangin	µM	0.13 ± 0.01	3.65 ± 0.150
Apigenin	µM	0.64 ± 0.11	1.12 ± 0.27
Quercetin	µM	2.44 ± 0.12	38.66 ± 1.20
Fisetin hydrate	µM	2.10 ± 0.09	>100
Morin hydrate	µM	5.88 ± 0.15	49.66 ± 0.56
Toxifolin	µM	65.06 ± 1.96	53.80 ± 3.91
Clorgyline	µM	0.0065 ± 0.0003	-
Deprenyl	µM	-	0.036 ± 0.0012
Harmine	µM	0.0039 ± 0.0003	27.50 ± 2.67

Source: Chaurasiya ND, Ibrahim MA, Muhammad I, Walker LA, Tekwani BL. Monoamine Oxidase Inhibitory Constituents of Propolis: Kinetics and Mechanism of Inhibition of Recombinant Human MAO-A and MAO-B. Molecules. 2014; 19(11):18936-18952. https://doi.org/10.3390/molecules191118936.

*The IC_{50} values computed from the dose response inhibition curves are Mean ± S.D. of triplicate observations. # *Retention time* (*Tr* values, indicate time for start and end for collection of the fraction.

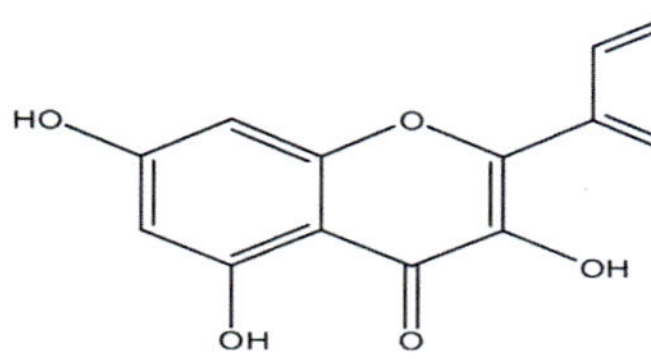

1. Galangin

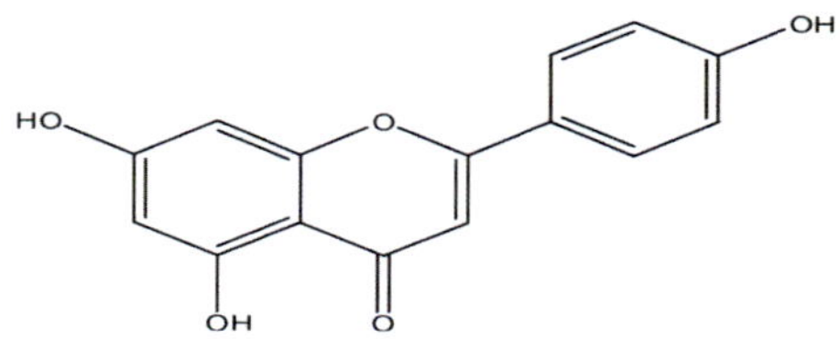

2. Apigenin

Figure 4.1. *Selection of MAO-B inhibitors according to PD related symptoms.*

Source: Chaurasiya ND, Ibrahim MA, Muhammad I, Walker LA, Tekwani BL. Monoamine Oxidase Inhibitory Constituents of Propolis: Kinetics and Mechanism of Inhibition of Recombinant Human MAO-A and MAO-B. Molecules. 2014; 19(11):18936-18952. https://doi.org/10.3390/molecules191118936.

i. **Improvement of Motor Symptoms:** MAO-B inhibitors are advised as first-line treatments for individuals with early-stage PD whose motor symptoms do not significantly impair their quality of life, according to the Guidelines for Adult Parkinson's Disease published by the National Institute for Health and Care Excellence (NICE) in 2017. When levodopa is not enough for Parkinson's disease patients with dyskinesia or motor fluctuations, MAO-B inhibitors may be chosen. The 2018 International Parkinson and Movement Disorder Society Evidence-Based Medicine Review's Treatments for the Motor Symptoms of PD suggests selegiline and rasagiline, two MAO-B inhibitors, as successful monotherapies for early-stage Parkinson's disease. However, rasagiline appears to be a clinically useful adjuvant to DA therapy for early/stable PD, while safinamide is not. There is insufficient evidence to support the use of selegiline in the treatment of motor fluctuations, but both rasagiline and safinamide work well. The fourth edition of the 2020 Chinese guidelines for the treatment of Parkinson's disease states that rasagiline is a better option than selegiline for addressing motor complications and that MAO-B inhibitors can be used in early PD patients and as add-on therapy in advanced PD patients (Gray and Ives, 2014).

ii. **Monotherapy in Early PD (First-Line Therapy):** The PD-MED study compared the long-term symptom control and quality of life improvement of patients with early PD treated with levodopa, DAs, or MAO-B inhibitors. It was a large, pragmatic, randomized controlled study (real-world study). Individuals receiving MAO-B inhibitors had a significantly higher chance of stopping their prescribed drug class for levodopa-sparing therapy than those receiving DAs (72% vs.50%). The primary reason for discontinuation was side effects, although a small percentage was attributed to lack of efficacy. Nevertheless, compared to initial treatment with DAs, after levodopa exposure, small but significantly better benefits were seen in PDQ-39 mobility scores (1.4 better), cognition, and the PDQ-39 summary index (0.8 better). However, the quality of life measured by the EuroQol EQ-5D scale was not improved. While motor fluctuations were greater in the DAs group, rates of dyskinesia were comparable between the MAO-B inhibitors and DAs groups. One plausible reason for the superior effectiveness of MAO-B inhibitors at lower levodopa equivalent doses (LED) in comparison to DAs (695 mg/day vs. 768 mg/day) may indicate that levodopa is not as effective as MAO-B inhibitors when added to DAs; however, more research is required to confirm this. Although DAs are typically thought to be more effective than MAO-B inhibitors, the PD MED study found that MAO-B inhibitors were at least as effective as DAs when used as initial levodopa-sparing therapy.

Patients with early Parkinson's disease may benefit from selegiline monotherapy, which can also postpone the need for levodopa therapy. Selegiline delayed the need for levodopa by 548.9 days compared to 312.1 days in patients treated with a placebo, according to a small-sample double-blind study. Two double-blind studies with 52 and 157 patients, respectively, were published in 1992 and 1998 for PD patients who had not received any treatment. In those trials, selegiline or a placebo was administered to the patients. Selegiline improved PD patients' motor symptoms when compared to placebo, and it also postponed the onset of disability and the need for levodopa. A 2017 Phase III 12-week randomized, double-blind study involving 292 Japanese patients with early PD showed that selegiline monotherapy was well tolerated and significantly improved the unified Parkinson's disease rating scale (UPDRS) score in patients with early PD ($p = 0.0005$).

In patients with early-stage Parkinson's disease, rasagline can reduce motor symptoms and may have disease-modifying benefits. A comparison of Americans, Europeans, and Asians has revealed similar outcomes. The effectiveness of Rasagiline was assessed in 2002 in the TEMPO study, which included patients with early Parkinson's disease from the USA and Europe. Following a 26-week course of therapy, the adjusted effect size for the total UPDRS showed improvements of -3.56 units for 2 mg of rasagiline and −4.20 units for 1 mg of rasagiline ($p < 0.001$) when compared to placebo. At the second year of follow-up in the TEMPO extension study, 46% of patients were under control with rasagiline monotherapy, negating the need for additional dopaminergic drugs.

In patients with early treatment-naive PD, the 2009 ADAGIO study assessed the disease-modifying effect of rasagiline monotherapy. By using a study design that involved starting rasagiline treatment early for 72 weeks, delaying treatment with a placebo for 36 weeks, and then starting 1 mg/2 mg of rasagiline for 72 weeks, three stratified primary endpoints based on UPDRS were set to determine the disease-modifying effect of 1 mg/2 mg of rasagiline. The study's primary objectives were to determine whether the 1 mg/2 mg rasagiline group's rate of total UPDRS change during a 12- to 36-week treatment period was superior to placebo; whether the early-start treatment group's UPDRS score changed more favorably between baseline and 72 weeks than the delayed treatment groups; and whether the early-start treatment group's rate of UPDRS change during 48 to 72 weeks was noninferior to that of the delayed treatment groups. The study's findings demonstrated that while the 2 mg rasagiline group did not meet all three stratified endpoints, the 1 mg rasagiline group did. Over the course of 12 to 36 weeks of treatment, the 1 mg and 2 mg rasagiline groups experienced significantly lower rates of weekly changes in UPDRS scores when compared to the placebo group (0.09±0.02 vs. 0.07±0.02 vs. 0.14±0.01, p = 0.01. At 72 weeks, the early-start group experienced a less severe overall UPDRS score change from baseline (1 mg) compared to the delayed-start group (2.82±0.53 vs. 4.50±0.56, p = 0.02), however there was no discernible difference between the 2 mg early-start and delayed-start groups (3.47±0.50 vs. 3.11±0.50, p = 0.60); with regard to the third stratified endpoint, the early-dose groups receiving 1 mg and 2 mg did not show a lower rate of improvement in UPDRS scores per week than the delayed-dose group (0.085±0.02 vs. 0.094±0.01 versus 0.085±0.02. p < 0.001, both 0.065±0.02). The disease-modifying effect of rasagiline was not conclusive because the 2 mg group did not meet the second endpoints. A longer-term study is needed to ascertain the disease-modifying effects of rasagiline in more motor and non-motor areas, and more sensitive evaluation scales and methods are required.

In Chinese patients with early PD, rasagiline's effectiveness was assessed in the 2018 CHORUS study. This randomized controlled study comprised 127 patients with PD who had not received any treatment prior to this point. The findings demonstrated that the 1 mg/day rasagiline group experienced a significantly higher decrease in total UPDRS scores than the placebo group (−3.18±0.95 vs. (p = 0.025), -0.18±0.98. Furthermore, after 26 weeks of treatment, rasagiline monotherapy significantly improved the MDS-UPDRS II + III scores compared with placebo (-6.39, 95% CI [-8.530, −4.250], p < 0.0001). This Phase III study assessed the safety and efficacy of rasagiline in 224 Japanese early PD patients. All of the patients (103 on rasagiline and 95 on placebo) who finished the randomized trial were enrolled in the second period's extension study and were given 1 mg of rasagiline for an additional 26 weeks. In both the placebo-rasagiline (95% CI [−4.05, −1.59] and rasagiline-rasagiline (95% CI [−4.57, −1.01] groups, the mean change in MDS-UPDRS (Part II+III) from baseline to 52 weeks was −2.8 points. This indicates that long-term treatment with rasagiline consistently improved motor symptoms in patients with good safety and tolerability, and that a late start to rasagiline did not compromise its efficacy in this study.

iii. **Symptomatic Adjunct Therapy in Early or Stable PD:** MAO-B inhibitors may alleviate symptoms and lower levodopa dosage in patients with early or stable PD. They may also improve neuroprotection, although further research is necessary due to insufficient data.

Selegiline The DATATOP study demonstrated that in patients with early-stage Parkinson's disease, treatment with selegiline alone or in conjunction with vitamin E may postpone the need for levodopa and the development of PD-related disability. Published in 1999, this 5-year prospective, randomized, double-blind, placebo-controlled study assessed the effectiveness of selegiline in patients with early Parkinson's disease as an adjuvant to conventional levodopa. Randomized to either a selegiline or placebo group were patients with Parkinson's disease who were not receiving levodopa treatment or who had been taking it for less than a year. Levodopa was titrated to each patient's specific requirements prior to the start of the study medication. The time at which levodopa needed to be increased by more than 50% of the titrated dose was the main outcome. The findings demonstrated that, in comparison to the placebo group, selegiline considerably shortened the median time to reach the primary endpoint (4.9 years vs. 2 + 6 years, p = 0 + 027). Over the course of the five years of treatment, the mean levodopa dose increased significantly in the placebo group but changed very little in the selegiline group. In contrast, the selegiline group experienced at least equal therapeutic efficacy with a lower levodopa dosage, suggesting that selegiline was useful as an adjuvant therapy with levodopa for the relief of motor symptoms. In a different study, patients treated with selegiline plus levodopa for five years had a markedly higher UPDRS score than patients treated with placebo plus levodopa. Additionally, the mean levodopa dosage with selegiline was 19% higher than that of the placebo group (p = 0.0002).

Studies have looked into the viability of taking DAs along with selegiline. When Nappi et al. investigated the effects of adding selegiline to lisuride therapy and discovered that the mean lisuride dosage could be decreased without the clinical effects getting worse. When L-deprenyl (10 mg daily) was added to low-dose bromocriptine (up to 25 mg daily) in 1995, Calzetti et al. found that the combination of selegiline and bromocriptine produced a stable clinical status for up to 12 months, a decrease in the number of patients requiring levodopa at 24 months, and a mildly significant improvement in most clinical rating scales. Both lisuride and bromocriptine, however, are ergot-related dopamine agonists, and prolonged use of bromocriptine increases the risk of fibrotic cardiac valvulopathies. Lyons with others. examined the impact of adding orally disintegrating selegiline on the reduction of DA-related adverse events (AEs) in PD patients with levodopa-induced motor fluctuations and pramipexole-related AEs of excessive daytime sleepiness, pedal edema, hallucinations, and impulse-control disorders. Findings revealed that most subjects' DA-related adverse events (AEs) had decreased or stopped by week 12, and UPDRS activities of daily living scores had significantly improved (p <0.005). This suggests that the addition of oral disintegrating selegiline along with DA dosage reductions primarily decreased DA-related AEs without compromising efficacy.

Rasagiline 1 mg of rasagiline or a placebo was administered to early PD patients whose conditions were not well controlled with their current DA treatment (ropinirole ≥ 6 mg/d or pramipexole ≥ 1.0 mg/d). The outcomes demonstrated that rasagiline adjunct therapy enhanced the overall UPDRS score (−3.6±0.7 vs. A UPDRS motor score of -3.4±0.5 compared to -1.2±0.7, p = 0.012). from baseline to week 18, with no increase in clinically relevant adverse reactions when compared to placebo (-1.6±0.5, p = 0.007). Another study assessed the effectiveness of rasagiline in patients with early treatment-naive PD when used as an adjuvant with pramipexole (P2B001, 0.3 mg pramipexole/0.75 mg rasagiline or 0.6 mg pramipexole/0.75 mg rasagiline). A total of 149 patients were randomly assigned to receive either a placebo or a 12-week supply of pramipexole/rasagiline at varying doses. Comparing the 0.3 mg pramipexole/0.75 mg rasagiline combination and the 0.6 mg pramipexole/0.75 mg rasagiline combination to the placebo group, significant improvements were observed in the total UPDRS score, PDQ-39, the UPDRS motor, and activities of daily living.

Safinamide Early PD patients who had previously received stable doses of a single DA were the subjects of a 2012 Phase III double-blind trial that examined the effectiveness of safinamide adjunct therapy. Patients were randomly assigned to groups that received 200 mg/day of safinamide, 100 mg/day of safinamide, or placebo. The findings demonstrated that when compared to a placebo, 100 mg/day of safinamide increased UPDRS III scores in patients with early Parkinson's disease (−6.0 vs. -3.0, p = 0.0419. However, patients in the 200 mg/day group did not show any improvement when compared to the placebo group (-3.9 vs. -3.0, p = 0.6404. During the extension phase of the aforementioned study, the time interval between baseline and additional intervention—such as raising the dosage of DA, adding a different PD treatment, or stopping therapy altogether—was the main measure of efficacy. While the rate of intervention was considerably lower in patients taking 100 mg of safinamide per day than in those on a placebo (25% vs. the median time from baseline to additional drug intervention (pooled safinamide vs. safinamide groups) did not reach statistical significance (51%, p < 0.05). placebo [559 as opposed to. 466 days, with p = 0.3342]. According to the 2018 MDS evidence-based recommendations, safinamide is "non-efficacious" and "not useful" when used in conjunction with DAs for early-stage PD without motor fluctuations.

iv. **Adjunct Therapy in Advanced PD:** Selenium Adjunctive selegiline therapy has not been well studied in advanced PD. A 6-week study with 96 PD patients who had noticeable symptom fluctuations revealed that a higher percentage of patients had improved gait (56% vs. 30.4%) and a higher degree of symptom score improvement (0.25 vs. 0.15) in the group taking 5 mg of bid selegiline as opposed to the placebo. Selegiline, however, was unable to increase the patient's "ON" time. In 1991, selegiline was added to the original regimen in a clinical study, which resulted in a significant reduction in the daily use of levodopa and a tendency to shorten the daily "OFF" time in seven PD patients with varying symptoms.

Rasagiline In the PRESTO trial, which was published in 2005, 472 PD patients from the USA and Europe were included. They had been prescribed levodopa and had a daily "OFF" time of less than 2.5 hours. The patients received one of three randomizations: 1 mg/day, 0.5 mg/day, or placebo. Following 26 weeks of treatment, compared to the placebo, the daily "OFF" time was decreased by 0.94 h (p<0.001) and 0.49 h (p=0.02) in the 1 mg/day and 0.5 mg/day groups, respectively. Additionally, improvements were observed in the motor performance during the "ON" time and in the activities of daily living during the "OFF" time. The same year, the LARGO study was published, demonstrating that 1 mg/day of rasagiline alleviated symptoms in patients who had received levodopa and experienced motor fluctuations. It also significantly decreased the mean daily "OFF" time when compared to a placebo (−1.18 h vs. −4.0 h, p = 0.0001), and a longer daily "ON" period without a significant amount of dyskinesia (0.85 h versus. p = 0.0005); 0.03 h. Rasagiline and entacapone demonstrated comparable efficacy. Furthermore, the LARGO study's sub-studies revealed that rasagiline had a trend toward lowering the UPDRS-ADL OFF score and significantly decreased the UPDRS motor OFF scores, while entacapone had no discernible impact (−1.95 vs. p = 0.14, 1.27).

In a 2013 randomized controlled study, the effectiveness of rasagiline as a supplement to levodopa treatment in Chinese patients with PD was examined. The results indicated that the mean adjusted total daily "OFF" time decreased more in the rasagiline group than in the placebo group (−1.75±1.69 h vs. -0. P < 0.001, h = 69±1.44. The 2018 CHORAL study also demonstrated that in Chinese patients receiving levodopa and experiencing motor fluctuations, rasagiline as an adjuvant was able to significantly reduce the mean total daily "OFF" time when compared with placebo (–1.25 h vs. (h = -0.76, p = 0.023). Patients tolerated it well, and it also enhanced their daily functioning and general health status.

Additionally, two 2019 studies on Japanese PD patients receiving levodopa and experiencing wearing-off phenomena revealed that patients treated with rasagiline 1 mg or 0.5 mg for 26 weeks had a decrease in "OFF" time of 0.84 h and 0.60 h when compared with placebo (p = 0.0006 and 0.0140, respectively), and patients treated with rasagiline 1 mg for 52 weeks had a decrease in "OFF" time from baseline (95% CI –1.376 to –0.399). Consequently, levodopa and rasagiline therapy as an adjuvant proved effective, and the results lasted for at least 52 weeks.

Safinamide Research revealed that safinamide and rasagiline, despite having distinct pharmacological mechanisms, were equally effective at blocking the action of MAO-B. Compared to placebo, both 100 mg/day and 50 mg/day of safinamide as an add-on treatment significantly prolonged the total "ON" time with no or non-troublesome dyskinesia in a Phase III multicenter, randomized, double-blind, 24-week trial published in 2014 (1.36±2.625 h vs. 1.37±2.745h compared to. 0.97±2.375 h. Furthermore, the safinamide group outperformed the placebo group in terms of improvement in the reduction of "OFF" time, UPDRS III assessment, and clinical global impression-correction scale (CGI-C) assessment. 2017 saw the publication of a randomized trial that demonstrated safinamide as an add-on therapy significantly prolonged "ON" time (1.42±2.80h vs. –1.56±2.35h vs. 0.57±2.47h, p<0.001), resulting in a decreased total daily "OFF" time. improved UPDRS III score rated during an "ON" phase (–3.43±7.72 vs. –0.54±2.21h, p<0.001). -1/83±8/23, p = 0.003) in contrast to the placebo. Additionally, a 24-week randomized, double-blind, placebo-controlled Phase II/III study revealed that adding 50 mg or 100 mg of safinamide daily improved the patients' symptoms and signs compared to placebo and increased the change in mean daily "ON" time by 1.39 h (p = 0.0002) and 1.66 h (p < 0.0001), respectively, for Japanese PD patients who did not respond well to levodopa.

v. **Non-Motor Symptoms:** Multiple types of non-motor symptoms, including sleep disturbance, fatigue, and neuropsychiatric symptoms, can arise at any stage of Parkinson's disease.

   i. ***Sleep Disturbance:*** The second most common non-motor PD symptom, subjective sleep discomfort affects about half of patients who are newly diagnosed. PD patients experience a variety of sleep disturbances, including restless legs syndrome, excessive daytime sleepiness, insomnia, and rapid eye movement behavior disorder. PD patients' sleep disorders have been linked to a number of factors, including the advancement of their disease, motor complications, dopaminergic medications, severe autonomic dysfunction, and the presence of hallucinations.

Amphetamine derivatives that metabolize selegiline may have adverse effects on sleep and sympathomimetic effects. Sleeplessness was one of the most frequent adverse events (AEs) when the AE data from the long-term studies were combined. Selegiline needs to be taken in the morning and at noon because it is assumed that amphetamine-like derivatives of selegiline worsen sleep quality, which is supported by the onset of insomnia during chronic selegiline intake in PD patients. Patients who experience excessive daytime sleepiness may try selegiline. Gallazzi and team stated that 10 mg of selegiline was given to 45 PD patients who had excessive daytime sleepiness, which typically developed after the introduction of DAs. The results showed a statistically significant improvement in somnolence but no change in the UPDRS III scores.

When used as monotherapy or adjunct therapy, risagiline helps patients with Parkinson's disease sleep better. In a 12-week prospective observational study, rasagiline added to levodopa as an adjunct resulted in better sleep outcomes than baseline and a reduction in mean sleep latency (-1.68±1.21 h vs. Significant differences were found in mean total sleep time (1.26±1.62 h vs. -0.55±0.69 h, p = 0.001). p = 0.026), or 0.32±0.70 h. Another randomized controlled trial revealed that rasagiline improved the quality of sleep as determined by polysomnography in patients with Parkinson's disease who experienced sleep disturbances. Additionally, compared to baseline, rasagiline treatment resulted in a significant reduction in the number of arousals, the percentage of light sleep, and the amount of time spent awake after sleep onset. It also improved daytime sleepiness as determined by the Epworth Sleepiness Scale. The lack of associations between motor function and the polysomnographic sleep parameters or the Parkinson's Disease Sleep Scale 2 (PDSS2) score suggests that the effects of rasagiline on sleep were unlikely to be linked to improvements in motor function.

The impact of safinamide on PD patients' sleep has only been documented in a small number of studies to date. A few researchers assessed how safinamide treatment affected PD patients' non-motor symptoms. Safinamide-treated patients had significantly lower ESS and PDSS2 scores. The SAFINONMOTOR study found that PD patients' sleep (NMSS-domain 2 and PSQI) significantly improved six months after starting safinamide. Future investigations into the effectiveness of safinamide in PD patients with sleep disorders are still necessary.

ii. ***Fatigue Symptoms:*** An overwhelming sense of exhaustion, lack of energy, and tiredness that is unrelated to physical activity is called fatigue. It is one of the most incapacitating symptoms of PD, affecting about half of patients even in the early stages and severely impairing quality of life. A post hoc analysis of the ADAGIO trial revealed that, in patients with PD who had not started treatment yet, fatigue symptoms increased more in the placebo group than in the groups receiving rasagiline 1 mg and 2 mg per day (0.17 vs. 0 against. –0.02), and rasagiline monotherapy considerably slowed the patients' weariness from developing. In a 2015 randomized controlled trial, patients with confirmed PD who reported moderate-to-severe fatigue benefited significantly from 1 mg/day of rasagiline compared with placebo from baseline to 12 weeks of treatment (12 vs. p = 0.003), or 8 points. Rasagiline is regarded as "efficacious" for treating fatigue in PD, according to the 2018 MDS Evidence-based review for updates on treatments for the non-motor symptoms. The limited sample size meant that the practice implication was only "possibly useful." De Micco et al. conducted a prospective cohort study. discovered that patients with motor fluctuating Parkinson's disease who received safinamide had significantly lower fatigue scores (p = 0.02). Safinamide treatment improved the sleep/ fatigue scores (–35.8%; p = 0.002) of PD patients in the open-label prospective study SAFINONMOTOR. This implies that safinamide may help PD patients feel less fatigued.

iii. ***Depression:*** PD patients frequently experience depression, which is characterized by apathy and anhedonia. The length of the disease, the intensity of the motor symptoms, the occurrence of motor complications, the anxiety, the sleep disturbance, the autonomic symptoms, the cognitive decline and dementia, etc. have been connected to a higher risk of depression in people with PD. A meta-analysis revealed that MAO-B inhibitors may lessen the intensity of depressive symptoms in PD patients, particularly in those who have the disease early. In a 1991 French multicenter, double-blind, randomized, controlled study, 93 patients with Parkinson's disease were randomly assigned to receive 10 mg/day of selegiline or a placebo for three months. The findings demonstrated that the selegiline group outperformed the placebo group in terms of improvement on the 90-day Hamilton Depression Rating Scale (HDRS) score and mental UPDRS Scale score (p = 0.005 and p < 0.001, respectively). In addition, the study showed that PD patients treated with selegiline adjunct with levodopa have significant improvement in MMSE and Beck Depression Inventory (BDI) scale scores than patients treated with levodopa only.

Furthermore, a 12-week, double-blind, placebo-controlled trial that evaluated the effect of 1 mg/day rasagiline on depression and cognition in non-demented PD patients with depressive symptoms found that rasagiline may significantly reduce the total BDI-IA score in week 4 compared with placebo (–5.46±0.73 vs. P = 0.026) and –3.22±0.67. Research has demonstrated that safinamide helped PD patients with their emotional disorders. Additionally, the study demonstrated that safinamide decreased the risk of adverse events (AEs) related to depression in PD patients treated with safinamide in addition to levodopa (p = 0.0444 and 0.005, respectively) and improved the emotional well-being score of the PDQ-39 questionnaire (p = 0.0067 and 0.0006, respectively), the GRID Hamilton Rating Scale for Depression (GRID-HAMD) score (P = 0.0408 and 0.0027, respectively), and the GRID-HAMD score at 6 months and 2 years, respectively. –0.3, p = 0.0731). On the other hand, a meta-analysis based on randomized controlled trials regarding the impact of MAO-B inhibitors on the reduction of depressive symptoms in PD revealed that while long-term evidence is lacking, MAO-B inhibitors are significantly effective in the short term in treating PD patients with depression.

iv. ***Bladder Dysfunction:*** One of the most prevalent autonomic dysfunctions in patients with PD is bladder dysfunction, which is thought to affect between 55 and 80% of patients. In 2014, a 2-month open-label study compared the urodynamic parameters of patients with early mild PD before and after they started receiving 1 mg/day of rasagiline. In 2021, a small retrospective analysis of urological symptoms in Parkinson's disease patients treated with safinamide revealed that subscale scores for micturition urgency, urinary incontinence, urinary frequency, and nocturia were significantly improved compared to baseline in patients receiving safinamide add-on therapy. These findings suggested that safinamide may help to improve PD patient urinary symptoms. The results also showed that rasagiline significantly improved bladder function, increased bladder capacity (16%), first micturition sensation (34%), and reduced residual urine volume (–53%) in PD patients.

v. ***Gait Disorder***: As the disease progresses, severe gait disorders can lead to disability and a decline in quality of life in PD patients. One common type of gait disorder in PD patients is freezing of gait (FOG), which is prevalent in Chinese patients with the disease. Studies have suggested that the MAO-B inhibitors selegiline and rasagiline can reduce the risk of developing FOG. Data from 800 early-stage PD patients in the DATATOP study showed that applying selegiline could reduce the risk of developing FOG by 53% ($p < 0.0001$). Furthermore, a post hoc analysis of the PRESTO and LARGO studies showed that adjunct therapy with rasagiline 1 mg/day improved UPDRS postural stability (–0.02 vs. placebo). -0.11, $p<0.05$) and the difference in gait score (0.01 vs. in PD patients (-0.10, $p<0.05$). Rasagiline significantly improved UPDRS III, FOG-Q, and PDQ-39 quality of life scores (all $p < 0.001$) for PD patients who had received stable treatment for at least 6 months and whose FOG duration was 3.3±1.8 years. In a pooled analysis of two randomized placebo-controlled studies, 100 mg/day safinamide significantly improved mean UPDRS III score (–5.15 vs. 3.0, $p = 0.003$) and the gait score (–0.56 vs. –0.34, $p = 0.0118$) from baseline in patients with advanced Parkinson's disease when compared to a placebo.

In summary, patients with both early and advanced Parkinson's disease respond well to treatment with MAO-B inhibitors. Rasagiline demonstrated strong evidence-based efficacy in both monotherapy and adjunct therapy for early and advanced PD and significantly reduced a variety of motor and non-motor symptoms in PD patients when compared to selegiline, which is primarily used in patients with early or stable PD, and safinamide, which is primarily used in patients with advanced PD. Binde and team presented a meta-analysis of 27 trials evaluating the best MAO-B inhibitors for early or later PD by assessing the UPDRS score and serious adverse events (AEs). They discovered that all of the included MAO-B inhibitors were effective when given as monotherapy when compared to placebo, but that selegiline outperformed other MAO-B inhibitors when combined with levodopa, regardless of whether the length of the disease was taken into consideration. A second meta-analysis of 79 publications was conducted later by Binde et al. included DAs (cabergoline, pramipexole, ropinirole, rotigotine) and MAO-B inhibitors in the comparison. Interestingly, they discovered that all the drugs under investigation were effective when given as monotherapy when compared with placebo, with the exception of safinamide; however, selegiline continued to be the best option when given in combination with levodopa. The conclusions drawn from meta-analyses still need to be validated in additional trials due to the lack of precise data from head-to-head RCTs that have compared one MAO-B inhibitor to another.

4.5.3. Safety of MAO-B Inhibitors

Evidence-based medicine recommendations suggest that dopamine agonists (DAs) have a higher risk of side effects and patient withdrawals due to poor tolerability compared to MAO-B inhibitors or levodopa in early Parkinson's disease. DAs are associated with excessive somnolence, hallucinations, and impulse-control disorders, while MAO-B inhibitors have a lower frequency of specific adverse events. In a study comparing rasagiline to placebo, rasagiline had slightly lower rates of treatment-emergent adverse events leading to withdrawal. Combination treatments with COMT inhibitors and DAs were found to significantly increase adverse event rates compared to placebo, as well as compared to MAO-B inhibitors. The PD-MED study showed similar rates of dyskinesia but higher rates of motor fluctuations in PD patients taking DAs compared to those taking MAO-B inhibitors. Overall, MAO-B inhibitors are recommended for long-term management of Parkinson's disease, as monotherapy in early stages and as adjunct therapy in advanced stages.

- ***Selegiline:*** There were concerns about the potential risks of combining selegiline with levodopa in treating PD patients due to reported "cheese reaction" and cardiovascular toxic effects that could lead to increased mortality. However, later meta-analyses have shown that the increased mortality associated with selegiline use is controversial, with no significant difference in mortality rates compared to control groups. Additionally, studies have shown that the combination of selegiline and levodopa may actually be more effective in improving clinical symptoms in PD patients without a significant increase in adverse events. Although some studies initially suggested a higher risk of mortality with selegiline plus levodopa therapy, these findings became statistically insignificant after excluding certain studies.

In addition, selegiline tends to cause hallucinations. A study examining the effects of selegiline in adjunct with levodopa on the cardiovascular system in patients with PD found that patients acutely loaded with selegiline in adjunct with levodopa had significantly higher plasma norepinephrine levels than patients receiving levodopa monotherapy and healthy controls ($p<0.001$). PD patients also experienced a higher incidence of orthostatic hypotension, though the difference between the groups was not statistically significant. The length of illness, the Hoehn and Yahr stages, and the levodopa dosages all had a significant impact on how severe the hallucinations were. A high dose of selegiline alone was sufficient to induce hallucinations in patients with PD, even in those with low levodopa dosages (≤300 mg/day), low Hoehn and Yahr stages, or short illness durations (≤8 years). The incidence of serotonin syndrome in 4568 patients receiving selective serotonin reuptake inhibitors (SSRIs) on selegiline treatment was found to be 0.24%, with 0.04% presenting with severe symptoms. As a result, patients on selegiline treatment should be advised to abstain from foods high in tyramine. Patients with PD who are on SSRIs, have postural hypotension, cardiovascular conditions, or experience hallucinations should be prescribed selegiline with caution.

- ***Rasagiline:*** Rasagiline is safe and well-tolerated both on its own and when used with levodopa. Common side effects include nasopharyngitis, falls, eczema, headaches, and bruising when used alone, and falls, nasopharyngitis, and dyskinesia when used with levodopa. Rasagiline does not interact with tyramine or have sympathomimetic effects, making it a safe long-term option for Parkinson's disease treatment. Studies have shown that rasagiline improves motor symptoms for up to 52 weeks. A retrospective analysis found that combining rasagiline with antidepressants, especially SSRIs, did not cause serotonin syndrome in PD patients. However, there is still a small risk associated with this combination.
- ***Safinamide:*** With similar incidences of TEAEs compared with placebo, most of which were mild to moderate doses, safinamide was well tolerated in various observational studies and randomized controlled trials. A long-term safety and efficacy study of safinamide as add-on therapy to levodopa enrolled 203 Japanese PD patients with wearing-off, 142 of whom completed 52 weeks of treatment. The incidence of adverse reactions was found to be 78.3%, according to the results. Nasopharyngitis (20%) and dyskinesia (17%) were the most common adverse reactions. Another randomized, double-blind, placebo-controlled Phase II/III study in Japanese Parkinson's disease patients revealed that the incidence of adverse reactions was 58%, 60%, and 61% in the placebo group, 50 mg/day and 100 mg/day safinamide groups, respectively, and that dyskinesia (2.1%, 8.3% vs. 10.6%) and visual hallucinations (1.4, 3 vs. 4.5%). A European real-world study conducted in 2021 to evaluate the safety of safinamide in patients with PD revealed that the majority of adverse events in treated patients were mild (62.0%) or moderate (28.0%), with only 2% being directly linked to safinamide. In most cases, these adverse events did not require treatment. Safinamide is safe and well-tolerated as an adjuvant therapy in patients with varying symptoms and in specific populations.

4.5.4. Future of MAO-B Inhibitors

In spite of multiple clinical trials, PD is still incurable. With the exception of the trial of rasagiline by delayed start design at a low dose of only 1 mg/day, clinical studies have not produced enough supporting results to support the goal of neuroprotection in PD, which has been to stop or reverse the cell death of nigrostriatal dopaminergic neurons and prevent the disease from progressing. In addition to the conventional oral dosage forms, other novel galenic forms of MAO-B inhibitors were investigated. These compounds have the potential to exhibit strong neuroprotective effects by controlling the mitochondrial apoptosis cascade, preserving mitochondrial function, and upregulating the gene coding expression of antioxidant enzymes, pro-survival neurotrophic factors, and anti-apoptotic Bcl-2. In addition, animal studies demonstrated that injectable rasagiline, based on an injectable long-acting formulation system, significantly increases dopamine levels in PD model rats ($p < 0.05$) and effectively improves motor symptoms. Encapsulating rasagiline in polycaprolactone microspheres prolonged drug release for 1 month by a single subcutaneous dose, and no significant difference was found with daily rasagiline administration in animal studies. Pharmacokinetic studies in healthy Chinese populations demonstrated that the transdermal rasagiline patch could prolong the duration of administration with good safety and tolerability.

The third generation of MAO-B inhibitors has evolved to have higher selectivity, reversible effects, wider safety margins, and potential for neuroprotection. It is worth investigating their clinical efficacy. Recent research indicates that monoamine oxidase is still a preferred molecular target in the study of neurodegenerative diseases. Numerous novel MAO-B inhibitors with high selectivity, reversibility, and fewer side effects are still being developed. Additionally, there are many selective MAO-B inhibitors in natural products that are still waiting to be discovered. These include flavonoids, xanthones, proanthocyanidins, iridoid, glucosides, curcumin, alkaloids, and their derivatives. Danshensu (3-(3,4-dihydroxyphenyl) -(2R)-lactic acid, salvianic acid A), which was isolated from several herbs, such as. Lilacin was discovered to suppress MAO-A and MAO-B activity. Danshensu treatment also markedly improved scopolamine and Aβ-induced cognitive impairments in mice. Furthermore, the creation of multitarget drugs based on MAO-B inhibitors in recent years—such as those that dual-inhibit MAO-B and cholinesterase—is anticipated to offer new hope for the treatment of neurodegenerative diseases like Parkinson's disease and Alzheimer's disease.

Apart from treating Parkinson's disease patients, MAO-B inhibitors have garnered significant interest in treating various aging and apoptotic diseases. In randomized controlled trials, patients with amyotrophic lateral sclerosis showed good tolerance to rasagiline. Rasagiline has the potential to protect patients with rapidly progressing amyotrophic lateral sclerosis, according to the results of a post hoc analysis. MAO-B inhibitors may also have potential anticancer activity, as they can inhibit glioma proliferation and significantly reduce glioma cell migration. Basic research has also demonstrated that rasagiline can inhibit the growth of melanoma (Agid et al, 1999; Rascol et al, 2002).

4.6. Anticholinergic Drugs Used in Parkinson's Disease

The first pharmacological treatments for Parkinson's disease were anticholinergic medications. They still have a role in the treatment of the condition, even though levodopa and other centrally acting dopaminergic agonists have largely replaced their use. These medications, which include benztropine, biperiden, diphenhydramine, ethopropazine, orphenadrine, procyclidine, and trihexyphenidyl, have minimal pharmacokinetic data as a therapeutic class. The majority of pharmacokinetic data comes from studies where young healthy volunteers receive single doses. Generally speaking, when given orally to humans, this class of medications is quickly absorbed. The range of oral bioavailability for various drugs is between 30% and 70%. All of the medications seem to have a high Vd in both humans and animals, and their distribution into tissues happens quickly. All of the medications exhibit comparatively low clearance in relation to hepatic blood flow, and they seem to undergo extensive metabolism, leading to the production of N-dealkylated and hydroxylated metabolites. Based on the information at hand, it appears that the parent drug and its metabolite are eliminated through the bile and urine. Although plasma concentration vs. the relationship between therapeutic effects and peripheral side effects has not been thoroughly investigated, there is some evidence that supports this theory. Compared to younger patients, elderly patients have poorer drug tolerance. The pharmacokinetic data for these medications in the elderly is noticeably lacking. The safe and efficient use of these medications in Parkinson's disease patients may be hampered by the lack of pharmacokinetic data for multiple dose administration and in the elderly.

The neurological condition known as Parkinson's disease (paralysis agitans) primarily affects middle-aged and older people. Parkinson's disease affects about 1 in 1000 people in the general population. According to estimates, the incidence is roughly 1% among those 65 years of age and older.

From a biochemical standpoint, Parkinson's disease is believed to be brought on by the degeneration of dopaminergic neurons in the neostriatum, a part of the brain's basal ganglia that is crucial for controlling the neural impulses that govern motor functions. The first medications used to treat Parkinson's disease had anticholinergic activity, even though the majority of the drugs used to treat the condition pharmacologically act as dopamine agonists either directly or indirectly. Levodopa, also known as L-dopa, was not widely used to treat Parkinson's disease until the late 1960s. Despite being a significant advancement in the treatment of Parkinson's disease, L-dopa is neither curative nor sufficient to fully alleviate the disease's symptoms, which usually include bradykinesia, muscular rigidity, involuntary resting tremor, and muscular weakness.

Additionally, dopamine's usefulness is restricted by a phenomenon known as "wearing off" that manifests after extended use. The development of pharmacological agents that modulate dopaminergic pathways has garnered significant attention from researchers and the pharmaceutical industry. However, the pharmacokinetics of drugs that act on the cholinergic system have received relatively less attention.

Despite their adjunct role, anticholinergic medications used to treat Parkinson's disease (ACP) are significant agents because they offer a different mechanism of action that may help with some of the disease's bothersome symptoms, particularly the involuntary resting tremor. In the early stages of the disease, they are used as monotherapy; in later stages, they work in concert with L-dopa.

ACPs have the potential to help postpone the need for L-dopa treatment because they are administered early in the course of the disease. This could enable the patient to get the most out of L-dopa later on in the illness. Furthermore, they might make it possible to lower the dosage of L-dopa needed in more severe situations, thus extending the drug's useful life. Another way that the ACP are clinically helpful is that they can lessen the extrapyramidal side effects that come with using antipsychotic medications.

4.6.1. Mechanism of Action of Anticholinergics Used in Parkinson's Disease

Muscarinic receptors are competitively antagonistic by the ACP. Trihexyphenidyl, benztropine, procyclidine, biperiden, ethopropazine, diphenhydramine, and orphenadrine are among the examples used in clinical settings. All of these medications are taken orally on a regular basis. For the treatment of muscle spasm, orphenadrine is also available as the citrate salt in oral and intravenous formulations. We don't know the ACP's precise mode of action. Parkinson's disease may be brought on by a lesion in the nigra striatum, which is thought to lower intranigral dopamine concentrations. Consequently, there is a disparity in the amount of dopamine and cholinergic neuronal pathways. It has long been thought that by lowering the level of neurotransmission mediated by neostriatal acetylcholine, anticholinergic medications can balance this imbalance in less severe forms of Parkinson's disease.

4.6.2. Current Status of Pharmacokinetic Knowledge of ACP

The current state of knowledge about the pharmacokinetics of the ACP is lacking. Others have already acknowledged this. For instance, "There is surprisingly little information on the pharmacokinetic properties of these anticholinergic drugs," to quote directly from Goodman and Gilman's Pharmacological Basis of Therapeutics, 8th edition. This statement is still relevant today even though it was written ten years ago. Pharmacokinetic data for these agents are probably lacking due to a number of factors, including the loss of patent protection and the introduction of newer, more potent anti-Parkinson treatments. A plausible rationale for the lack of pharmacokinetic information could be the extremely low dosages of various widely utilized ACPs. This leads to correspondingly low plasma concentrations, which could lead to sensitivity issues in the analysis. In fact, the highest clinically advised dosages for procyclidine HCl, trihexyphenidyl HCl, and benztropine mesylate are just 6 mg, 10 mg, and 20 mg daily, respectively. Orphenadrine HCl and diphenhydramine HCl, two structurally related H1-antagonist antihistamine compounds, are typically used at clinically higher doses of at least 100 mg daily. Additionally, ethopropazine, an anticholinergic phenothiazine compound, is used at much higher dose levels, ranging from 50 to 600 mg daily. The relative potency of the various agents in binding to muscarinic receptors appears to be connected to the variation in dose levels between them. For instance, the IC50 values for atropine, benztropine, procyclidine, trihexyphenidyl, and orphenadrine in rat brain muscarinic receptors were determined to be 0.0022, 0.018, 0.026, 0.070, and 0.37 mM, respectively. There is some pharmacokinetic information about the anticholinergic medications used in Parkinson's disease, albeit it is sparse and shallow. The majority of these studies consist of limited reports of pharmacokinetic data from analytical methods papers, or Phase I evaluations using single doses in young, healthy volunteers. Additionally, there is some pharmacokinetic data pertaining to these agents in animal models.

4.6.3. Pharmacokinetic Properties of the ACP

- ***Absorption:*** ACPs are all administered as the HCl salt, except for benztropine, which is administered as the mesylate salt. The other ACPs are absorbed rather quickly, except for benztropine mesylate, following oral administration of solid formulations. Usually, it takes less than 2.5 hours to reach maximal plasma concentrations (Grimaldi, 1986) (Table 4.5).

Table 4.5. *Main Findings of Retrieved Studies on Anticholinergic Medications*

Ref (Name, Year)	Country	Study Design	Population	Mean Age (yrs) ± sd	Psychiatric Comorbidity	Medical Comorbidity	Route of Adminis-tration and Dosage	Physical Symptoms	Psychiatric Symptoms	Polyabuse	Outcome	Notes
ATROPINE												
Taylor et al., 2007	North Carolina (USA)	Case report	$N = 1$; F	29	None	None	IM, 4 mg	Tachycardia, tachypnoea, dilatated pupils, dry mucous membranes, dry skin, urinary retention	Anxiety	30 meloxicam tablets, alcohol	Activated charcoal with sorbitol, IV fluids	Symptoms resolved over a 6 h period of observation
Wang, 2002	Pennsylva nia (USA)	Case report	$N = 1$; F	41	· Depression; · SUD (heroin addiction)	None	Oral	Pupils dilated, dry skin, sinus bradycardia, ataxia. After IV naloxone: tachycardia, tachypnoea, hypertension	Slurred speech. After IV naloxone: agitation, delirium, disorientation	Codeine and morphine mixed with atropine	IV Naloxone, IV Lorazepam, rapid-sequence intubation, orogastric lavage, and activated charcoal	During hospitali-zation: persistent agitation refractory to benzodi-azepine, pneumonia, and stress gastritis
Weiner et al., 1998	Connecticut (USA)	Case report	$N = 1$; M	39	· SUD (alcohol and cocaine abuse)	None	Nasal	Tachycardia, hypertension, warm and dry skin, facial flushing, dilated pupils minimally reactive to light, absence of bowel sounds	Agitation, intermittent delirium; disorientation	Cocaine	IV Lorazepam 1 mg, activated charcoal 50 g, cathartic mixture	Patient ingested cocaine adulterated with atropine
BENZHEXOL/ TRIHEXYPHE-NIDYL (THP)												

Crawshaw et al., 1984	New Zealand	Observational study	*N* = 21; M = 17	21 ± 6	• Antisocial personality disorder or socialized conduct disorder (*N* = 8) • Schizophrenia (*N* = 7) • Borderline personality disorder • Depression • Bipolar disorder • SUD (Alcohol dependence and multiple substance abuse) • Adjustment disorder	Extra-pyramidal side-effects of neuroleptic medication in patients with schizophrenia	Oral, 15–60 mg	Dehydration, tachycardia, pronounced thirst, and blurred vision	Toxic-confusional state with psychosis and visual hallucinations, illusions, and distorted time sense (*N* = 10); difficulties in recent memory and new learning were associated with problems of attention and concentration (*N* = 6)	Alcohol, cannabis (*N* = 12), hallucinogens (*N* = 10), opiates (*N* = 10), amphetamines (*N* = 9), benzodiazepines (*N* = 7), cough-mixtures, solvents, cocaine, and various neuroleptics	NA	
Deutsch et al., 1992	New York (USA)	Case report	*N* = 1; F	33	• Adjustment disorder with depressed mood	Cerebral palsy	Oral, maximum 105 mg (21 tablets) in a few hours in each time	Dry skin, dry mouth, and blurred vision	Restlessness, depression, confusion, disorientation, and auditory and visual hallucinations	None	IV lorazepam	Anticholinergic psychosis with hallucinosis

Fisch et al., 1987	Israel	Case series	*N* = 14; M = 5	21–30	• Borderline personality disorder (*N* = 2); • Mixed personality disorder (*N* = 1); • Heroin dependence (*N* = 1); • Methadone dependence (*N* = 1); • Chronic schizophrenia (*N* = 3); • Residual schizophrenia (*N* = 6)	None	Oral, 20–60 mg	None	1. Took THP regularly to achieve a state of hallucinosis; severe paranoid psychosis following the ingestion of 25 mg THP; 2. Sedative and anxiolytic effect; 3. Mildly psychedelic, euphorigenic, and sedative effect; 4. Relieve withdrawal symptoms; euphorigenic effect and hypomanic state; 5. Euphoric and energizing effect; 6. Euphorigenic, stimulating, and socializing effect	Heroin, diazepam	NA	One patient feigned extrapy-ramidal symptoms in order to obtain THP
Goggins et al., 1979	Norway	Case Report	*N* = 1; M	40	• Depression • Obsessions	Weight loss	Oral 35–40 mg/die	Tachycardia and nausea	Restlessness, euphoria	None	NA	
Harrison, 1980	England (UK)	Case Report	*N* = 1; M	19	• Anxiety • Depression	NA	Oral	Swollen abdomen	Euphoria	NA	NA	

Kajimura et al., 1993	Japan	Case report	*N* = 1; M	55	None	Essential tremor	Oral, 20 mg/day for 18 years	Headache, tachycardia, and general fatigue	Memory loss, cognitive impairment. On withdrawal: anxiety, irritability, insomnia, perspiration, and anorexia	None	After stopping THP, clotiazepam and flunitrazepam were used to manage withdrawal	
Kaminer et al., 1982	Israel	Case report	*N* = 1; M	30	• Chronic paranoid schizophrenia	None	Oral, 30–40 mg/die	Dystonic reaction, withdrawal symptoms, and tachycardia	Acute: auditory hallucinations Chronic: anxiety reduction, sleep disturbance, and euphoria	Cannabis, LSD, amphetamines, barbiturates, and alcohol	Treated with haloperidol 10 mg	The patient used to mix drugs and THP
Keshavan et al., 1985	England (UK)	Case report	*N* = 1; M	38	• Schizoaffective disorder	None	Oral, 70 mg	NA	Euphorigenic effect, auditory and visual hallucinations	Pimozide 8 mg, lorazepam 2,5 mg day	Admitted to psychiatric ward, gradually reduction of benzhexol with withdrawal symptoms, agitation, depression, and exacerbation of auditory halluci-nations	
Lo et al., 1996	Taiwan	Case report	*N* = 1; M	35	• Chronic schizophrenia	None	Oral, 200 mg/day for 2 years	None	Delusion of reference, thought broadcasting, loosening of association, paralogical thinking, auditory hallucination	None	Decreased dosage of THP and clonazepam	Patient feigned extrapy-ramidal syndrome to obtain biperiden injection
Macvicar, 1977	California (USA)	Case report	*N* = 1; M	30	• Paranoid schizophrenia	None	Oral 24–30 mg/die	Dry mouth and constipation	Toxic psychosis, hallucinations, euphoria, and talkativeness	NA	NA	
Mahal et al., 2018	Delhi (India)	Case series	*N* = 2; M	32	• Delusional Disorder	1st case: headache, recurrent abdominal pain; 2nd case: none	Oral, 40–60 mg	1st case: headache, sweating, and tachycardia; 2nd case: none	Drug abuse aimed to obtain relaxation; withdrawal symptoms were restlessness, irritability, and aggressiveness	1st case: nicotine and alprazolam; 2nd case: nicotine and opioid	NA	History of multiple prescription drug misuse

McInnis et al., 1984	Iceland	Case series	*N* = 2; M = 1	25 and 35	• Drug and alcohol abuse • Schizophrenia	None	Oral, 40 mg	Ataxia, headache, visual difficulties, and photophobia	Confusion, self-harm, disorientation, agitation, bizarre behavior with difficulties of speech, and reduced concentration	Haloperidol, benzodiaz-epines, alcohol; perfenazine (100 mg IM every 2 weeks), chlor-promazine 50 mg, and clomipramine	NA	
Michael et al., 1984	Karnataka (India)	Case series	*N* = 2; M	28 and 30	• Schizophrenia	None	Oral, 6 mg	None	None	Trifluo-perazine 15–20 mg, chlor-promazine 300–600 mg	Withdrawal symptoms- including agitation, tachycardia, restles-sness, aggres-siveness, lethargy, giddi-ness, sweating, and craving	
Mohan et al., 1981	Delhi (India)	Case report	*N* = 1; M	35	• Chronic depression	None	Oral 120–140 mg/die	NA	Visual hallucinations, paranoid ideas, and ideas of reference	NA	NA	
Nappo et al., 2005	São Paulo (Brazil)	Survey	*N* = 37; M = 29	20–30 yy =14; 30–40 yy =18; >40 yy = 5	None	NA	Oral, from one-half to four pills (3–8 mg)	Dry mouth, gastritis, vomiting, tachycardia, urinary retention, and dental caries	Euphoria, hallucinations, delirium, nervousness, aggressiveness, memory loss, decreased attention, loss of appetite, insomnia, and depression	Alcohol, coffee, nicotine	NA	THP was neither the initial drug in the substance user's career nor their main drug
Petkovic et al., 2012	Serbia	Case report	*N* = 1; F	59	• Persistent delusional disorder	None	Oral, 15 mg	NA	NA	None	Death	THP blood and urine concentrations were those associated with fatalities

Qureshi, 1992	Saudi Arabia	Observational study	N = 14; M = 13	27.93 ± 6.55	• Schizophrenia (N = 9) • Schizoaffective disorder (N = 1) • Mood disorder (N = 3) • Factitious disorder (N = 1)	NA	Oral	Tardive dyskinesia, extrapyramidal symptoms	Symptoms of withdrawal included palpitations, restlessness, body aches, lethargy, irritability, aggression, discomfort, craving, and anxiety	Polydrug abuse (57.14%)	THP on a prophylactic basis with improvement in negative symptoms	
Qureshi et al., 1997	Saudi Arabia	Case control	N = 30; M = 25	33.83 ± 7.4	• Drug abuse (N = 23) • Unspecified mental disease (N = 18) • Schizoid (N = 16)	NA	Oral	Dyskinetic movements	Drug abusers were characterized by less negative symptoms	Some 53% abused beverages, amphe-tamines, and benzo-diazepines	NA	
Rao et al., 2014	Karnataka (India)	Case report	N = 1; F	55	• Psychotic disorder	None	Oral	NA	Increased speech output, psychomotor agitation, and reduced need for sleep	None	Treated with clonazepam, haloperidol 10 mg/day, and THP 4 mg/day	
Rubinstein, 1979	California (USA)	Case series	N = 8 (N = 6 related to THP), 4 M, 2 F	25–32	• Schizoaffective disorder • Schizophrenia	None	Oral, 15–250 mg/die	Eye-rolling and finger stiffness	When recorded (cases 2–3), bizarre and violent behavior, difficulty in speech, and hallucinations were described; in some cases, high-dosage THP was taken to get high	Diazepam, LSD, amphe-tamines, thiothixene, cannabis, and PCP	Case 5 was treated with diazepam and fluphenazine for PCP-induced toxic psychosis	Most of the patients contin-ued to ask for THP during the hospit-alization
Sofair et al., 1983	New York (USA)	Case report	N = 1; M	24	• Chronic depression	None	Oral, 60 mg/die	Dry mouth, constipation	Relaxation and impaired concentration	THP addiction	Abrupt cessation of THP	

Thunyapipat et al., 2018	Thailand	Case series	N = 27, M = 15	14.2 (range 10.6–21)	• Mental health comorbidity • ADHD • Conduct disorder • Learning and intellectual disability	NA	Oral, from 1 to 50 tablets once	No peripheral anticholinergic symptoms	Agitation, hallucination	Unspecified drug abuse (63.6%)	Motivational interviewing in 68.4% of hospitalized cases	Of those who received motivational interviewing, all discontinued abusing THP at a monthly follow-up visit
Torrents et al., 2018	France	Cohort study	N = 69; M = 67, F = 2	36	• Unspecified psychiatric disorder (N = 4)	NA	Oral	NA	The abuse aimed to reach anxiolytic, sedative, and stimulating effects or to control the use of another drug; reported side effects were behavioral disorders such as aggressiveness, agitation, and paranoia	Tobacco (72%), benzo-diazepines, cannabis, alcohol	Not reported	
Younis et al., 2009	United Arab Emirates	Observational study	N = 190	29.5 (19–52)	• Intermittent explosive disorder • OCD	NA	Oral	NA	The abuse aimed to relax and control aggressive outbursts	Alcohol, cannabis, cocaine, and opioids	95 patients had difficulty stopping taking benzhexol	
Zemishlany et al., 1996	Israel	Case control	N = 14; M = 11	34 ± 5.3	• Antisocial personality disorder (N = 3)	NA	Oral, >20 mg	NA	Thinking disturbance, withdrawal retardation, hostile suspiciousness, anxious depression	Cannabis and alcohol	Neuroleptic treatment	
BENZTROPINE												
Craig et al., 1981	Colorado (USA)	Case series	N = 2; M = 1	19 and 22	NA	None	Oral, 120–140 mg	1st case: dilated pupils, dry skin, urinary retention; 2nd case: tachycardia, fever, hypertension, dilatated pupils, warm and dry skin	1st case: agitation, bizarre behavior, altered mental status; 2nd case: hallucinations, flight of ideas, agitation, combativeness	1st case: abuse of sedative-hypnotics and oral narcotics; 2nd case: speed, LSD, alcohol	1st case: treated with physos-tigmine, dischar-ged 18 h later; 2nd case: treated with physos-tigmine	Diagnostic trial of physostigmine

Esang et al., 2021	Penn-sylvania (USA)	Case report	*N* = 1; M	67	• Schizophrenia	Benign prostatic hyperplasia; essential hypertension	Oral	Hematochezia, abdominal pain, constipation, and difficulty with urination	None	None	Spontaneous remission of symptoms after returning to therapeutic doses	
Isbister et al., 2003	Australia	Case report	*N* = 1; M	33	• Schizophrenia • Borderline personality disorder • Recorded recreational use of benztropine	Hypertension; epilepsy; cluster headache	Oral, 27 tablets (2 mg each) during the previous 6 days	Abdominal pain, distention, drowsiness, hypertension, tachycardia, blurred vision, anticholinergic-induced ileus with absent bowel sound	Confusion, hallucinations, delirium	NA	IV fluids, meperidine, IV neostigmine 2 mg + 2.5 mg	
Rubinstein, 1979	California (USA)	Case report	*N* = 8 (*N* = 2 were related to benztr-opine, M)	26 and 28	Schizophrenia	NA	Oral/IM	Stiffness and eye rolling	Nervousness	Drug abuse (heroin, alcohol, unspecified)	Treated with thioridazine and diazepam	
BIPERIDEN												
Affaticati et al., 2015	Italy	Case report	*N* = 1; M	27	None	Withdrawal syndrome symptoms, e.g., headache	Oral 16 mg/die	Urinary retention	Mild confusional state with temporal, spatial disorientation, impairment of attention and concentration, psychomotor agitation	Trihexy-phenidyl, cocaine, alcohol, cannabis	Biperiden gradually tapered; the patient was also treated with quetiapine, 50 mg/d	After 6 months, he stopped using biperiden
Ozucelik et al., 2007	Turkey	Case report	*N* = 1; M	52	• Chronic psychosis	None	120 mg IM (60 biperiden tablets)	Swelling and pain caused by an abscess in injection site. Mildly elevated hepatic function tests	NA	NA	General surgery for abscess drainage and antibiotics	
DICYCLOMINE												
Sinha et al., 2020	Chandigarh (India)	Case report	*N* = 1; M	30	None	Dysmenorrhea, headache	Oral 10–15 tablets per day, 50–75 mg/day	Tachycardia, palpitation, sweating	Withdrawal symptoms, anxiety	Dicyclomine and mefenamic acid	Reversion to normal physiological state in a week after being treated with fluoxetine 20 mg per day and clonazepam 0.5 mg per day	

Das et al., 2013	Bengal (India)	Case report	N = 1; F	18	None	None	IM	Weakness, palpitation, fever, blurred vision, sweating, dry skin	Confusion, withdrawal reaction, anxiety, depression, anorexia	None	Treated with IV physo-stigmine with remission in a week	Drug use began with drug treatment for enterocolitis
GLYCOPY-RRONIUM TOSYLATE												
Tarr et al., 2021	Bronx (USA)	Case report	N = 1; F	14	• ADHD	Acne vulgaris	Topical	Progressive myopia, dry mouth, anhidrosis, urinary hesitancy, and chronic constipation	None	None	Discharged at home after monitoring spontaneous remission	Patient would possibly have access to other medication when unsupervised
ORPHENADRINE												
Nissen et al., 1987	Norway	Case report	N = 1; F	26	• Psychosis (alcohol-induced psychotic reactions)	None	Oral, 800 mg	Dry and warm, pupils dilated, asymmetrical abdominal reflexes	Disorientation, clouding of consciousness, agitation, aggressivity, pressured speech and laughing with loosening of associations, psychosis with mystic-megalomanic delusion and visual hallucinations	Levodopa 2000 mg; benserazide chloride 400 mg; alcohol	Admitted to psychiatric ward	
Schifano et al., 1988	Italy	Case report	N = 1; M	24	• SUD (amphetamines and cocaine abuse)	Not reported	Oral, up to 1250–1500 mg/day over a period of 2 months	Dizziness, tremor	Euphoria, visual hallucinations, mood enhancement, unpleasant misperceptions	NA	Drug stopped because difficult to obtain	Haloperidol and orphenadrine prescribed for hallucinations
OXYBUTYNIN												
Balasar et al., 2016	Turkey	Case series	N = 2; M	27 and 45	• SUD (alcohol and substance abuse)	overactive bladder	Oral, 100–150 mg/day and 300–400 mg/day	Xerostomia, constipation, urinary arrest	Relief from the need of using drugs and alcohol	None	NA	
PENTOLATE, PRISOLINE, AND NAPHCON-A (OPHTHALMIC DRUG)												

Al-Khalaileha et al., 2019	Jordan	Observational study	*N* = 140; M:79; F: 51	<20 yy: 13; 21–40 yy: 81; 41–50 yy: 29; 50–60 yy: 5; >60 yy: 2	NA	NA	Topical	Conjunctivitis, eczematoid blepharoco-njunctivitis, and conjunctival hyperemia	The abuse was aimed to relax, get high, induce pleasure, and boost energy	NA	NA	*N* = 19 cases have been suspected for abuse
PROCYCLIDINE												
Coid, 1982	England (UK)	Case report	*N* = 1; M	36	• Antisocial personality disorder	None	Oral 40 mg	NA	Disinhibition, mania, aggressiveness	Physeptone® -(methadone), alcohol		
SCOPOLAMINE/ SCOPOLAMINE N-BUTYLBR-OMIDE												
Jalali et al., 2014	Iran	Cross-sectional case series	*N* = 36; M	27–42	None	None	Smoked tablets	Dry mouth, dry throat, bowel movement, palpitation, blurred vision, flushing	Insomnia, irritability, inability to concentrate, incoherent speech, slurred speech, amnesia, illogical thinking and hallucinations	Substance abuse (on methadone)	Not reported	
Kummer et al., 2015	Germany	Case series	*N* = 2; M	16 and 15	None	None	Oral 40 mg una tantum	Flushed and dry skin, tachycardia	1st case: severe agitation, disorientation, intermittent aggressive behavior, nonsensical speech; 2nd: partial amnesia	None	Transferred to intensive care unit, he was treated with midazolam and haloperidol; both were discharged from hospital 2 days later	
Strano-Rossi et al., 2021	Italy	Case report	*N* = 1; M	41	SUD	Multiple traumas from aggression	Smoked tablets	Cerebral and lung edema	NA	Cannabis	Death	Other drugs identified in urine and blood included benzodiazepines, antipsychotic drugs in therapeutic or subtherapeutic concentrations

TROPICAMIDE												
Bozkurt et al., 2014	Turkey	Case series	N = 2; 1 M; 1 F	37–38	None	None	IV	1st case: decreased appetite, weight loss, and blurred vision; 2nd case: palpitations and sweating	1st case: the patient experienced relief and relaxation mixing tropicamide and heroin; hallucinations and dissociation were recorded; 2nd case: dissociation, anxiety, and concentration problems	1st case: cocaine, clonazepam, ecstasy, cannabis, and heroin; 2nd case: alprazolam, codeine, cocaine, and ecstasy	1st case: treated with naloxone and opioid withdrawal symptoms; discharged after 14 days of hospita-lization; 2nd case: discharged with quetiapine 100 mg/day treatment	Tropicamide was mixed with heroin
Spagnolo et al., 2013	Italy	Case report	N = 1; F	22	None	None	IV	Palpitations, hypertension, tachycardia, fever, mydriasis, warm and flushed skin, and xerostomia	Euphoria, hallucinations	Heroin	Treated with diazepam	
UNSPECIFIED ANTI-CHOLINERGIC DRUGS												
Wells. et al., 1990	Tennessee USA)	Controlled prospective study	N = 21; M = 14	33.6 ± 6.1	• Mood disorder (N = 3) • Schizophrenia (N = 15) • chizoaffective disorder (N = 2) • chizophr-eniform disorder (N = 1)	NA	NA	Dehydrated skin, tachycardia, blurred vision, and thirst	Relaxation (N = 17), elevated mood (N = 15), energy (N = 14), reduced concentration (N = 11), visual hallucinations (N = 4), confusion (N = 3), and auditory hallucinations (N = 3)	Antipsy-chotics	NA	

Source: Chiappini S, Mosca A, Miuli A, Semeraro FM, Mancusi G, Santovito MC, Di Carlo F, Pettorruso M, Guirguis A, Corkery JM, et al. Misuse of Anticholinergic Medications: A Systematic Review. Biomedicines. 2022; 10(2):355. https://doi.org/10.3390/biomedicines10020355.

Abbreviation: ADHD—attention deficit hyperactivity disorder; F—female; M—male; DPT—drug provocation tests; HC—healthy control; IM—intramuscular; IV—intravenous; LSD—lysergic acid diethylamide; N/A—not applicable; PCP—phencyclidine; SD—standard deviation; SUD—substance use disorder.

Generally speaking, the dose given seems to have an impact on the variations in the Cmax values obtained with these agents following oral administration. For instance, following single oral doses of 2, 4, and 15 mg, respectively, of trihexyphenidyl HCl, the Cmax of trihexyphenidyl in humans has been reported to be 10 ng/mL (n=1 subject); 7.15±2.58 ng/ml (n=8 subjects); and roughly 50 ng/mL (n=2 subjects). Following a single oral dosage of 2 mg of benztropine mesylate, the subjects' observed mean Cmax was only about 1.5 ng/mL (n = 5). A portion of these concentrations were determined through the use of radioimmunoassay methods, which, while highly sensitive, raise certain concerns about the specificity of the assay. After taking 4 mg of the HCl salt orally once, biperiden reaches a Cmax of about 4 ng/mL. One oral dose of 100 mg of the HCl salt results in much higher plasma concentrations of orphenadrine, with a mean±SD of 147±39 ng/mL. Procyclidine offers a notable deviation from trihexyphenidyl, biperiden, and benztropine in that it produces comparatively elevated mean plasma concentrations of 113 ng/mL upon a single oral dosage of 10 mg. At 100 mg, the Cmax is comparable to orphenadrine, the higher dosage level. The pharmacokinetic characteristics of ethopropazine, a phenothiazine derivative, in humans are not known from published research.

There are no reported human absolute bioavailabilities (F) for any of the ACPs. The absolute oral bioavailabilities of procyclidine, biperiden, and diphenhydramine are 0.75, 0.33, and 0.72, in that order. Ethopropazine has an extremely low oral F of less than 5% in rats. It has been observed that rats absorb orphenadrine in their stomachs.

- **Distribution:** Each of these drugs that have been administered intravenously has shown a volume of distribution larger than total body water. In the post-distributive phase, plasma concentrations of ACP seem to decrease slowly, leading to extended terminal half-life values. The relatively low plasma clearance and volume of distribution values seem to be the reason for the higher procyclidine plasma concentrations compared to other ACPs.

Biperiden, orphenadrine, and ethopropazine rapidly enter the brain, the intended site of action. Rats received a brief intravenous infusion of biperiden, and within 3–10 minutes, maximal brain concentrations were reached. The half-life of ethopropazine in brain tissues following intravenous bolus doses is less than half an hour. After being administered intraperitoneally, radiolabelled orphenadrine and its main N-demethylated metabolite, tofenacine, reached their maximum concentrations in the rat brain in less than 15 minutes and 60 minutes, respectively. These medications' high lipophilicity may be the cause of their high concentrations in brain tissue. ACP uptake may be aided by the high concentrations of lipophilic biomolecules found in brain tissues, such as phosphatidyl choline and sphingomyelin. A recent study found that intralysosomal drug uptake promoted high tissue uptake of both biperiden and trihexyphenidyl.

It is unclear how much ACP binds to plasma proteins in humans. Ethopropazine exhibits nonlinearity in both its pharmacokinetics and binding, and it is highly bound (>95%) in rats.

- **Metabolism and Excretion:** Overall, it appears that all ACP compounds are extensively metabolized in both humans and animals. They contain an aliphatic tertiary amine group that can undergo N-dealkylation and N-oxidation. Hydroxylation of the alicyclic groups has been observed in compounds like procyclidine and trihexyphenidyl. Benztropine has been found to undergo N-oxidation, N-dealkylation, and ring hydroxylation in rats. The clearance of ACP is low compared to hepatic blood flow, suggesting that a high hepatic first-pass effect is not expected after oral administration.

This class of drugs includes several chiral medications. None of these compounds' stereoselectivity in human metabolism has been formally evaluated. Rat plasma concentrations of ethopropazine enantiomers are known to be nonstereoselective.

N-demethylorphenadrine, the N-demethylated metabolite of orphenadrine, seems to obstruct the parent drug's metabolism. It is well known that orphenadrine interferes with P-450 isoenzymes. It has been demonstrated that unchanged ACPs and their metabolites are eliminated through the bile and urine systems.

4.6.4. Therapeutic Considerations

- **Current Guidelines for Dosage Titration:** The majority of ACP dosage regimens are empirical in nature, with dose titration based on the degree of symptom alleviation and the occurrence of dose-limiting side effects, which are mainly caused by peripheral anticholinergic activity (e.g., constipation, hazy vision, and dry mouth). Despite a few attempts to identify the type or existence of a plasma concentration vs. data regarding the toxicological effect relationship following single doses; however, none exist for the therapeutic effects in Parkinson's disease (e.g., decrease in tremor). Following oral and IV administration, changes in salivary flow and pupil diameter seem to be correlated with changes in procyclidine and biperiden plasma concentrations.

The relationship between serum trihexyphenidyl concentrations and therapeutic activity has been studied in patients with torsion dyskinesia. No relationship was seen between therapeutic effect and serum concentration, although a relationship was present between age and side effects. This study was deficient in several respects. At the time it was believed that the $t_{½}$ of trihexyphenidyl was 3.5 h. Later work using more sensitive assay methodology has indicated that the $t_{½}$ is a much longer value of 33 h. Given that the drug follows multicompartmental kinetics, the earlier study, which used a less sensitive assay, may have actually reported a distribution phase as being the terminal phase t½. Furthermore, doses and intervals were not standardized and the number of patients studied was quite small.

- **Consideration of Dosage Adjustment in the Elderly:** Older patients do not tolerate the ACP class of medications as well as younger patients do. Compared to younger patients, elderly patients appear to be more vulnerable to the peripheral anticholinergic side effects (e.g., constipation, tachycardia, urine retention, and impaired vision), as well as to centrally mediated effects like mental disorientation. Because of this, some medical professionals advise against using ACP in older patients and instead to use L-dopa or other dopaminergic medications.

It is noteworthy that the pharmacokinetics of anticholinergic medications in the elderly are the subject of relatively few reports in the literature, despite the fact that the elderly's poor tolerability of these medications is a clinically significant observation. This is especially evident given that middle-aged and older patients are the majority affected by Parkinson's disease. Certain of these medications (e.g., orphenadrine) are metabolized to a significant degree, and that a decrease in blood flow, liver mass, and the level of mixed function oxidase enzyme activity may be linked to aging. Additionally, the ACP group appears to have a Vd greater than the total amount of body water. Procyclidine, diphenhydramine, and biperiden have Vds of 12.1, 40.5, and 24 L/kg following intravenous dosing, respectively. Based on their Vd/F values and assuming moderate to complete bioavailability, trihexyphenidyl and orphenadrine also seem to have a relatively high Vd following oral dosage. Senior patients may have a higher volume of distribution than younger patients because they have a larger percentage of body fat in their bodies. To demonstrate this, in a study on the effects of intravenously given biperiden on rats, older rats exhibited a steady-state volume of distribution that was 80% higher than that of younger rats, as well as a CL that was 39% lower. Ultimately, this led to increased levels of biperiden in the aged animals' brain and plasma. The lower tolerability of anticholinergics in elderly patients may be related to pharmacokinetic differences, assuming that these findings can be generalized to other anticholinergics and between species.

Age-related variations in the pharmacokinetics of diphenhydramine in humans have been studied. When compared to a group of younger subjects, the elderly group of subjects showed a significantly higher AUC and $t_{1/2}$ as well as a lower CL/F. In addition, the Cmax was greater in the older participants than in the younger ones. The authors discovered—perhaps surprisingly—that as people aged, the Vd of diphenhydramine dropped. In contrast to these findings, a different study found no discernible difference in Cmax or AUC between a group of subjects who were older and a group of young adults. The older cohort that Simons et al. studied was different from this one. were five years older than the group Scavone and colleagues studied. In addition, a greater dosage was used in the Simons et al. study. which could have made it possible to characterize the terminal phase $t_{1/2}$ more accurately.

- **Chirality and the AntiParkinsons Anticholinergic Drugs:** The fact that the majority of ACPs—procyclidine, ethopropazine, biperiden, orphenadrine—are chiral and are used as the racemate in clinical settings is a significant factor in their pharmacokinetics. There is no published data on the stereospecific pharmacokinetics of these agents, with the exception of ethopropazine in rats. This makes evaluating their pharmacodynamic and pharmacokinetic characteristics more difficult. It has been shown that in order to precisely define the relationship between plasma concentrations and pharmacological effect, drugs with stereoselective pharmacodynamics require an examination of the enantiomers' pharmacokinetics. In fact, it has recently been demonstrated that the enantiomers of some anticholinergics exhibit significant stereoselectivity in terms of receptor binding affinities for a variety of distinct muscarinic receptor subtypes. For rat striatal muscarinic receptors, for instance, the R-enantiomer of trihexyphenidyl has an affinity that can be up to 427 times higher than the S-enantiomer.

The R-enantiomer exhibits 69 to 525-fold higher binding affinities than its antipode in five cloned human muscarinic receptor subtypes. Regarding procyclidine, its R-enantiomer exhibits a 126-fold higher affinity for striatal muscarinic receptors than its antipode. In a mouse model of 6-hydroxydopamine, procyclidine R-enantiomers were administered intraperitoneally or intracerebroventricularly. Despite these pharmacological differences, the degree of stereoselectivity observed was less than expected based on the binding affinities of the R-enantiomers. It was suggested that stereoselectivity in the R-enantiomer metabolism could be the reason for this discovery (Agid et al, 1999; Rascol et al, 2002).

A Closer Look

Dyskinesias

Dyskinesias, aberrant and involuntary movements, emerge as a complication of long-term treatment with levodopa in PD. Despite its effectiveness in managing motor symptoms, levodopa administration can lead to motor fluctuations, where patients cycle between periods of adequate symptom control (on periods) and periods of excessive movement (dyskinesias). These dyskinetic movements encompass chorea, dystonia, or athetosis, involving unpredictable and often disabling writhing or twisting motions affecting the limbs, trunk, or face. The pathophysiology of dyskinesias in PD is multifactorial, stemming from the complex interplay of dopamine depletion, pulsatile stimulation of dopamine receptors, and alterations in basal ganglia circuitry. Factors such as disease duration, age at onset, severity of motor symptoms, and cumulative levodopa dose contribute to the risk of developing dyskinesias. Management strategies for dyskinesias are varied, involving adjustments to levodopa dosages, incorporation of adjunctive therapies like dopamine agonists, and consideration of advanced interventions such as deep brain stimulation (DBS). Physical therapy and exercise regimes also play a crucial role in improving motor function and minimizing the impact of dyskinesias on daily activities. Despite these interventions, achieving an optimal balance between symptom control and dyskinesia mitigation remains a significant clinical challenge in PD management. Continued research efforts are essential to uncover the underlying mechanisms of dyskinesias and to develop more targeted and personalized treatment approaches to enhance the quality of life for individuals living with Parkinson's disease.

Summary

- The treatment of PD involves a multidisciplinary approach aimed at managing symptoms, improving quality of life, and slowing disease progression.
- Dopaminergic (relating to dopamine) therapy lies at the crux of PD treatment. Dopaminergic medications fall into four main categories, listed in declining order of dopamine potency.
- Levodopa, or L-dopa, is the most effective drug for minimizing PD symptoms and is the initial medication in the majority of people with PD.
- Dopamine agonists are medications that stimulate dopamine receptors (docking sites) in the brain.
- MAO-B inhibitors block or decrease monoamine oxidase B. This enzyme breaks down dopamine in the brain.
- Amantadine is an antiviral drug believed to work by increasing dopamine's effects in the brain. It may also block glutamate docking sites in the brain.
- Anticholinergic drugs decrease the action of acetylcholine, a brain chemical that helps regulate movement. Anticholinergics should be avoided in older individuals due to potential side effects, especially constipation, retaining urine, and thinking/memory problems.
- A COMT inhibitor is an add-on levodopa therapy to manage "off" periods in advanced Parkinson's. It works by preventing the breakdown of dopamine.
- Nourianz (istradefylline) is a pill approved as an add-on treatment to levodopa in people with PD experiencing "off" periods.
- Chronic drug treatment of Parkinson's can eventually lead to motor complications, namely "off" periods and levodopa-induced dyskinesia.

References

1. Agid, Y., Ahlskog, E., Albanese, A., et al. (1999). Levodopa in the treatment of Parkinson's disease: a consensus meeting. *Movement Disorders, 14*, 911–913.
2. Bohnen, N. I., Kaufer, D. I., Ivanco, L. S., et al. (2003). Cortical cholinergic function is more severely affected in parkinsonian dementia than in Alzheimer disease: an *in vivo* positron emission tomographic study. *Archives of Neurology, 60*, 1745–1748.
3. Brooks, D. J. (1997). Advances in imaging Parkinson's disease. *Current Opinion in Neurology, 10*, 327–331.
4. Brooks, D. J., & Sagar, H. (2003). Entacapone is beneficial in both fluctuating and non-fluctuating patients with Parkinson's disease: a randomized, placebo-controlled, double-blind, six-month study. *Journal of Neurology, Neurosurgery & Psychiatry, 74*, 1071–1079.
5. Calne, D. B., Teychenne, P. F., Claveria, L. E., Eastman, R., Greenacre, J. K., & Petrie, A. (1974). Bromocriptine in parkinsonism. *BMJ, 4*, 442–444.

6. Cohen, G., & Spina, M. B. (1989). Deprenyl suppresses the oxidant stress associated with increased dopamine turnover. *Annals of Neurology, 26*, 689–690.

7. Eshel, Y., & Korczyn, A. D. (1979). Amantadine antagonism of oxotremorine effects. *Journal of Neural Transmission, 46*, 79–83.

8. Factor, S. A., & Molho, E. S. (1999). Transient benefit of amantadine in Parkinson's disease: the facts about the myth. *Movement Disorders, 14*, 515–516.

9. Fernandez, H. H., Friedman, J. H., Jacques, C., & Rosenfeld, M. (1999). Quetiapine for the treatment of drug-induced psychosis in Parkinson's disease. *Movement Disorders, 14*, 484–487.

10. Ferreira, J. J., Thalamas, C., Montastruc, J. L., et al. (2001). Levodopa monotherapy can induce "sleep attacks" in Parkinson's disease patients. *Journal of Neurology, Neurosurgery & Psychiatry, 248*, 426–427.

11. Finberg, J. P., Wang, J., Bankiewicz, K., et al. (1998). Increased striatal production from L-DOPA following selective inhibition of monoamine oxidase B by R (+)-N-propargyl-1-aminoindan (rasagiline) in the monkey. *Journal of Neural Transmission, 52*, 279–285.

12. Frucht, S., Rogers, J. D., Greene, P. E., et al. (1999). Falling asleep at the wheel: motor vehicle mishaps in persons taking pramipexole and ropinirole. *Neurology, 52*, 1908–1910.

13. Gancher, S. T., Nutt, J. G., & Woodward, W. R. (1995). Apomorphine infusion therapy in Parkinson's disease: clinical utility and lack of tolerance. *Movement Disorders Society, 10*, 37–43.

14. Giladi, N., Shabtai, H., Gurevich, T., Benbunan, B., Anca, M., & Korczyn, A. D. (2003). Rivastigmine (Exelon) for dementia in patients with Parkinson's disease. *Acta Neurologic Scandinavica, 108*, 368–373.

15. Gray, R., Ives, N., Rick, C., Patel, S., Gray, A., Jenkinson, C., McIntosh, E., Wheatley, K., Williams, A., & Clarke, C. E. (2014). Long-term effectiveness of dopamine agonists and monoamine oxidase B inhibitors compared with levodopa as initial treatment for Parkinson's disease (PD MED): A large, open-label, pragmatic randomized trial. *The Lancet, 384*, 1196–1205.

16. Grimaldi, R., Perucca, E., Ruberto, G., Gelmi, C., Trimarchi, F., Hollman, M., & Crema, A. (1986). Pharmacokinetic and pharmacodynamic studies following the intravenous and oral administration of the anti-Parkinsonian drug biperiden to normal subjects. *European Journal of Clinical Pharmacology, 29*, 735–737.

17. Jenner, P. (1995). The rationale for the use of dopamine agonists in Parkinson's disease. *Neurology, 45*, S6–S12.

18. Kakish, J., Tavassoly, O., & Lee, J. S. (2015). Rasagiline, a suicide inhibitor of monoamine oxidases, binds reversibly to α-synuclein. *ACS Chemical Neuroscience, 6*, 347–355.

19. Korczyn, A. D. (1973). Pathophysiology of drug-induced dyskinesias. *Neuropharmacology, 11*, 601–607.

20. Korczyn, A. D. (1990). Autonomic nervous system disturbances in Parkinson's disease. In M. B. Streifler, A. D. Korczyn, E. Melamed, & M. B. H. Youdim (Eds.), *Advances in Neurology: Parkinson's Disease: Anatomy, Pathology Therapy* (pp. 463–468). New York, NY: Raven Press.

21. Korczyn, A. D. (1994). Parkinson's disease. In K. L. Davis (Ed.), *Psychopharmacology; The Fourth Generation of Progress* (pp. 1479–1485). New York, NY: Raven Press.

22. Korczyn, A. D. (2001). Hallucinations in Parkinson's disease. *The Lancet, 358*, 1031–1032.

23. Korczyn, A. D. (2002). COMT inhibitors in Parkinson's disease. In S. A. Factor & W. J. Weiner (Eds.), *Parkinson's Disease* (pp. 379–397). New York, NY: Demos.

24. Korczyn, A. D. (2003). Dopaminergic drugs in development for Parkinson's disease. In A. Gordin, S. Kaakkola, & H. Teravainen (Eds.), *Advances in Neurology, 91. Parkinson's Disease* (pp. 267–271). Philadelphia, PA: Lippincott Williams & Wilkins.

25. Korczyn, A. D., Brunt, E. R., Larsden, J. R., et al. (1999). A 3-year randomized trial of ropinirole and bromocriptine in early Parkinson's disease. *Neurology, 53*, 364–370.

26. Korczyn, A. D., Keren, O., & Eshel, Y. (1982). Effect of amantadine on pupillary diameter in mice. *Israel Journal of Medical Sciences, 18*, 145–147.

27. Lange, K. W. (1998). Clinical pharmacology of dopamine agonists in Parkinson's disease. *Drugs & Aging, 13*, 381–389.

28. Ling, L. H., Ahlskog, J. E., Munger, T. M., et al. (1999). Constrictive pericarditis and pleuropulmonary disease linked to ergot dopamine agonist therapy (cabergoline) for Parkinson's disease. *Mayo Clinic Proceedings, 74*, 371–375.

29. Lund, B. C., Neiman, R. F., & Perry, P. J. (1999). Treatment of Parkinson's disease with ropinirole after pergolide-induced retroperitoneal fibrosis. *Pharmacotherapy, 19*, 1437–1438.

30. Marsden, C. D., & Parkes, J. D. (1976). "On-off" effects in patients with Parkinson's disease on chronic levodopa therapy. *The Lancet, 1*, 292–296.

31. Montastruc, J. L., Rascol, O., & Rascol, A. (1989). A randomized controlled study of bromocriptine versus levodopa in previously untreated Parkinsonian patients: a 3-year follow-up. *Journal of Neurology, Neurosurgery & Psychiatry, 52*, 773–775.

32. Olanow, C. W., & Schapira, A. H. V. (2000). Waking up to sleep episodes in Parkinson's disease. *Movement Disorders Society, 15*, 212–215.

33. Olanow, C. W., & Stucchi, F. (2004). COMT inhibitors in Parkinson's disease: can they prevent and/or reverse levodopa-induced motor complications? *Neurology, 62*, S74–S82.

34. Ondo, W., Hunter, C., Almaguer, M., et al. (1999). A novel sublingual apomorphine treatment for patients with fluctuating Parkinson's disease. *Movement Disorders, 14*, 664–668.

35. Pal, S., Bhattacharya, K. F., Agapito, C., et al. (2001). A study of excessive daytime sleepiness and its clinical significance in three groups of Parkinson's disease patients taking pramipexole, cabergoline and levodopa mono and combination therapy. *Journal of Neural Transmission, 108*, 71–77.

36. Parkinson's Disease Study Group. (1993). Effects of tocopherol and deprenyl on the progression of disability in early Parkinson's disease. *New England Journal of Medicine, 178*, 125–183.

37. Rabey, J. M., & Korczyn, A. D. (1992). Efficacy of memantine, an NMDA receptor antagonist, in the treatment of Parkinson's disease. *Journal of Neural Transmission, 4*, 277–282.

38. Rabey, J. M., Treves, T. A., Neufeld, M. Y., Orlov, E., & Korczyn, A. D. (1995). Low-dose clozapine in the treatment of levodopa induced mental disturbances in Parkinson's disease. *Neurology, 45*, 432–434.

39. Rajput, A. H., Martin, W., Saint Hilaire, M. H., et al. (1997). Tolcapone improves motor function in parkinsonian patients with the "wearing off" phenomenon: a double-blind, placebo-controlled multicenter trial. *Neurology, 49*, 1066–1071.

40. Rascol, O., Blin, O., Thalamas, C., et al. (1999). ABT-431, a D1 receptor agonist prodrug, has efficacy in Parkinson's disease. *Annals of Neurology, 45*, 736–741.

41. Rascol, O., Brooks, D. J., Korczyn, A. D., et al. (2000). A 5-year study of the incidence of dyskinesias in patients with early Parkinson's disease who were treated with ropinirole or levodopa. *New England Journal of Medicine, 342*, 1484–1491.

42. Rascol, O., Goetz, C., Koller, W., Poewe, W., & Sampaio, C. (2002). Treatment interventions for Parkinson's disease: an evidence-based assessment. *The Lancet, 359*, 1589–1598.

43. Rinne, U. K. (1983). Problems associated with long-term levodopa treatment of Parkinson's disease. *Acta Neurologica Scandinavica, 95*, 19–26.

44. Roberts, J. W., Mouradian, M., Ho Sohn, Y., et al. (1994). D2 agonist N-0923 in the treatment of Parkinson's disease. *Neurology, 44*, 244.

45. Schapira, A. H. (2000). Sleep attacks (sleep episodes) with pergolide. *The Lancet, 355*, 1332–1333.

46. Shaunak, S., Wilkins, A., Pilling, J. B., & Dick, D. J. (1999). Pericardial, retroperitoneal, and pleural fibrosis induced by pergolide. *Journal of Neurology, Neurosurgery, and Psychiatry, 66*(1), 79–81.

47. Stern, M. B. (2001). The early treatment of Parkinson's disease: levodopa, DA agonists or both. *Parkinsonism & Related Disorders, 7*, 27–33.

48. Treves, T. A., Paleacu, D., Rabey, J. M., & Korczyn, A. D. (1995). Depression inventories in Parkinson's disease. In H. Przuntek, P. H. Kraus, P. Klotz, & A. D. Korczyn (Eds.), *Instrumental Methods and Scoring in Extrapyramidal Disorders* (pp. 31–43). Vienna, Austria: Springer.

49. Van Camp, G., Flamez, A., Cosyns, B., et al. (2004). Treatment of Parkinson's disease with pergolide and relation to restrictive valvular heart disease. *The Lancet, 363*, 1179–1183.

50. Verhagen Metman, L., Del Dotto, P., van den Munckhof, P., et al. (1998). Amantadine as treatment for dyskinesias and motor fluctuations in Parkinson's disease. *Neurology, 50*, 1323–1326.

Chapter 5

NON-MOTOR FEATURES OF PARKINSON'S DISEASE

Contents

Introduction

PD is a neurodegenerative condition characterized by stiffness, bradykinesia, and rest tremor in the motor domain. Due to their acknowledged role in exacerbating the disease and contributing to disability, non-motor aspects of PD have drawn increased attention in the last twenty years. These include autonomic abnormalities, sleep disturbance, depression, dementia, and hyposmia and other sensory abnormalities.

Orientation and Directional Terms:

Term	Definition	Illustration
Akathisia	Akathisia is a clinical syndrome in PD that's characterized by an inner feeling of restlessness and the need to move, while also being unable to remain still.	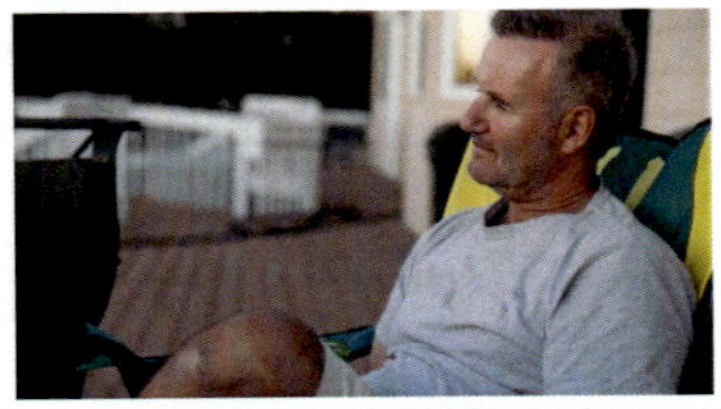
Olfactory dysfunction	Olfactory dysfunction is common and highly prevalent in PD and accurate clinical testing is now possible.	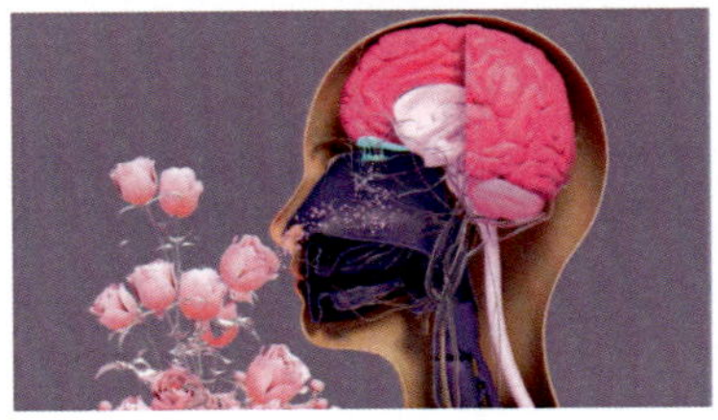
Pain	Pain is also a common, often under-explored and undeclared non-motor symptom of PD related also to non-motor fluctuations in PD.	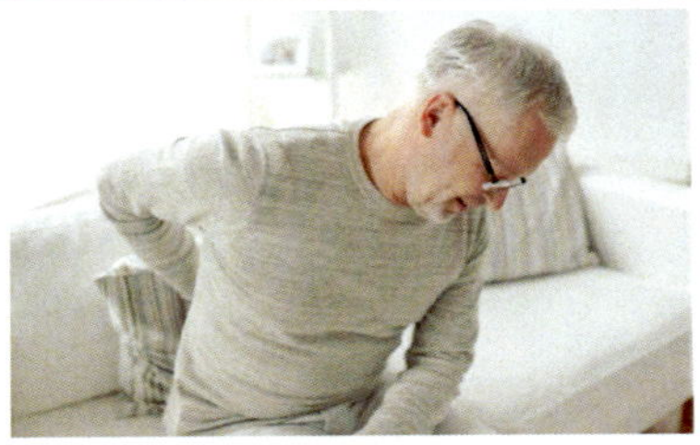
Psychiatric disorders	Psychiatric disorders in PD, especially depressive disorders, are treatable conditions that, when treated deliberately and assiduously, respond effectively to medications, behavioral treatments, or a combination of these. The goal of treatment is remission of the psychiatric syndrome.	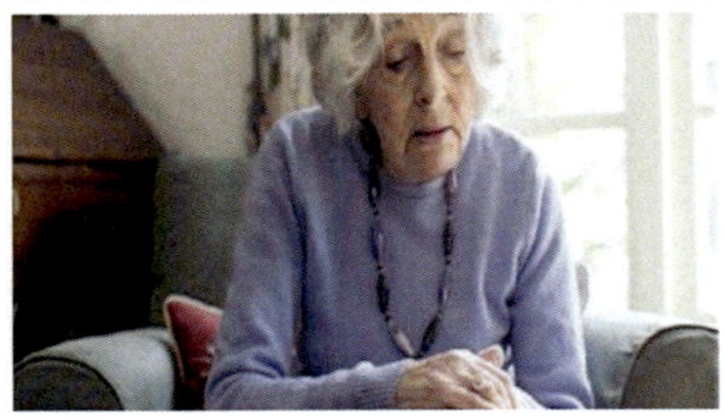
Psychosis	Psychosis in PD typically occurs later in the course of the illness and common symptoms include visual hallucinations and delusions, which are present in up to 40% of cases of PD.	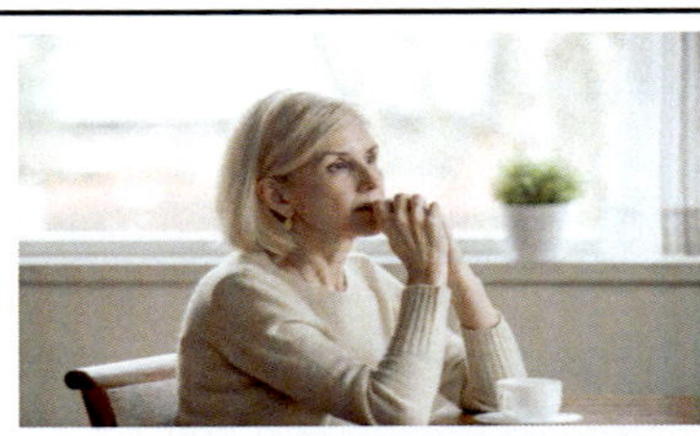
Sleep disturbances	Disturbances in sleep and wakefulness affect most of the PD patient population and their prevalence increases with the duration of disease.	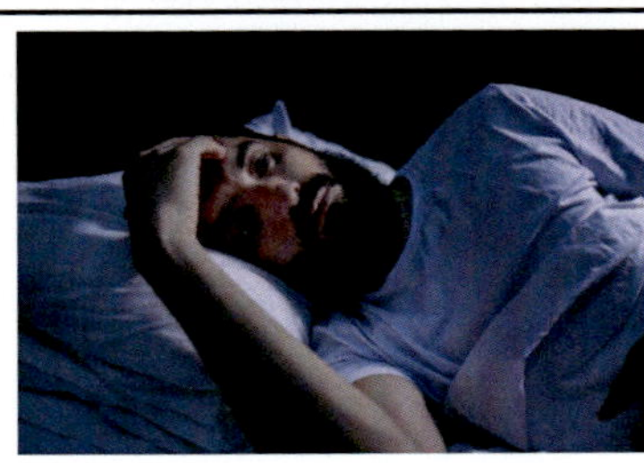

5.1. Sensory Features

One common non-motor feature of PD is sensory symptoms, specifically pain. In fact, almost every PD patient has at least one sensory symptom during their prodrome, and as the disease worsens, the frequency and intensity of these symptoms rise.

5.1.1. Olfactory Deficits

One early and defining characteristic of PD is impairment of smell. Smell deficiencies can occur years before clinical motor symptoms appear, and hypo- or anosmia are now thought to be biomarkers for Parkinson's disease before symptoms appear. Since the 1970s, almost all studies have demonstrated olfactory disturbances, including abnormalities in olfactory threshold and discrimination in PD. Some data show that over 95% of patients with PD may present with detectable olfactory loss; however, the prevalence rates vary depending on the tests and parameters used. According to published data, between 45 and 90% of people with Parkinson's disease have olfactory dysfunction. Evidence of significant olfactory loss (hyposmia and anosmia) was found in 96.7% of patients (at all stages) in a recent multicenter study involving 400 PD patients; however, when age was taken into account, this percentage dropped to 74.5%. Furthermore, regardless of the olfactory test used for diagnosis, over 80% of PD patients with smell loss were either severely hyposmic or functionally anosmic.

1. **Premotor Stage:** It is now accepted that impaired olfaction poses a risk for the development of motor PD, and a number of studies have examined the relationship between hyposmia and the likelihood of developing PD in the future using various methodologies. These studies suggest that idiopathic hyposmia may suggest a prodromal period of 2–10 years when combined with other markers like abnormal dopamine transporter single photon emission computed tomography scan or transcranial sonography (TCS) of substantia nigra (SN) hyperechogenicity (Norcliffe-Kaufmann, Lucy, Kaufmann & Horacio, 2013) (Figure 5.1).

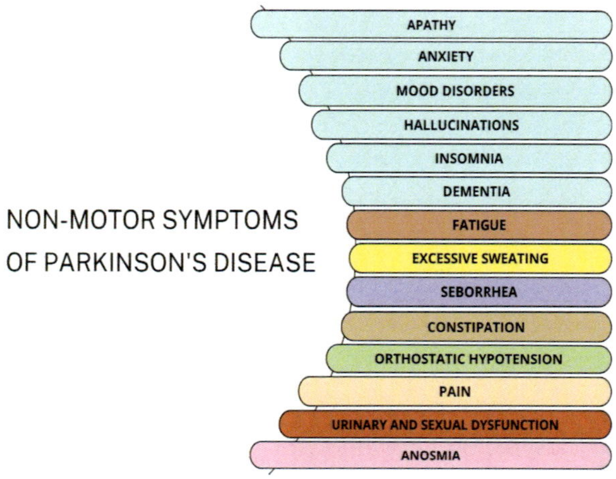

Figure 5.1. *Studies showing impaired olfaction as a risk factor for development of motor Parkinson's disease.*

Source: Bej E, Cesare P, Volpe AR, d'Angelo M, Castelli V. Oxidative Stress and Neurodegeneration: Insights and Therapeutic Strategies for Parkinson's Disease. Neurology International. 2024; 16(3):502-517. https://doi.org/10.3390/neurolint16030037.

2. **Pathophysiology:** Braak and team presented a novel idea of a six-stage pathological process of Parkinson's disease. This process states that olfactory dysfunction is caused by Lewy bodies that first develop in the anterior olfactory nucleus and olfactory bulb (OB).

Lewy body formation was found in the OB as well as other olfactory-related brain regions, including the entorhinal cortex, the amygdaloid complex, the anterior olfactory nucleus, and the hippocampal formation, according to postmortem study results. In patients with Parkinson's disease, Westermann et al. discovered altered hippocampal formation and amygdaloid complex neuronal activity during olfactory stimulation, and they postulated that structural abnormalities related to olfaction are linked to the pathophysiology of olfaction in PD.

The cause of olfactory dysfunction in Parkinson's disease is not fully understood, but certain studies suggest that it may be linked to shrinkage in olfactory areas of the limbic and paralimbic cortices. These issues with smell have been associated with changes in the structure and function of the olfactory bulb and sulcus. MRI studies have shown that analyzing the volume of the olfactory bulb could aid in distinguishing and diagnosing Parkinson's disease early on. However, there is conflicting data, with one recent study revealing a decrease in olfactory system size in Parkinson's patients compared to healthy individuals, while other studies did not find notable differences in bulb size between the two groups. Furthermore, Huisman et al. discovered an increase in dopaminergic neurons in the olfactory bulb of Parkinson's patients.

According to some recent research, cholinergic denervation of the limbic archicortex, rather than nigrostriatal dopaminergic denervation, is a more significant predictor of hyposmia in PD patients, and deficits in odor identification are linked to a higher degree of cognitive impairment. These results are based on a study that used 11C-methyl4-piperidinyl propionate acetylcholinesterase as a cholinergic ligand during PET scans on 58 patients with Parkinson's disease. The results of the odor identification test showed a positive correlation with acetylcholinesterase activity in the neocortex ($r = 0.46$; $p = 0.0003$), amygdala ($r = 0.50$; $p < 0.0001$), hippocampal formation ($r = 0.56$; $p < 0.0001$), and neocortex ($r = 0.46$; $p < 0.0001$), as well as with verbal learning episodic learning ($r = 0.30$; $p < 0.05$). In addition, compared to normal controls, patients with PD also had a higher frequency of rhinorrhea, a finding that is likely unrelated to olfactory loss or motor deficits.

Another theory that links olfaction to the pathophysiology of Parkinson's disease is the "dual-hit" hypothesis put forth by Hawkes et al. According to the infective basis for PD it is postulated that a viral neurotropic agent may enter the brain via the nasal route, and undergo anterograde transmission by extensive existing connections of the olfactory bundle to the temporal lobe and other cortical areas, thus causing olfactory dysfunction. There has also been evidence of a retrograde transmission, whereby the pathogen may enter the medulla through vagal neurons and the Meissner's plexus.

3. Methods of Detection

- ***Nonspecific Patient-Based Assessment:*** The PD non-motor group created the NMSQuest, a 30-item self-completed screening tool with a "yes/no" response format that has undergone extensive field validation and specifically addresses hyposmia. This tool was intended to empower the patient and caregiver to declare non-motor symptoms (NMS) in the clinic.
- ***Psychophysical Assessment:*** There are forty "scratch and sniff" odor strips in the University of Pennsylvania Smell Identification Test (UPSIT). Scratching the strip with the tip of a pencil releases the scents, which should be sniffed right away. Four multiple-choice answers that describe the possible smell

of the odor are available for the subject to select from.

The Sniffin' Sticks test assesses olfactory discrimination, identification, and threshold simultaneously. There are three separate olfactory function tests in the test kit. The test's results are displayed as a "transition dyspnea index (TDI) score," which is the total of the identification, discrimination, and threshold scores. The olfactory function degree is estimated by this score.

- ***Imaging Studies:*** Deeb and team have revealed that, when it comes to predicting PD, a simple smell test is just as sensitive as a dopamine transporter scan (the sensitivities of the UPSIT and dopamine transporter scan are high at 86 and 92%, respectively). While the dopamine transporter scan is better for "localization," a smell test is much "cheaper" and neither is disease specific.

Using diffusion tensor imaging of the SN and anterior olfactory structures in addition to olfactory testing (OT), Rolheizer et al. compared recently diagnosed PD patients with a matched control group.

Olfactory testing in the patient group showed a significant impairment. Significant group differences were seen in the SN and anterior olfactory region by diffusion tensor imaging, with fractional anisotropy of the olfactory region clearly differentiating the PD subjects from controls.

Metaiodobenzylguanidine myocardial scintigraphy, TCS, and OT have recently been combined to serve as a PD diagnostic tool. The authors demonstrated that the TCS of the SN and OT together significantly raised the sensitivity to a level that was adequate for separating PD patients from controls. TCS, OT, and metaiodobenzylguanidine myocardial scintigraphy had diagnostic sensitivity of 78.8%, 84.8%, and 60.6%, respectively.

4. **Confounding Conditions:** Olfactory impairment can occur in multiple system atrophy (MSA), dementia with Lewy bodies, progressive supranuclear palsy (PSP), and corticobasal degeneration (CBD), but it is less common in these conditions than in idiopathic PD. There has been evidence of varying degrees of olfactory impairment in patients with idiopathic PD, MSA, PSP, and CBD. In Parkinsonian patients, preserved or mildly impaired olfactory function is more likely to be associated with atypical Parkinsonism, such as MSA, PSP, or CBD, whereas significantly reduced olfaction is more suggestive of PD. Patients with Parkinson's disease and Alzheimer's disease perform worse on odor identification and recognition tasks than on odor detection thresholds tasks, according to a meta-analysis. Furthermore, compared to patients with Alzheimer's disease, PD patients have greater impairments on detection thresholds.
5. **Treatment:** Anecdotal evidence suggests that deep brain stimulation of the subthalamic nucleus could aid in Parkinson's disease patients' cognitive processing of olfactory information. Hummel et al. found that in patients with hyposmic Parkinson's disease, deep brain stimulation improved odor discrimination but not odor thresholds.

5.1.2. Pain

One common NMS of PD is pain, which can be more distressing for some patients than their motor disability in certain cases, especially if the pain is severe or unmanageable. Pain associated with PD varies widely, and in as many as 25% of patients, the onset of motor symptoms or the commencement of anti-Parkinsonian therapy is preceded by chronic pain.

Pain in one or both shoulders, initially misdiagnosed as bursitis, arthritis, or rotator cuff injury, frequently occurs years before motor symptoms (usually ipsilateral to the affected shoulder).

But even though it's practically universal, pain in people with Parkinson's disease is frequently underreported and mismanaged. In one study, 34% of PD patients took analgesics despite the fact that 83% of them reported having pain.

Determining the precise cause of pain in PD patients can be challenging due to comorbidity and the exacerbation of an unrelated primary osteoarthritis pain, for instance, by PD-related problems like dyskinesias or rigidity. Further complicating matters, pain categories may overlap. For instance, dopaminergic treatment may be effective for secondary orofacial pain. Consequently, in order to distinguish and measure the relative contributions of PD and comorbidities to the pain syndrome that a given patient experiences at any given time, validated scales or questionnaires must be developed (Buhmann et al, 2020).

Many authors have tried to categorize pain in PD based on the site, nociceptive versus neuropathic pain, and underlying etiology; the Wassner-Deuschl and Chaudhuri-Schapira classifications (Table 5.2) attempt to incorporate all of these factors.

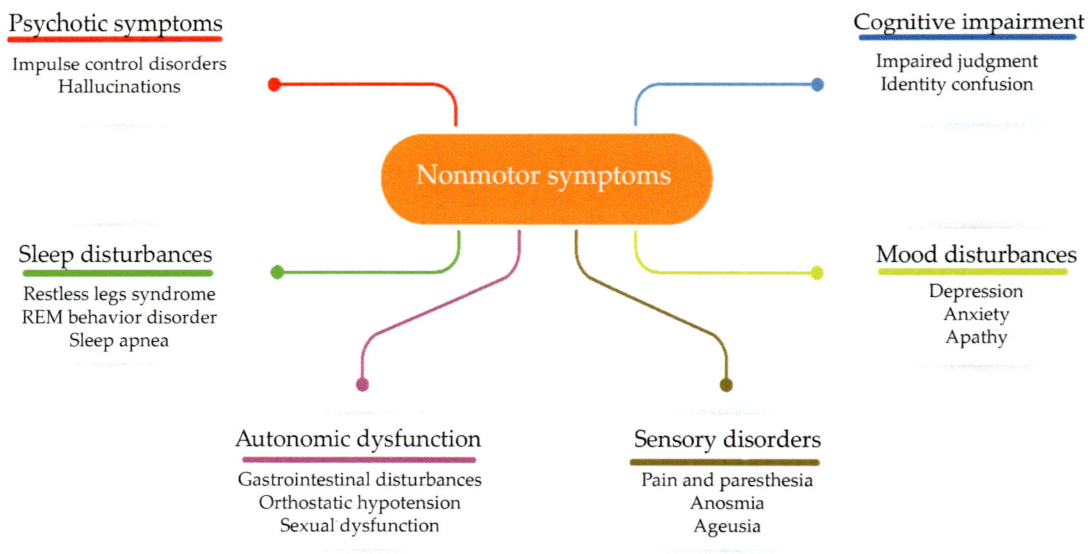

Figure 5.2. *Pain in Parkinson's disease*

Source: Váradi C. Clinical Features of Parkinson's Disease: The Evolution of Critical Symptoms. Biology. 2020; 9(5):103. https://doi.org/10.3390/biology9050103.

1. **Pathophysiology:** PD-related pain may originate from malfunctioning dopaminergic-dependent centers, which control autonomic function and suppress pain, as opposed to comorbidity. Levodopa normalizes the over-activation of multiple nociceptive cerebral areas in Parkinson's disease patients in response to painful stimuli, as revealed by PET and functional MRI studies. Studies reveal that PD patients' pain threshold to cold was significantly lower during "provoked off" states compared to "on" states, and that "off" periods exhibit abnormal sensitivity to pain. Peripheral mechanisms, such as pain resembling cramps associated with dystonia, could potentially be accountable.
2. **Epidemiology***:* It is difficult to estimate the prevalence of pain syndromes among PD patients with accuracy because few epidemiological surveys define "pain" precisely or include a control group. According to overall prevalence statistics, 60–80% of PD patients report having pain. The majority of complaints (70%) were related to musculoskeletal pain, which was followed by dystonic pain (40%) radicular or neuropathic pain (20%) and central neuropathic pain (10%). Analgesics were only given to 34% of patients. After adjusting for osteo-articular comorbidities, the DoPaMiP study found that pain was twice as common in PD patients than in patients without the disease. It also found that chronic pain was common but underreported in PD patients.
3. **Treatment:** By optimizing anti-Parkinsonian treatment, pain related to motor symptoms, dopamine responsiveness, and fluctuations—such as "off" or "early morning" dystonias and pseudo-neuropathic syndromes during off periods—may be reduced. Peak-dose dyskinesias-induced osteoarticular pain exacerbations can be mitigated with antidyskinetic strategies.

There is growing evidence that treatments involving dopaminergic systems may be helpful in managing pain. A noteworthy improvement in pain, as assessed by a Likert scale, was observed in PD cases treated with rotigotine patch in the double-blind, placebo-controlled RECOVER study when compared to placebo. With pain being a significant component of nonmotor fluctuation in PD, this finding may support the value of longer-acting therapies in the condition by helping to even out motor and nonmotor response fluctuations. In PD patients, levodopa infusion therapies also seem to help with pain; however, an imaging study did not find any evidence of apomorphine's analgesic effects.

To assess the risk-benefit ratios of analgesics for a variety of pain syndromes in patients with Parkinson's disease, more research is required. Nevertheless, doctors should think about prescribing anti-inflammatory medications and analgesics in accordance with the WHO's "ladder" if changing dopaminergic therapy is ineffective or inappropriate in treating pain. PANDA is a large-scale, multinational, randomized, placebo-controlled study that uses oxycodone to treat pain in Parkinson's disease patients.

5.1.3. Akathisia and Restless Legs Syndrome

Another common source of discomfort for patients with PD is akathisia, which is defined as a subjective inner restlessness accompanied by an inability to stay still and a constant need to move or change positions. Akathisia has been found to correlate with age at onset and severity of PD, and it may affect 45% of patients. Severe symptoms may mimic restless legs syndrome (RLS), but RLS is distinguished by an urge to move the legs, especially at night, as opposed to generalized restlessness. While some studies have found a relatively high frequency (~20%) of RLS in PD, case-control studies have found a relatively low prevalence of RLS in Singapore's Chinese and Indian populations (Jankovic, 2013) (Table 5.1).

Table 5.1. *Restless Leg Syndrome in Parkinson's Disease—An Example**

	PwPD + RLS N = 35	**PwPD – RLS N = 96**	***p*-Value**
Motor symptoms			
MDS-UPDRS III	36.45 (±11.02)	31.17 (±14.22)	**0.009**
MDS-UPDRS IV	3.46 (±2.61)	3.44 (±3.27)	0.114
H&Y	2.42 (±0.60)	2.38 (±0.79)	0.415
SCOPA-Motor	24.97 (±7.19)	21.61 (±9.34)	0.009
Non-motor symptoms			
IRLSSG	14.74 (±6.10)	–	<0.001
PDQ 39	27.83 (±12.54)	23.34 (±15.09)	**0.046**
ISI	12.68 (±5.98)	9.8 (±5.91)	**0.016**
PDSS 2	31.43 (±10.18)	20.84 (±9.91)	**<0.001**
ESS	10.71 (±4.91)	8.43 (±5.61)	**0.02**
MMSE	27.54 (±2.33)	27.19 (±3.69)	0.786
MoCA	23.71 (±4.7)	23.33 (±5.8)	0.938
HADS Depression	16.91 (±6.89)	13.40 (±7.85)	**0.013**
HADS Anxiety	6.55 (±3.71)	4.97 (±3.76)	**0.027**
HADS Total	10.35 (±3.61)	8.43 (±4.50)	**0.016**

Source: Diaconu Ş, Irincu L, Ungureanu L, Ciopleiaş B, ***în*** *D, Falup-Pecurariu C. Restless Legs Syndrome in Parkinson's Disease. Journal of Personalized Medicine. 2023; 13(6):915. https://doi.org/10.3390/jpm13060915.*

ESS: Epworth Sleepiness Scale; H&Y: Hoehn & Yahr; HADS: Hospital Anxiety and Depression Scale; IRLSSG: International Restless Legs Syndrome Study Group rating scale; ISI: Insomnia Severity Index; MMSE: Mini-Mental State Examination; MoCA: Montreal Cognitive Assessment; PD: Parkinson's disease; PDQ-39: Parkinson's Disease Questionnaire; PDSS-2: Parkinson Disease Sleep Scale – 2; PwPD: people with Parkinson's disease; RLS: restless legs syndrome; SCOPA: Scales for Outcomes in Parkinson's disease; MDS-UPDRS: Movement Disorders Society Unified Parkinson's Disease Rating Scale. Bold values denote statistical significance ($p < 0.05$).

*Main characteristics regarding motor and non-motor symptoms between the two groups (PwPD + RLS vs. PwPD – RLS; Mann–Whitney U Test).

Nonetheless, a recent Korean study found that RLS was highly prevalent in PD patients and proposed that long-term anti-Parkinsonian therapy, not the disease itself, may be responsible for RLS development.

5.1.4. Other Sensory Abnormalities Associated with PD

Patients with Parkinson's disease also experience other sensory abnormalities. For instance, color discrimination, contrast sensitivity (particularly in the blue-green axis), visual speed, visual construction, and visual memory may all gradually deteriorate in certain Parkinson's disease patients. Non-motor tasks were impacted by visual or visuospatial impairment, according to an analysis of 81 PD patients. Symptoms like double vision, visual hallucinations, difficulty estimating spatial relations, and bumping into objects were frequently reported. Freezing of gait was the only motor symptom connected to visuospatial functioning, and 44% of the patients reported experiencing this. Prolonged visual evoked potential latencies and aberrant electroretinographic patterns have been found during electrophysiologic testing, indicating that retinal ganglion cell impairment may contribute to the acuity loss experienced by individuals with Parkinson's disease.

When comparing patients with PD to healthy controls, age-dependent high-frequency hearing loss has been observed. While brain stem auditoryevoked potentials were normal in every patient, pure tone audiometry scores correlated with Hoehn and Yahr scale scores. Presbycusis may be predicted by the natural aging process interacting with intrinsic neurodegenerative changes in PD to disrupt cochlear transduction mechanisms.

5.2. Cognitive and Behavioral Abnormalities in Parkinson's Disease

The classic neuropsychiatric condition is PD. Cognitive and behavioral abnormalities are prominent features of PD, despite the disease being primarily defined by motor abnormalities. They impact almost all patients and are often more significant than motor impairments in terms of the disease's burden. Distinguishing primary motor features of PD on the mental status examination from features of mental disorders can be challenging due to the overlap of motor, cognitive, and psychiatric characteristics. A depressive disorder's blunted affect, frontal-subcortical impairment-related abulia, facial masking, anticholinergic medication-induced inattention and confusion, or any combination of these conditions could be represented by restricted emotional reactivity. This uncertainty plays a role in the underdiagnosis or undertreatment of neuropsychiatric disorders. A conscious, continuing search for and treatment of neuropsychiatric disorders is part of optimal PD management (Trojano & Costanza Papagno, 2018) (Figure 5.3).

Neuropsychiatric disorders in Parkinson's disease are caused by several factors. Anxiety, depression, or demoralization can be reactive feelings brought on by fears of Parkinson's disease. But the majority of problems seem to be directly linked to the neurobiology of Parkinson's disease or its treatment. PD affects the frontal and limbic dopamine systems, which are involved in cognitive and emotional processes, in addition to nigrostriatal dopaminergic degeneration. Cognitive and psychiatric pathologies are also influenced by neuronal degeneration that is serotonergic, noradrenergic, and cholinergic. Treatment for PD is linked to additional disturbances, like emotional instability brought on by "on-off" motor fluctuations. Psychiatric symptoms can be brought on by anti-Parkinsonian drugs, dopaminergic drugs, or neurosurgical procedures. Anticholinergic drugs, for instance, frequently cause delirium, psychosis, or cognitive impairment (also referred to as an encephalopathy). Many cognitive and behavioral symptoms have been linked to deep brain stimulation, especially when bilateral subthalamic nuclei are targeted, according to a substantial body of research. These include a rise in the likelihood of suicide as well as a deterioration or emergence of language, cognitive, and affective dysfunction.

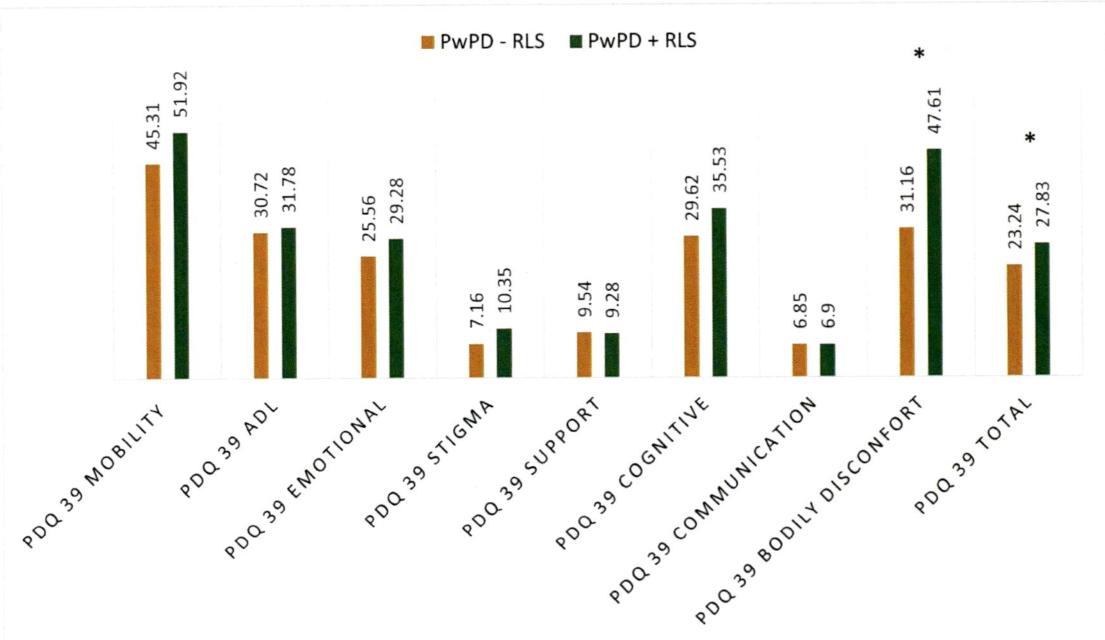

Figure 5.3. *Overlapping or common clinical features of major depression and Parkinson's disease.*

Source: Diaconu Ș, Irincu L, Ungureanu L, Ciopleiaș B, Țînț D, Falup-Pecurariu C. Restless Legs Syndrome in Parkinson's Disease. Journal of Personalized Medicine. 2023; 13(6):915. https://doi.org/10.3390/jpm13060915.

Complications of Parkinson's Disease, like imbalance, can lead to a series of psychiatric issues. This can include developing phobic anxiety about falling or experiencing delirium with agitated behavior due to a subdural hematoma from a fall. Additionally, depressive and anxiety disorders are frequently present before a Parkinson's Disease diagnosis is made. Therefore, these affective disorders could be seen as potential risk factors or early symptoms of Parkinson's Disease.

Neuropsychiatric disorders in Parkinson's Disease go beyond just the symptoms, significantly impacting the quality of life and functional ability more than the physical motor issues like dyskinesias or fluctuations. Depression, in particular, has a major impact on quality of life and is also linked to more severe cognitive and motor deficits, impaired daily activities, other mental and medical health issues, as well as increased burden and depression for caregivers.

5.2.1. Prevalence

Cognitive disorders, affective disturbances, psychosis, and behavioral disorders are the primary subtypes of neuropsychiatric disturbances in PD (Figure 5.4). The definition of "caseness," the population sampled, the diagnoses examined, and the variability in the presentation and progression of neuropsychiatric disorders all influence the prevalence data. However, they are visible at all phases of Parkinson's disease, even before symptoms appear. Every patient has some degree of cognitive changes. Dementia typically progresses at different rates over time. Depression is the most common psychiatric disorder, after cognitive disorders. The "gold-standard" for making psychiatric diagnoses is clinical interviewing with standardized diagnostic criteria. In addition, self-report or clinician-rated psychiatric symptom rating scales with specific cutoff scores to indicate "caseness" are used to estimate prevalence. Although this method is useful for measuring prevalence, it underrepresents rates because there is a wide range of illness severity, symptoms can recur or persist over time, and symptom profiles can change, particularly in response to treatment (Riedel, 2010) (Table 5.2).

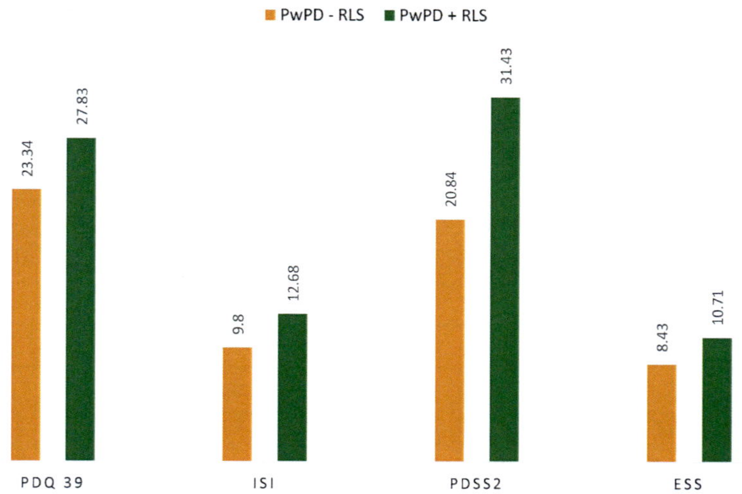

Figure 5.4. *Psychiatric disturbances in Parkinson's disease.*

Source: Diaconu Ș, Irincu L, Ungureanu L, Ciopleiaș B, Țînț D, Falup-Pecurariu C. Restless Legs Syndrome in Parkinson's Disease.Journal of Personalized Medicine. 2023; 13(6):915. https://doi.org/10.3390/jpm13060915.

Table 5.2. *Prevalence of Neuropsychiatric Disturbances in Parkinson's Disease: The Scores of Specific Items of MDS-NMS in the Two Groups (PwPD + RLS vs. PwPD – RLS), Mann–Whitney Test*

	PwPD + RLS		**PwPD – RLS**		
	Mean	**Std. Deviation**	**Mean**	**Std. Deviation**	***p***
MDS-NMS A. Depression domain total score	3.629	3.5570	3.629	3.5570	0.058
MDS-NMS B. Anxiety total score	4.000	5.5572	4.000	5.5572	0.126
MDS-NMS C. Apathy total score	1.886	2.0113	1.886	2.0113	0.183

MDS-NMS D. Psychosis total score	0.314	0.8668	0.314	0.8668	0.953
MDS-NMS E. Impulse Control Disorders total score	0.029	0.1690	0.029	0.1690	0.463
MDS-NMS F. Cognition total score	6.514	8.1615	6.514	8.1615	0.850
MDS-NMS G. Orthostatic hypotension total score	3.229	6.2830	3.229	6.2830	0.703
MDS-NMS H. Urinary total score	7.029	6.2755	7.029	6.2755	0.314
MDS-NMS I. Sexual total score	0.314	1.5295	0.314	1.5295	0.191
MDS-NMS J. Gastrointestinal total score	2.000	2.4254	2.000	2.4254	0.941
MDS-NMS K. Sleep total score	15.229	10.3216	15.229	10.3216	**<0.001**
Restlessness fr x sev	3.057	3.0673	3.057	3.0673	**<0.001**
Periodic limb movements fr x sev	1.343	2.1955	1.343	2.1955	**<0.001**
Snoring, difficulty breathing fr x sev	2.000	2.1693	2.000	2.1693	**<0.001**
MDS-NMS L. Pain total	11.743	8.4029	11.743	8.4029	**0.003**
Other types of pain (nocturnal, orofacial) fr x sev	3.714	3.6346	3.714	3.6346	**0.002**
MDS-NMS M. Other non-motor symptoms total	11.086	7.9164	11.086	7.9164	0.177
Physical fatigue fr x sev	5.771	4.2084	5.771	4.2084	**0.007**
MDS-NMS total	67.000	35.4119	67.000	35.4119	**0.007**

Source: Diaconu Ş, Irincu L, Ungureanu L, Ciopleiaș B, Țînț D, Falup-Pecurariu C. Restless Legs Syndrome in Parkinson's Disease. Journal of Personalized Medicine. 2023; 13(6):915. https://doi.org/10.3390/jpm13060915.

fr: frequency; MDS-NMSS: International Parkinson and Movement Disorder Society Non-Motor Rating Scale; PD: Parkinson's disease; PwPD: people with Parkinson's disease; RLS: restless legs syndrome; sev: severity. Bold values denote statistical significance ($p < 0.05$).

5.2.2. Clinical Characteristics of Psychiatric Syndromes in PD

- **Cognitive Disorders:** It is not always evident that PD patients have cognitive impairment, which can vary from mild selective disturbances to total dementia. Even for those who have dementia, results on dementia screening exams, like the Mini-Mental State Examination, are frequently within the normal range. It is advised to use more sensitive (Level I) tools. Selective impairments in executive and visuospatial functions, memory, and attention are observed early in PD. Data processing (e.g., verbal fluency) and cognitive speed are also impacted. The primary focus of memory impairments is on explicit recall, with recognition memory remaining largely intact and the "rapid forgetting" or aphasia associated with Alzheimer's disease (AD) absent. These deficiencies can impact work or independent living and show up as issues with planning, prioritizing, forgetting, and being easily distracted.

Dementia typically manifests as one of three categories of global impairments that prevent independent living and usually develop later in life. Selective deficiencies are exacerbated in the first, especially in memory and information processing. Although the clinical course of this second group differs from AD's, it exhibits broader involvement of cortical functions, such as apraxia, aphasia, and memory. The third group has severe language impairments and PD and AD characteristics. Dementia with Lewy bodies (DLB) and PD share numerous characteristics. In people with DLB, dementia symptoms either appear before Parkinsonism or appear a year after the onset of motor symptoms. Moreover, florid hallucinations, which are typically visual, and erratic attentional states are features of DLB. Levodopa therapy may be effective in treating Parkinsonism in DLB patients, but side effects—particularly psychosis—may be more severe.

Delirium is a common cause of global cognitive impairment in PD, so it is always worth considering a diagnosis. The majority of the time, comorbid medical conditions (e.g., pneumonia, UTIs), however psychoactive drugs for PD or mental illnesses (e.g., benzodiazepines, anticholinergics, dopamine agonists, hypnotics, and painkillers) are often the culprits. Delirium frequently coexists with dementia as well as milder cognitive impairment, exacerbating the baseline cognitive impairment. The predominant characteristics are disorientation and confusion. On-off motor fluctuations can cause confusion with mental state fluctuations, such as lucidity in the morning and confusion and agitation in the evening, particularly in advanced Parkinson's disease and dementia (Saadat P & Faramarzi, 2020).

- **Affective Disorders:** Affective disorders are characterized by long-lasting mood swings, prominent somatic complaints and signs, cognitive abnormalities, and vegetative symptoms (disturbances in sleep and appetite) that are similar to those of Parkinson's disease. Therefore, in order to identify affective disorders, direct investigation into mood phenomena is essential. If not, these diagnoses go unnoticed. Conclusions that affective disturbances are "understandable" may result from advanced patient age or the difficulties associated with Parkinson's disease. Affective disorders, like other medical conditions, are characterized by a constellation of signs and symptoms with a generally predictable course and prognosis, in contrast to emotional reactions to particular concerns or circumstances.

Compared to other chronic illnesses, PD is more likely to cause depressive disorders, such as dysthymia, major depression, and minor depression. Age of onset, duration, severity of PD or PD stage or subtype, timing of depression onset, and depression severity are not consistently correlated with PD. More troubling than the motor impairment, depression in patients with mild PD can be severely disabling. When a patient's self-reported disability surpasses what is anticipated based on the examination, a diagnosis of depression should be taken into consideration. Fears about the implications of a depressive diagnosis can make patients or doctors reluctant to consider one; however, undiagnosed and untreated mental disorders are ultimately more problematic. Focusing on emotional symptoms instead of neurovegetative ones aids in diagnosis. Core characteristics of major depression include a pervasive and persistently low mood, diminished ability to enjoy otherwise enjoyable activities (anhedonia), or a decline in interest from one's usual baseline. These characteristics are similar to those of major depression in patients without neurological disease. PD patients without depression may restrict their activities (e.g., woodworking) due to motor symptoms, but a patient with depression from Parkinson's disease will not look for enjoyable hobbies. Patients with Parkinson's disease who exhibit nonsomatic depressive traits, such as extreme pessimism, negative ruminations, tearfulness, hopelessness, and guilt, can be distinguished from those who do not. According to certain research, PD patients with major depression are less likely to experience suicidality, delusions, self-blame, and a negative attitude toward themselves. These phenomena, though, are still possible. Nonmajor forms of depression exhibit similar phenomena, albeit with fewer and milder symptoms. Even "subsyndromal" depressions are a serious cause of distress.

Coping difficulties are a critical indicator. Unremitting mood disorders make effective coping and adaptation nearly impossible. People with PD adjust to and overcome its challenges after treatment, which indicates that the mood disorder is improving. Many patients report, "I can cope with PD, but not when depressed." Clinicians ought to ask openly about thoughts of death, suicide, or homicide, as well as feelings of powerlessness and hopelessness.

The term "pathological laughter and crying" or "emotional incontinence" refers to pseudobulbar affect, which is characterized by excessive, uncontrollably occurring, inappropriate, and transient crying or laughing in the absence of feelings of sadness or mirth. In PD, pathological tearfulness is more common. Distress, embarrassment, or social dysfunction may result from the symptoms. Increased emotionality frequently happens when there isn't a dominant mood disorder. However, in these situations, patients may believe that they have a depressive illness due to their frequent crying in response to upsetting or moving events. One man, for instance, used to cry every time he remembered how much he loved his family. He could not talk about his family or accept gifts from his grandchildren without crying and feeling ashamed. Moreover, delirium and benzodiazepines are linked to pseudobulbar affect. Other Parkinsonian disorders, such as progressive supranuclear palsy, should be taken into consideration in the differential diagnosis when pseudobulbar affect is a prominent feature, especially at the onset of the motor disturbance.

Apathy is a disorder that can occur alone or as a feature of depressive disturbances. It is characterized by decreased motivation and self-initiated goal-directed emotional, cognitive, and behavioral activity. While in most cases apathy does not react to medication or surgical (*i.e.,* apathy may arise from the reduction of dopaminergic medications following subthalamic nucleus stimulation in deep-brain stimulation) therapies. This could be the outcome of a dopaminergic withdrawal syndrome. Affected patients participate in few activities, such as impromptu conversation, and exhibit little goal-directed interest in their environment or in themselves. Even though apathetic patients don't often complain, their actions worry families because they might mistakenly believe the patient's actions to be intentional. Clinical outcomes are exacerbated by apathy because apathetic people are less likely to exercise, adhere to treatment plans, or practice self-care.

Mania and hypomania are not well defined phenomena in Parkinson's disease. Some patients experience depressive and hypomanic or manic episodes of bipolar disorder, a chronic affective disorder, long before PD. However, dopaminergic drugs or neurosurgical procedures are the most common causes of isolated manic phenomena. In the "on state," certain patients exhibit hypomanic traits, such as heightened irritability and goal-directed behavior. Mania and hypomania present similarly to non-PD patients, with the exception of varying mood states in certain patients. Features include irritability, hyperactivity, elevated mood and sense of self, increased goal-directed activity, including dangerous behaviors and psychotic phenomena that are mood-congruent.

Anxiety syndromes consist of physical, emotional, and cognitive symptoms. The physical symptoms, like shaking, sweating, stomach issues, rapid heartbeat, and other autonomic symptoms, are similar to those seen in Parkinson's disease, making diagnosis more challenging. Focusing on emotional symptoms can help in identifying anxiety disorders. It can be tough to differentiate between pathological anxiety in Parkinson's disease and regular anxiety caused by certain situations, like feeling anxious while crossing a street due to slowed movements. However, anxiety disorder symptoms are typically repetitive and seen as excessive. Panic disorder, generalized anxiety disorder, and social phobia are the most common anxiety disorders in Parkinson's disease. Many anxiety issues in Parkinson's disease don't fit neatly into existing diagnostic categories. Anxiety disorders in Parkinson's disease often coexist with depression and can present as episodic, situational, or chronic conditions.

Episodic attacks characterized by an abrupt onset of severe unprovoked anxiety and fear are a feature of panic disorder. Patients often fear they are going to die, are having a heart attack, or are losing their sense of self. Chest pain, dyspnea, gastrointestinal distress, dizziness, paresthesias, and autonomic symptoms (e.g., seizures) are examples of physical symptoms. g. tachycardia, flushing of the face). Some patients claim to have daily panic episodes linked to motor impairments. While claustrophobia, social phobia, and other phobias are unprovoked, panic attacks involve intense fear brought on by particular situations. Anxiety that is noticeably elevated may manifest as panic symptoms.

With generalized anxiety disorder, a person experiences excessive, ongoing worry and anxiety about a variety of life circumstances. There is weariness, difficulty concentrating, and tenseness in the muscles. Most anxiety disorders are accompanied by disturbed sleep. One more subdued aspect of anxiety that is sometimes difficult to identify is avoidance. For instance, avoiding autonomous walking may result from fears of falling even in the absence of prior falls.

Drug-induced or erratic mood states are specific to PD and are somewhat correlated with "on-off" times associated with anti-Parkinsonian medication. Individuals who experience levodopa-related motor fluctuations are typically more nervous than those who do not. Severe anxiety or even panic attacks can sometimes strike during off-peak hours. When "off," "non-motor" fluctuations are also common and typically involve intense panic attacks, noticeable melancholy, or agitation; however, these symptoms may also linger even after motor function returns to normal.

Less frequently, during the "on" state, improved wellbeing, if not hypomania, happens. Motor impairments are also made worse by extreme situational anxiety.

For instance, even in cases where PD symptoms were otherwise mild, one person who was nervous about answering the phone would become akinetic whenever it rang. Frequent severe mood swings are a feature of both the dopamine dysregulation syndrome (DDS) and the dopamine agonist withdrawal syndrome (DAWS), which are classified under behavioral disturbances.

- **Psychotic Disorders:** In PD, delusions and hallucinations are examples of psychotic phenomena. Concurrent dopaminergic therapies are linked to psychosis. Interestingly, though, dopaminergic drugs are not the only cause of psychosis in people with Parkinson's disease. Cognitive impairment, particularly dementia, and sleep deprivation are attributed to significant risk factors. Even though delirium is not usually present when PD-related psychotic symptoms manifest, it is always important to take delirium into account when a patient exhibits newly onset or worsening psychotic phenomena.

The most prevalent psychotic phenomenon in PD is visual hallucinations, which can range from brief, basic images like shadows to intricate scenes with fully realized people. Scenes and other aspects of hallucinations are usually the same each time. Many patients are fully or partially aware that their experience is hallucinatory. Without understanding, though, patients may grow wary, become agitated about alleged intruders, or try to feed imaginary houseguests. Other forms of visual hallucinations are experienced by up to half of patients. About 10% of patients experience auditory hallucinations; other forms of hallucinations are less frequent. Major depressive disorder or manic episode are present in psychotic affective disorders. When dopaminergic medication is not administered and hallucinations persist, DLB should be taken into account.

Delusions tend to manifest in patients who have previously experienced hallucinations, even though the specific details of each may not be connected. Typical delusional themes include paranoid thoughts, like suspicions of a partner being unfaithful, belief in conspiracies, or fear of being poisoned. Some delusions may also be strange or bizarre in nature. Delusional paranoia can lead to risky behaviors.

- **Behavioral Disorders Specific to PD:** In PD, anti-Parkinsonian therapy—particularly dopamine agonists—and neurosurgical intervention are linked to impulse control disorders, or ICDs. On the other hand, PD is not linked to a higher risk of ICD. Pathological gambling, compulsive shopping, hypersexuality, compulsive eating, and paraphilias are examples of common ICDs; many patients will have more than one ICD. While mood disorders or psychosis may also be present, ICDs are not signs of mania or hypomania; in fact, many people who have ICDs describe their behaviors as unlike anything they would normally do. It is unknown what factors make some people more susceptible to ICDs than others. Male sex, younger age, younger age-onset PD, pre-PD ICD(s), bipolar disorder, impulsive personality traits, and a personal or family history of substance abuse have all been identified as risk factors for ICDs. Absence of awareness of the severity of their issue and the actions they take may have serious negative effects on the law, the economy, and society. Therefore, before beginning dopamine agonist therapy in particular, clinicians should advise patients and their families about the possibility of ICDs. Collateral data can be useful when patients are hesitant to divulge sensitive information.

Certain individuals may develop Dopamine Dysregulation Syndrome (DDS), which involves an unhealthy habit of consuming excessive amounts of dopaminergic medication beyond what is necessary to manage motor symptoms. This compulsive drug consumption often includes behaviors typically associated with addiction, such as craving and seeking out the drug. Abusing dopaminergic medication can result in severe motor side effects and mental health issues, including drug-induced dyskinesias, difficulty in reducing dosage, agitation, feelings of euphoria, withdrawal symptoms like depression and anxiety, and impairment in work and social relationships.

DAWS is frequently misdiagnosed and can be extremely difficult to treat. Withdrawing or attempting to withdraw from dopamine agonists can cause severe psychological and physical dependence symptoms, which are commonly seen in people with ICDs. Psychiatric features include drug craving and its associated behaviors, marked anxiety, panic attacks, agitation, irritability, depression and dysphoria. Physical signs of drug withdrawal include generalized pain, insomnia, fatigue, and autonomic phenomena, including orthostatic hypotension, dizziness, nausea and diaphoresis.

Punding is a syndrome that was first identified in amphetamine addicts. It is characterized by complex, meaningless stereotyped behaviors, like repeatedly handling or sorting objects, disassembling them, and then trying to reassemble them. Patients can disassemble and reassemble appliances or flashlights, catalog jewelry, figure out amounts on a calculator, or shelve and reshelve books at home. It's possible that patients won't identify these repetitive behaviors as abnormal. Additionally, patients are less likely to seek assistance for the behaviors because many of them claim to be calming. Instead, they are more likely to upset other people, particularly if the patient refuses to stop and the behaviors cause them to neglect important tasks like eating or sleeping.

Excessive involvement in intricate activities, typically related to novel interests or pastimes, is known as hobbyism and is a behavioral disorder that can significantly impact individuals with Parkinson's disease. The patient's pastime eventually takes up the majority of their waking hours. In one study, 31.2% of the population had both punding and hobbyism, while 18.5% of the PD cohort only showed punding (70%) or hobbyism (110.5%).

5.2.3. Treatment

Neuropsychiatric disorders in Parkinson's disease are difficult to treat. In PD, psychiatric conditions are treatable, particularly depressive disorders. Additionally, they respond well to drugs, physical therapies, psychotherapies, rehabilitative therapies, or a mix of these when given thoughtful, diligent treatment. Remission of the psychiatric syndrome, along with enhanced function and overall well-being, are the objectives of treatment. Restoring cognitive function to premorbid levels or getting rid of mood swings or hallucinations might not be achievable. A recovery-oriented approach, on the other hand, places more emphasis on optimism, hope, and the pursuit of meaningful goals for that person. It also highlights the value of autonomy and social supports, as well as individual strengths and resilience.

- **Cognitive Dysfunction:** Drugs prescribed for AD have been the focus of clinical trials for the treatment of cognitive dysfunction in PD. The only approved cholinesterase inhibitor, rivastigmine, is a reasonably safe and effective treatment for global status, cognitive dysfunction, behavioral disorders, and everyday living activities. Lower initial doses may reduce adverse effects related to the gastrointestinal tract and motor system. There is evidence to support the benefit of memantine in PD dementia. Patients without dementia may benefit from atomoxetine, a norepinephrine-reuptake inhibitor, if they have cognitive deficits. Early research on cognitive rehabilitation points to potential advantages, but it's unclear if these will last. Speech, physical, and occupational therapy help define functional abilities and offer strategies to enhance function or lessen the effects of executive dysfunction and other disorders.

- **Affective Disorders:** "Watchful waiting" and problem-solving techniques are a reasonable plan with a follow-up in two to three weeks when life stressors are the main issue. Social workers, home care services, and occupational, physical, and speech therapists can all be of assistance in this area. It is advisable to promote physical activity, constructive mental pursuits, and proper sleeping habits.

When depressive disorders continue to cause substantial distress or dysfunction, antidepressant medications may be indicated. Although they are frequently used, selective serotonin-reuptake inhibitors (SSRIs) are not always effective. There is no evidence to support worries that SSRIs exacerbate Parkinsonism. Treatment options for major and non-major depression in PD include antidepressant medication and cognitive behavioral therapy (CBT), which have been shown in recent randomized single-site and multisite controlled trials. Dopamine agonists lessened depressive symptoms, and nortriptyline, venlafaxine, desipramine, paroxetine, and citalopram demonstrated greater efficacy than placebo for major depression, though study results are not consistent. When compared to other antidepressant classes, tricyclic antidepressant treatment was linked to a delayed initiation of dopaminergic therapy, according to a patient-level meta-analysis involving 2064 participants from studies on early PD patients. The analysis revealed no correlation between the delay and motor status, indicating that the antidepressant medication may have a moderating effect on the disease.

Ensuring appropriate management of depressive disturbances requires longitudinal follow-up, targeted monitoring of depressive symptoms, and treatment modifications. Generally speaking, even patients who respond well to antidepressant treatment still have residual symptoms that need to be managed with further medication adjustments until the depressive disorder goes away. The 10-week CBT trial for PD-depression showed 56% improvement in symptom severity compared to 8% for the control group, with some patients already on antidepressants. As is the case with the general population, remission may need to be attained through rigorous measurement-based and stepped-care approaches that involve several months' worth of medication trials in addition to psychotherapy.

When a quick response is required for severe depression, such as for psychosis related to depression or severe vegetative symptoms, electroconvulsive therapy is a useful treatment option for PD depression. Other signs include intolerance to medication and insensitivity to antidepressants.

Studies on apathy treatment in PD patients without a depressive illness are lacking. The most crucial thing is to teach caregivers how to handle a patient who lacks motivation and how a daily routine can optimize function and activity level.

Dopaminergic or noradrenergic drugs, including amphetamines, modafanil, levodopa, amphetamine reuptake inhibitors (SNRIs), and dopamine agonists, have been linked to improved function. Indirect benefits of cognitive-enhancing drugs may be seen in apathy.

- **Anxiety Disorders:** Regarding anxiety in Parkinson's disease, there are no published controlled treatment trials. Indicated for idiopathic anxiety disorders, SSRIs, SNRIs, and CBT seem to be beneficial in Parkinson's disease. Nortriptyline at a low dose (e.g., 10 mg each night) can assist with anxiety during the day and sleeplessness at night. Because of the potential for negative cognitive effects, falls, drug tolerance, and dependence, benzodiazepines should be avoided. Low starting dosages (e.g., lorazepam 0–25 mg) should be weaned as soon as feasible and used temporarily or sporadically in cases of elevated anxiety symptoms. Atypical antipsychotics can be beneficial when taken in small doses (e.g., starting at 6.25 mg of quetiapine before bed) or occasionally spaced out throughout the day. When selegeline, a monoamine oxidase-B inhibitor, is taken with SSRIs or tricyclic antidepressants, serotonin syndrome may occur, but clinical experience indicates that these combinations are well tolerated. Antidepressant dosages should be modest to begin with because they can exacerbate anxiety.
- **Psychotic Disorders:** The initial step in treatment involves addressing potential contributors to psychosis, such as medical or medication-related factors. It is recommended to gradually eliminate medications one by one. Cognitive-enhancing drugs may also be considered to help reduce psychotic symptoms. When psychotic symptoms become problematic or lead to agitated or aggressive behavior that impacts caregiving or safety, clozapine and quetiapine are the only suggested antipsychotic medications due to their dopamine-blocking properties. Clozapine is supported by strong data, with effective doses typically starting at 6.25 mg at bedtime and advancing to at least 25 mg daily for most patients. Quetiapine is commonly used as a first-line antipsychotic in the USA, as it does not require hematological monitoring like clozapine. Although its efficacy data is not as robust, it is often effective in practice. New antipsychotic medications that do not cause motor side effects are currently being studied in clinical trials.
- **Behavioral Disorders:** It is difficult to treat behavioral disorders in PD, such as ICDs, DDS, DAWs, punding, and hobbyism. Since many patients have multiple behavioral disorders in addition to other psychiatric comorbidities (such as psychosis, depressive disorder, and cognitive dysfunction), the situation is frequently chaotic. Furthermore, because problem behaviors are frequently covert, treatment

engagement is compromised by the conditions themselves. The recommendations ought to be adhered to, with a focus on stopping dopamine agonist treatment. Some patients may not be able to handle this because of DAWS or worsening motor symptoms; in these cases, deep brain stimulation or a gradual dopaminergic medication taper may be necessary. To stabilize behavior and start treatment, hospitalization might be required. Nartrexone and other drugs are being tested in treatment for addictive behaviors. Clozapine or quetiapine may be beneficial for controlling symptoms or in cases where psychosis is present. Treatment is necessary for other psychiatric comorbidities, particularly depression. Families frequently have to restrict their patient's access to money in order to prevent catastrophic financial losses, particularly in cases where the patient is prone to compulsive gambling. Support groups and behavioral psychotherapies are beneficial but insufficient unless the offending medications are stopped. Modifications in Parkinson's disease medication may mitigate the severity of punding behaviors when they become troublesome. Programs or structured activities during the day can lessen the chance of repetitive behaviors occurring and even improve nocturnal sleep. Sleep aids such as quetiapine or trazodone can help. SSRIs have the potential to lessen OCD symptoms.

5.3. Sleep Disturbances

Patients with Parkinson's disease often experience sleep disturbances. Patients may experience insomnia and/or nighttime restlessness due to depression and/or hallucinations. Male patients with advanced disease, cognitive impairment, drug-induced psychosis, and orthostatic hypotension are more likely to experience pathologic sleep. Patients may experience frequent nighttime awakenings due to either body rigidity or urgent urination even after they have fallen asleep. They consequently struggle to get a good night's sleep.

Rapid eye movement behavior sleep disorder (RBD) is a common occurrence characterized by a lack of muscle paralysis during REM sleep, leading to increased movements while dreaming. This disorder is strongly linked to neurodegenerative conditions like PD. Recent research indicates that RBD may develop before PD symptoms appear. About half of individuals with RBD eventually go on to develop PD, making RBD a potential early sign of the disease.

During REM sleep, movements do not exhibit signs of Parkinsonism, possibly due to motor signals from the cortex bypassing the extrapyramidal system. In managing this disorder, it is important to adjust dopaminergic medications to lower doses, particularly at night. Long-acting dopamine agonists could be a potential option to consider. While Clonazepam is commonly used, it is important to monitor for side effects like excessive sedation.

Oversleeping during the day (EDS) is prevalent. Lack of sleep during the night creates a vicious cycle for poor sleep hygiene in addition to the exhaustion that many PD patients experience. This extreme drowsiness, which frequently resembles the levels seen in sudden-onset sleep disorders like narcolepsy and cataplexy, can be incapacitating. Studies using polysomnography have demonstrated a brief transition from wakefulness to stage II sleep. Dopaminergic medications, particularly dopamine agonists, can also exacerbate drowsiness and the abrupt onset of sleep. Management typically involves changing the timing of medication or assisting patients in ending the vicious cycle by enhancing their quality of sleep at night. Modafinil might provide EDS relief. Even though this medication does not worsen Parkinson's disease symptoms, multiple randomized controlled trials found that it either had no discernible benefit or only slightly improved symptoms.

Restless leg syndrome (RLS) can cause sleep disturbances for a significant number of patients. It is characterized by an uncomfortable sensation in the legs that prompts patients to move. This sensation usually occurs when patients are at rest, especially at night. Moving or walking can provide temporary relief. RLS often occurs alongside periodic limb movement during sleep, which involves repetitive jerking movements of the limbs while asleep. Both conditions greatly impact the quality of sleep. RLS is more common in PD patients compared to those without PD. The exact cause is not fully understood, but it is believed to involve certain dopamine systems in the brain. Dopamine agonists like ropinirole and pramipexole are effective in managing RLS symptoms. Levodopa can also help, but the risk of augmentation limits its use as a first-line treatment. Other medications such as gabapentin, clonazepam, and opiates have shown to be helpful. Some studies have even suggested that deep brain stimulation of the subthalamic nucleus can improve RLS symptoms.

5.4. Autonomic Dysfunction in Parkinson's Disease

Patients with PD nearly always have autonomic dysfunction, which can include abnormalities of the gastrointestinal tract, cardiovascular system, respiratory system, bladder, and sexual system in addition to problems with perspiration and thermoregulation.

Patients' levels of autonomic dysfunction vary widely; some have very mild symptoms, while others have severe and incapacitating symptoms. The heterogeneous nature of PD with its multitude of etiologies is highlighted by the phenotypic variation. Rarely, years before motor abnormalities manifest, isolated severe autonomic failure may be the first clinical sign of PD.

PD is included in the category of degenerative illnesses known as "autonomic synucleinopathies," which impact autonomic neurons and are linked to the deposition of a-synuclein in either neurons, glia, or both. Other autonomic synucleinopathies are pure autonomic failure (i.e., without a motor phenotype), dementia with Lewy bodies, and multiple system atrophy (MSA). While autonomic dysfunction is rare in patients with other neurodegenerative disorders, such as tauopathies, it is present in the majority of synucleinopathy patients.

5.4.1. Pathology

Even though PD is regarded as a CNS disorder, peripheral postganglionic autonomic neuron degeneration is the primary cause of autonomic impairment in these patients.

The knowledge that PD's pathological feature was peripheral sympathetic denervation was largely driven by *in vivo* studies employing fluorodopamine-based PET or myocardial scintigraphy with ^{123}I-metaiodobenzylguanidine (^{123}I-MIBG). These investigations revealed decreased amine uptake in the heart of PD patients, but not in those with progressive supranuclear palsy or MSA, two other types of Parkinsonism. The observation in postmortem studies of cardiac tissues of patients with PD of a marked reduction of tyrosine hydroxylase positive fibers as well as synuclein deposits in surviving sympathetic fibers in epicardial nerves has now confirmed this notable cardiac denervation.

Neuropathological studies conducted on cohorts of elderly people without neurological impairments have demonstrated that Lewy body (LB) pathology affects the peripheral autonomic ganglia, the enteric nervous system, the dorsal motor nucleus of the vagus, and the autonomic nuclei of the spinal cord early on, before lesions in the substantia nigra are discovered.

These elderly, neurologically intact people with "incidental" LB disease—which is regarded as presymptomatic Parkinson's disease—also exhibit a marked decrease in α-synuclein deposits and tyrosine hydroxylase positive heart fibers. The possibility that erectile dysfunction and constipation can manifest years before PD motor symptoms is explained by the early involvement of peripheral autonomic neurons.

5.4.2. Systems Affected

Drooling, dysphagia, constipation, and urinary dysfunction were listed as prominent clinical features in James Parkinson's initial report. Abnormalities related to the heart, sex, and thermoregulation are also common. Typically, as the illness worsens, the autonomic impairment gets worse. Medication frequently prescribed for PD may make autonomic symptoms worse.

5.4.3. Cardiovascular System

One particular concern is orthostatic hypotension. The symptoms include exhaustion, fainting, and position-related dizziness. For PD patients, position-related dizziness frequently results in falls. It might be a mild symptom in the early stages of Parkinson's disease and not become a significant issue until later on. Usually, dopaminergic drugs don't make a big difference. They might even make the symptoms worse, particularly if you use dopamine agonists. Orthostatic hypotension is primarily treated symptomatically. Striking a balance between Parkinson's disease medications and regular antihypertensive medications is recommended for patients who take them. Patients are advised to increase their salt intake and drink the recommended amounts of water. To avoid the abrupt drop in blood pressure that occurs with positional changes, they should be trained to slowly rise from a sitting position and to wait a little period of time before starting their gait. Additionally, compression stockings might help the situation. Antihypertensive drugs might be required in more extreme situations to treat the symptoms of orthostatic hypotension. The two most often prescribed medications are midodrine, a selective alpha-adrenergic agonist with peripheral action, and fludrocortisone, a mineralocorticoid that retains salt. 9.1% of Parkinson's disease patients needed such drugs to treat orthostatic hypotension, according to an epidemiologic study.

- **Orthostatic Hypotension:** When standing, vascular resistance does not increase and blood pressure (BP) decreases when sympathetic nerves are not fully activated or defective, causing insufficient release of norepinephrine. Orthostatic hypotension (OH) affects 30–40% of Parkinson's disease patients.

Standing-related vertigo or lightheadedness is the hallmark symptom of OH and is caused by cerebral hypoperfusion. Additional symptoms that are frequently linked to OH include fatigue, weariness, impaired cognitive function, blurred vision, and pain in the shoulders and back of the neck (also known as the "coat-hanger" distribution). Even though neurogenic OH is highly prevalent in PD patients, it's crucial to determine for each patient whether the drop in blood pressure during standing is, in fact, neurogenic (i.e., because of compromised sympathetic activation), or if the issue is being caused by other modifiable, non-neurogenic factors. Common non-neurogenic causes include varicose veins, anemia, dehydration, and, often, a-blockade for the treatment of benign prostatic hypertrophy in men. All of these conditions can aggravate or cause pre-existing OH. Possible systemic, endocrine, and cardiac causes should also be addressed during the history-taking process. OH can get worse when taking levodopa or direct dopaminergic agonists.

One way to determine if orthostatic hypotension is caused by neurogenic factors is to conduct a simple laboratory test called the Valsalva maneuver with beat-to-beat blood pressure monitoring. In this test, the patient is instructed to exhale forcefully for 15 seconds with a closed glottis while maintaining an expiratory pressure of 40 mmHg. Typically, blood pressure will increase from baseline after the strain is released. However, if there is a lack of sympathetic activation, this increase in blood pressure during Phase IV of the Valsalva maneuver will be missing.

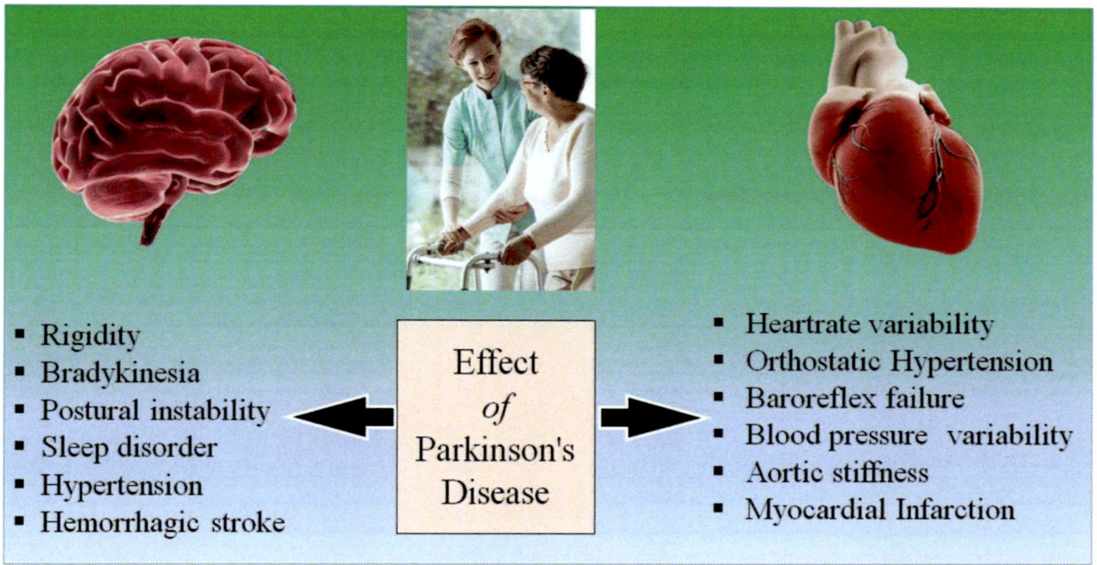

Figure 5.5. *Heart issues in Parkinson's disease and autonomic failure.*

Source: Suri JS, Paul S, Maindarkar MA, Puvvula A, Saxena S, Saba L, Turk M, Laird JR, Khanna NN, Viskovic K, et al. Cardiovascular/Stroke Risk Stratification in Parkinson's Disease Patients Using Atherosclerosis Pathway and Artificial Intelligence Paradigm: A Systematic Review. Metabolites. 2022; 12(4):312. https://doi.org/10.3390/metabo12040312.

When OH occurs in patients with cardiovascular autonomic failure, it usually manifests more prominently in the morning and right after meals. Because recumbency during the night raises blood pressure and causes pressure natriuresis, which lowers intravascular volume overnight and exacerbates OH in the morning, the symptoms of OH are more severe in the morning.

Even in those with PD who do not experience OH, postprandial hypotension is frequently seen. Often, the apparent worsening of Parkinsonian symptoms after meals is due to postprandial hypotension. Patients often go undiagnosed because they seem confused or "frozen," which could indicate a "off" state brought on by erratic levodopa responses.

- **Orthostatic Hypotension and Cognition:** When it comes to older adults, OH is a reliable indicator of cognitive decline. According to recent research, patients with PD who also have OH are more likely to experience cognitive impairment. It is hypothesized that OH may cause silent ischemic lesions that impair cognition, even though association does not prove causation. This is debatable because it's generally accepted that OH should only be addressed when symptoms appear. It's unclear if more intensive care to possibly maintain perfusion needs to be looked into. As an alternative, the correlation between OH and cognitive decline may be attributed to the gradual build-up of LB in cortical, basal ganglia, and autonomic neurons over time, as well as the overlap of motor, autonomic, and cognitive phenotypes that make up the spectrum of LB disorders.
- **Treatment of Orthostatic Hypotension:**

a. ***Nonpharmacological Interventions:*** Drugs like diuretics and antihypertensives (especially α-blockers) that can exacerbate OH should be stopped. Sometimes it helps to give extra carbidopa to make sure peripheral dopamine production isn't making OH worse.

Patient education is essential to the management of overdose headache (OH), and nonpharmacological treatments are the initial line of treatment. Salt in the diet should be liberalized and water intake should be increased in order to increase plasma volume. Although waist-high graded compression stockings are useful in lowering venous pooling, many Parkinson's disease patients find them uncomfortable to wear and impractical to put on by themselves. In order to maintain blood pressure and cerebral perfusion, physical countermanoeuvres such as leg crossing and tensing the muscles in the buttocks, legs, and abdomen are useful in lowering venous pooling and raising cardiac filling.

In patients with autonomic failure, consuming half a liter of water rapidly can have a significant pressor effect. This is likely due to the remaining sympathetic nerves being activated through a local spinal reflex. Elevating the head of the bed to a 15–30° angle while you sleep decreases pressure natriuresis during the night and increases plasma volume in the morning.

b. ***Pharmacological Interventions:*** Some PD patients still experience OH symptoms in spite of nonpharmacologic treatments, necessitating pharmacological management. There are two basic types of common medications used to treat OH: those that raise vasoconstrictor tone and those that increase plasma volume. Furthermore, treating anemia when it exists can greatly enhance OH.

c. ***Volume Expansion:*** Fludrocortisone, a synthetic mineralocorticoid, increases plasma volume while retaining sodium. In about 7 days, the maximum clinical response happens. Ankle edema and weight gain are typical indicators of volume expansion. Because hypokalemia can occur, salt intake should be increased and potassium levels should be watched. Fludrocortisone exacerbates supine hypertension by raising peripheral vascular resistance and improving norepinephrine responsiveness. These effects last even when the medication is stopped. Moreover, fibrosis is produced by activation of mineralocorticoid receptors in the kidney and heart, which can speed up the development of end-organ target damage in OH patients.

Desmopressin, a synthetic vasopressin analog, has been shown in small trials to lessen postural drop in the morning, minimize overnight water loss, and reduce nocturnal polyuria. The risk of hyponatremia needs to be carefully considered.

d. ***Increasing Vascular Resistance:*** Midodrine, an α-1-adrenoreceptor agonist, acts in the peripheral vasculature to elevate blood pressure without passing through the blood–brain barrier. After oral ingestion, it has a peak pressor effect within one hour, and its half-life is roughly four hours.

Droxidopa, or $_L$-threo-2,3-dihydroxphenylserine, is an artificial amino acid that, upon oral administration, is catalyzed by the enzyme dopa-decarboxylase to yield norepinephrine in a single step. Blood pressure rises and circulating norepinephrine levels rise following the administration of droxidopa. When standing, the pressor effect starts after one hour, peaks after three and a half hours, and lasts for six hours. Droxidopa produced clinically meaningful and statistically significant improvements compared with placebo in dizziness/lightheadedness at week 1 (1.0 unit change; p = 0.018), the primary end point, as well as in several secondary end points, including beneficial effects on falls, in a Phase III trial evaluating the drug for the treatment of symptomatic neurogenic OH associated with Parkinson's disease. The majority of adverse events were mild to moderate, and one of them was supine hypertension.

According to recent reports, norepinephrine-reuptake inhibitors may also be helpful in raising standing blood pressure and improving norepinephrine bioavailability in the periphery, particularly in cases where postganglionic sympathetic neuron loss is incomplete. Pyridostigmine, an acetylcholinesterase inhibitor, has a slight pressor effect and enhances cholinergic transmission in autonomic ganglia. Clinical experience, however, has yielded erratic outcomes.

It is necessary to carefully titrate pressor drugs. It is important to adjust medication schedules so that each drug's peak effect occurs at the same time that orthostatic hypotension symptoms are at their worst. 24-hour ambulatory blood pressure monitoring is frequently helpful in detecting hypotensive episodes that might not be evident in the workplace, such as in the morning, following a meal, or following physical activity.

e. ***Correcting Anemia:*** Anemia must be treated since it can make OH worse. Recombinant erythropoietin treatment raises blood pressure by inhibiting nitric oxide, increasing red blood cell mass and blood viscosity. Patients with hypotensive Parkinsonian anemia may benefit from a 6-week course of recombinant erythropoietin (4000 units twice-weekly) administered subcutaneously.

- **Pharmacological Strategies for Postprandial Hypotension:** Large meals high in carbohydrates should be avoided because they make postprandial hypotension worse. It has been demonstrated that medications that block α-glucosidase, such as acarbose and vogibose, are useful in treating postprandial hypotension. By inhibiting α-glucosidase in the small intestine's brush border, these medications lessen the breakdown of complex carbohydrates. Lessening the postprandial drop in blood pressure is probably achieved by slowing down the absorption of glucose and the release of vasodilatory hormones. Octreotide, a somatostatin analog, can cause splanchnic vasoconstriction and may be helpful in treating postprandial hypotension in patients.
- **Cardiac Denervation in PD:** One distinctive feature of PD diagnosis is loss of cardiac sympathetic neurons. The fatigue that many patients describe may be a result of sympathetic denervation of the heart, which may occur before motor features. A recent small study found that the I-MIBG heart-to-mediastinal uptake ratio was significantly lower in PD patients who reported feeling fatigued (123) than in patients who did not report fatigue. Research conducted on heart transplant recipients indicates that exercise capacity is negatively impacted by cardiac denervation. In fact, patients with PD had lower heart rates (HRs) and blood pressure (BPs) during exercise stress testing than controls, and a retrospective analysis of these tests revealed that the maximal HR increase was attenuated in patients who later developed Parkinson's disease.

In genetic PD, the degree of cardiac denervation varies. Patients with PD who also have the LRRK2 mutation, for instance, seem to have less cardiac sympathetic denervation than patients with PD who also have the synuclein gene mutation E46K or who have PD but no known genetic mutation.

- **Supine Hypertension:** In addition to OH, arterial hypertension is common in supine patients with PD and autonomic failure. Even though it doesn't cause any symptoms, nighttime hypertension speeds up the damage to end organ targets. Drugs that lower blood pressure can exacerbate orthostatic hypotension, making treatment challenging. This problem can be partially resolved by sleeping with the head of the bed raised. Administering short-acting vasodilators (hydralazine, nitrates) while supine at night is another option, but caution must be exercised as they have the potential to significantly worsen OH.

5.4.4. Gastrointestinal

Perhaps the most prevalent sign of autonomic impairment in PD patients, constipation is a powerful predictor of the disease's future course. LB is found in enteric neurons throughout the gastrointestinal tract (GI tract) in patients with PD. This includes the esophagus, stomach, small intestine, and colon. In particular, LB is found in neurons of the Auerbach plexus in the lower esophagus, primarily in vasoactive intestinal polypeptide-containing neurons. Remarkably, at three months of age, transgenic mice expressing mutant human α-synuclein displayed distinct abnormalities in the function of the enteric nervous system and immunoreactive aggregates of synuclein in the enteric ganglia.

- **Drooling:** Overdrooling of saliva is typical in Parkinson's disease patients. Rather than excessive salivation, this is the result of not swallowing. Anticholinergics are generally ineffective and have a side effect of decreasing gut motility, which, along with cognitive impairment, limits their clinical usefulness as a drooling therapy. Botulinum toxin injections directly into the salivary glands are becoming more and more common; however, the toxin may migrate into neighboring muscles and cause dysphagia.
- **Gastroparesis and Constipation:** Patients with PD frequently experience gastroparesis, or the slow emptying of the stomach. In order to prevent malnutrition, it is important to carefully manage common symptoms of gastroparesis, such as nausea and the sensation of fullness soon after starting a meal. Additionally, gastroparesis may impede levodopa's therapeutic effect and absorption in the duodenum.

Patients with PD frequently experience constipation, either as a result of impaired gut motility or abnormal control of the pelvic floor muscles used in defecation. There have been reports of megacolon and pseudo-obstruction in PD patients.

Stool softeners and diet adjustments are helpful. Patients with PD cannot take methoclopramide because it centrally blocks dopamine receptors by crossing the blood-brain barrier. In cases of gastroparesis, dopamine blockers like domperidone—which hardly passes the blood–brain barrier—are frequently administered. Injections of botulinum toxin and apomorphrine into the external sphincter or puburectalis muscle have reportedly been helpful in treating pelvic floor muscle dyssynergia.

A marked or very marked improvement was reported by 16 out of 25 (64%) subjects receiving lubiprostone, which locally activates intestinal ClC-2 chloride channels and increases intestinal fluid secretion without changing serum electrolyte levels, versus five of 27 (18.5%) subjects receiving placebo in a randomized, placebo-controlled study involving 54 subjects with PD and constipation ($p = 0.001$).

5.4.5. Respiratory

Autonomic dysfunction may not be the only cause of respiratory issues linked to PD. In PD, respiratory dyskinesias, restrictive disorders, upper airway obstruction, and other drug-related respiratory disorders can occur. Additionally, some PD patients have sleep apnea and irregular breathing, which may be related to autonomic nervous system involvement.

5.4.6. Bladder Dysfunction

For both men and women with PD, the most prevalent urinary symptom is frequent urination caused by hyperactive detrusor muscle. Urinary incontinence can happen, but it is more common in MSA patients, which should raise concerns regarding the diagnosis. Because the symptoms of an enlarged prostate can be very similar, it is important to take this condition into account when diagnosing bladder dysfunction in older men. To diagnose neurogenic bladder and differentiate it from benign prostatic hypertrophy, urodynamic studies may be required. The urethral sphincter is constricted by the dense innervation of α-receptors at the urethral outlet.

Bladder and urethra outlet dilatation is made possible by α-adrenergic blockade, which also makes it easier to empty the bladder. These medications should be used cautiously in PD patients since they may exacerbate or cause OH. Subcutaneous apomorphine and detrusor muscle injections with botulinum toxin are other methods. Reducing fluid intake in the evening and sleeping with the head and torso raised to lessen supine hypertension are two ways to lessen the frequency of nocturia.

5.4.7. Sexual Dysfunction

PD patients frequently experience sexual dysfunction. Men frequently experience erectile dysfunction, decreased sexual arousal, low sex drive, and inability to achieve an orgasm. In women with Parkinson's disease, the frequency of sexual dysfunction is frequently underreported. Sexual dysfunction may be caused by a variety of factors, including a dopamine deficiency. Prior to treating sexual dysfunction, the patient and spouse must have a conversation. One should think about potential drug side effects as a potential source of sexual dysfunction. Although severe OH limits the usefulness of sildenafil (Viagra, Pfizer, NY, USA) in certain patients, it is frequently effective in improving erectile dysfunction in male patients. Patients need to be aware of this risk and refrain from having sex while standing. Apomorphine can boost libido and cause a penile erection. Despite erectile dysfunction, high dosages of anti-Parkinson medications can cause an increase in sexual drive. For female PD patients experiencing sexual dysfunction, there are currently no proven treatments. (Kinateder & Marinho, 2022)

5.4.8. Thermoregulation and Sweating

Thermoregulatory and sudomotor abnormalities in Parkinson's disease patients lack a distinct phenotype. It has been documented that hyper- and hypo-hydrosis, as well as normal sweating function, exist. Sweating profusely when taking medication that inhibits dopaminergic activity (i.e., off periods) is most likely the most typical sudomotor complaint in patients with "on/off phenomena." Thermoregulation abnormalities have the potential to be fatal. According to recent research from France, summertime heat increases the risk of death for patients with Parkinson's disease and OH.

5.4.9. Dermatological

PD patients frequently experience seborrhea. Its intensity varies widely. One possibility for its mechanisms is aberrant skin autonomic innervation. It is unknown whether skin deposition of synuclein contributes to seborrhea. For the treatment of this PD-related dermatologic issue, intracutaneous botulinum toxin injection may be useful in addition to standard dermatological therapies.

5.4.10. Scales of Autonomic Dysfunction

A self-administered questionnaire called the autonomic scale for outcomes in Parkinson's disease (SCOPA-AUT) is used to screen for autonomic dysfunction and determine its severity. With 25 questions covering orthostatic, gastrointestinal, urinary, thermoregulatory, pupillomotor, and sexual topics, it is simple to use. It might not be as sensitive in identifying orthostatic symptoms.

Recently, the validity of the OH questionnaire was confirmed with the aim of evaluating the degree of OH symptoms and their influence on day-to-day activities. It works well for determining how well treatments are working. It does not, however, address the non-cardiovascular components of autonomic dysfunction.

5.5. Biomarkers for Parkinson's Disease

Biomarkers are traits that can be objectively measured and serve as markers for either pathophysiology or normal physiological function.

Biomarkers may help with prognosis, diagnosis, and therapy response prediction. Imaging biomarkers that measure the dopaminergic system's integrity have been thoroughly studied in relation to Parkinson's disease. There is a significant unmet need for the development of biomarkers that evaluate the state of α-synuclein pathology or that target particular disease mechanisms. These biomarkers may hasten the identification of therapies that alter the course of disease (Emamzadeh et al. 2018).

5.5.1. Importance of Biomarkers for Parkinson's Disease

These could be conducted on blood, cerebrospinal fluid (CSF), or other tissues using biochemical assays, structural or molecular imaging studies, or other techniques. Biomarkers may help with diagnosis as well as prognostic and therapy response prediction.

The significance of biomarkers in PD cannot be overstated, as the disease can be challenging to diagnose in its early stages and its gradual progression over time makes it challenging to assess treatment efficacy or disease activity. Imaging biomarkers that evaluate the level of dopaminergic integrity have been studied in great detail. For instance, striatal dopamine transporters (DATs) can now be purchased commercially using single-photon emission computed tomography (SPECT) scan imaging. Important areas of ongoing research include the development and validation of biomarkers that measure the state of α-synuclein (α-syn) pathology or that record response to potentially disease-modifying treatments.

5.5.2. Biomarker Definitions and Conceptual Framework

The working group on NIH biomarkers definitions has created a standard set of definitions for biomarker-related terms and positioned them within a theoretical framework that takes into account the connection between biomarkers and significant clinical outcomes as well as physiological aspects of disease activity. This framework's primary definitions are:

- A biological marker (biomarker) is a characteristic that is objectively measured and evaluated as an indicator of normal biological processes, pathogenic processes, or pharmacologic response to a therapeutic intervention;
- A clinical end point is defined as a characteristic or variable that reflects how a patient feels, functions or survives. In a clinical trial, changes ina clinical end point may reflect the effect of a therapeutic intervention. For the purpose of understanding the usefulness of a drug in a clinical setting, clinical end points are the most credible measure that can be assessed in a clinical trial;
- A surrogate end point is a biomarker that is intended to substitute for a clinical end point. A surrogate end point is expected to predict clinical benefit or harm, or lack of benefit or harm based on epidemiologic, therapeutic, pathophysiologic or other scientific evidence. Surrogate end points are a subset of biomarkers. The NIH

> working group discouraged the use of the term 'surrogate marker' because it suggests the substitution is for a marker rather than for a clinical end point.

There are several applications for biomarkers in clinical care and research. Biomarkers provide a biological activity indication and can be employed as clinical trial outcome measures in the drug development process. Biomarkers are helpful in clinical care as prognosticators, treatment response monitors, and supplements to clinical diagnosis. When a biomarker's activity offers a window into a physiological or clinical process that is challenging to observe directly, it is almost always most helpful. Variations in a biomarker, for instance, could reveal whether a medication is attaching to its target or changing a physiological function. This kind of data is useful for early-stage clinical trials. The use of biomarkers for clinical processes can provide insight into future events, such as anticipated disease activity or treatment response (Wu et al., 2011).

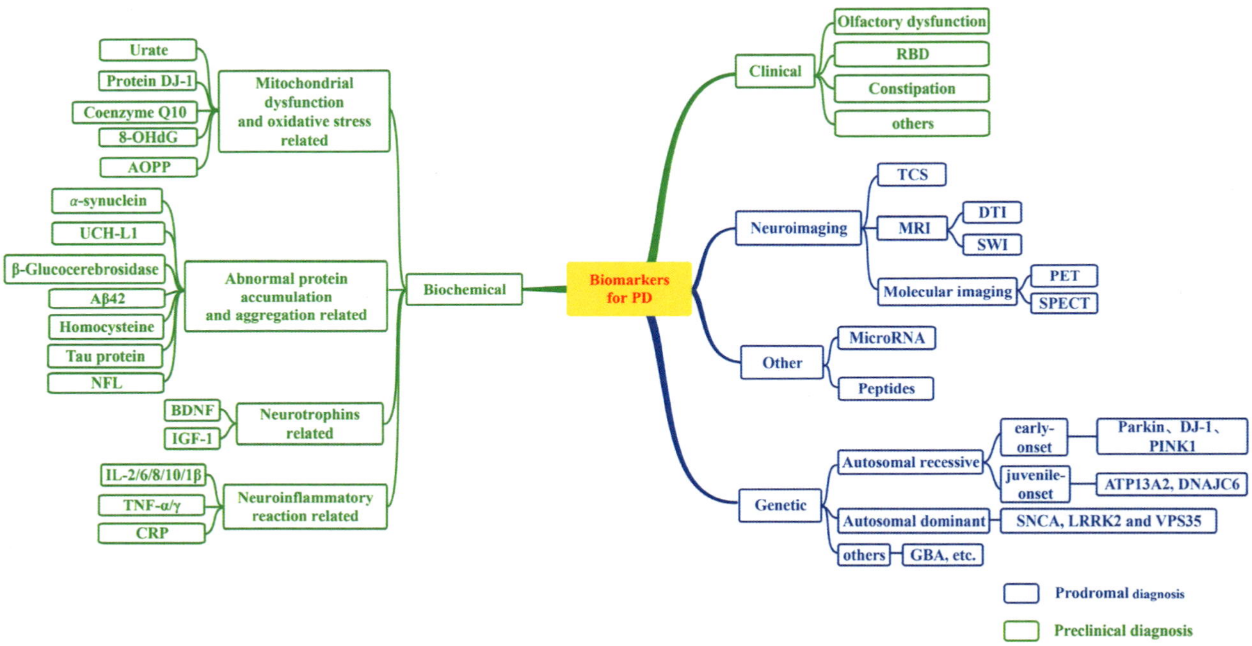

Figure 5.6. *Types of biomarkers for PD.*

Source: He R, Yan X, Guo J, Xu Q, Tang B and Sun Q (2018) Recent Advances in Biomarkers for Parkinson's Disease. Front. Aging Neurosci. 10:305. doi: 10.3389/fnagi.2018.00305.

Only a tiny portion of all biomarkers are surrogate end points. The effect that would be seen on a pertinent clinical end point would be perfectly captured by an ideal surrogate end point. Because regulatory bodies may accept evidence of a significant effect on a surrogate end point as adequate proof of a therapy's efficacy, surrogate end points are especially valuable. It can be difficult to determine a legitimate surrogate end point measure, and there aren't many instances of legitimate surrogate end points. As of right now, no biomarkers for Parkinson's disease are recognized as surrogate end points. Examples of surrogate end points from other medical specialties include blood levels of cholesterol as a proxy for the impact of lipid-lowering therapy on cardiovascular outcomes, such as stroke and death, and HIV viral load as a measure of antiretroviral therapy efficacy. It is necessary for a surrogate end point to fully capture the net effect of treatment on the clinical outcome as well as correlate with the true clinical outcome. When a biomarker is not directly linked to the mechanism through which a therapy affects a disease, or when a therapy has multiple mechanisms of action (or toxicity), then the biomarker may not be a valid surrogate end point.

Apart from the previously mentioned categorization scheme, biomarkers can also be defined as indicators of a state or a trait. A state biomarker assesses the disease's current state. One type of state biomarker is DAT imaging, which is subject to change over time in tandem with the physiology it measures. Trait biomarkers quantify an attribute, like a genetic mutation, that remains constant over time. The best use cases for trait biomarkers are in diagnosis; they can also serve as disease risk markers. State biomarkers may be helpful in monitoring changes in the disease over time and the effectiveness of treatment in addition to being helpful in diagnosis.

5.5.3. Biomarkers for PD: Biochemical Biomarkers

Components that are measured in blood or other bodily fluids or tissues (biopsy or pathology specimens) are known as biochemical biomarkers. Because standardized quantitative analysis is frequently possible and biochemical biomarkers have the potential to be relatively inexpensive and scalable, they are especially valuable. Inexpensive, scalable biomarkers include basic blood tests and genetic tests based on single-nucleotide polymorphism.

Although many entities have been studied in the highly active field of searching for biochemical biomarkers for PD (Figure 5.6), no reliable and clinically valid biochemical markers have yet to be found (Delenclos , 2016).

A large portion of the search for biochemical biomarkers for PD has been directed towards α-syn protein since it seems to be crucial to the disease's pathophysiology. One can measure α-syn in various tissues such as blood, CSF, saliva, and biopsy samples taken from the brain or peripheral areas (e.g., stomach or salivary organs). Thus far, these investigations have failed to yield a α-syn-based biomarker that exhibits a strong correlation with the severity of the disease or is capable of accurately differentiating PD patients from controls. Certain studies have reported higher levels of soluble α-syn in plasma; however, these findings have not been reliably repeated. Reduced levels of α-syn in the CSF have been linked to an increased risk of PD, but not to the extent that measuring α-syn in the CSF would be a helpful PD diagnostic test. Furthermore, there isn't any solid proof as of yet that CSF α-syn levels vary over time. There is still hope that studying pathological forms of α-syn, such as aggregated or phosphorylated forms, will prove more beneficial than studying total α-syn.

Apart from α-syn, several other plausible biochemical biomarkers have been investigated. A rare cause of familial PD is mutations in DJ-1, which is a component of the cellular defense against oxidative stress. Research on DJ-1 in blood and CSF that tried to differentiate PD patients from controls produced mixed results; no correlation with the severity of the disease has been shown. Another candidate PD biomarker that has been explored is the presence of urea in the plasma or CSF. Higher plasma uric acid levels have been linked to a lower risk of PD in epidemiological studies. Furthermore, a small number of studies in clinical trial cohorts have shown that elevated blood or CSF uric acid levels are linked to a slower rate of progression of PD motor feature development. An ongoing clinical trial of inosine, which raises uric acid levels, is investigating whether an intervention to raise uric acid levels will slow the progression of PD. More, independent studies are required to validate these findings.

Biomarker discovery techniques such as transcriptomics (measuring mRNA expression), proteomics (assays of large panels of proteins), and metabolomics (studies of large panels of cellular metabolites using spectroscopy) are now feasible due to advancements in high-throughput screening technology and computing power. These methods employ fluid samples from sizable patient and control cohorts to search a comparatively large panel of potential analytes for group differences. These methods have the potential to uncover new biomarkers and disease mechanisms because it is not always clear which analytes will provide useful information. False discovery is a serious risk, though, so findings from "-omics" research must be confirmed in different cohorts.

Biomarkers could be used to monitor particular PD characteristics. Numerous research have looked into the CSF's biochemical biomarkers as potential indicators of cognitive decline. Patients with demented PD have been found to have lower concentrations of CSF amyloid-β, an established biomarker for Alzheimer's disease, when compared to nondemented PD patients. Elevations of p-Tau and total Tau, which are also indicative of Alzheimer's disease, are less reliable, though. Lower serum EGF levels in patients with PD were linked to a faster rate of cognitive decline in a proteomics study with independent replication.

To sum up, biochemical biomarkers have great potential for use in PD diagnosis, prognosis, and treatment response. Because α-syn-based biomarkers are likely linked to central disease mechanisms, they are especially appealing. Nevertheless, research has not yet found a biochemical biomarker in CSF or blood that is sensitive enough or specific enough to be helpful as a diagnostic tool. Furthermore, there is currently insufficient data to support the use of these markers as indicators of the course of the disease or the effectiveness of treatment. To find biochemical biomarkers that are clinically useful, more research will be required. Although more successful, attempts to find biomarkers of cognitive decline in PD have not addressed all of the mechanisms causing cognitive decline and may not apply to everyone who does not exhibit cognitive symptoms (Wu et al, 2011).

A Closer Look

Biomarkers for PD: Imaging Biomarkers

Imaging biomarkers for PD range from molecular imaging techniques using either positron emission tomography (PET) or SPECT to structural imaging with MRI or transcranial ultrasound. In contrast to the situation with biochemical biomarkers, several imaging biomarkers have shown the potential to be useful as diagnostics, and one is available for clinical practice. The role of these modalities in prognosis and response to therapy is less well defined.

Author	Year	Objective	Algorithm	Result	Pros	Cons
Nunes et al. [12]	2019	To discriminate PSD, HC and Alzheimer's disease data using retina texture biomarkers	SVM	Classification of PSD, HC, and Alzheimer's disease accuracy = 82.9%	Classify PSD, AD and HC from the data	Lower Accuracy
Pereira et al. [13]	2019	To classify the PSD patient using medical imaging	AI algorithms	Classification accuracy of PSD and HC subject accuracy = 65.7%	Classify PD, and HC subject from SPECT and MRI images	Lower accuracy
Mangesius et al. [14]	2020	Proposed decision algorithm to classify parkinsonism with imaging biomarkers	Decision tree algorithm	Classification of parkinsonism accuracy = 83.7%	Classify PD, MSA and PSP from MRI imaging biomarker	Does not given the classification of HC subject
Lin et al. [15]	2020	To detect the disease progression of PSD patient	Biomedical method to extract the data	-	Provide a disease progression of 3-year data of PSD patient	Does not given a classification of HC subject
Kathuria et al. [16]	2021	To classify and diagnosis of PSD patient from atypical parkinsonism and HC using MRI and F-DOPA PET imaging	Biomedical method to extract the features from imaging modality	MRI_VenoBOLD Accuracy: 95% Sensitivity: 88.4% Specificity: 66.7%, MRI_SWI Sensitivity: 93% Specificity: 80%	Diagnosis of idiopathic PSD and atypical parkinsonism with nigrosome imaging	Small sample size of atypical parkinsonism subject.
The proposed scheme	2021	Classification of PSD and HC patients using imaging biomarkers data	Stacked ML model	Accuracy = 92.5%, F1_score = 98%, Precision = 98% and Recall = 97%	Diagnosis of PSD and HC using imaging biomarkers, Measures the disease progression of PSD patient	-

Source: Hathaliya J, Modi H, Gupta R, Tanwar S, Alqahtani F, Elghatwary M, Neagu B-C, Raboaca MS. Stacked Model-Based Classification of Parkinson's Disease Patients Using Imaging Biomarker Data. *Biosensors.* 2022; 12(8):579. https://doi.org/10.3390/bios12080579.

Dopaminergic imaging is currently the most well-established category of biomarker for PD and related disorders. Dopaminergic degeneration is central to the pathological process in PD, and changes can be measured with imaging in a way that corresponds well to accepted concepts of PD pathology. Longitudinal studies show that dopaminergic imaging leads to an earlier accurate diagnosis of a Parkinsonian syndrome. However, one key limitation of dopaminergic imaging is that it is abnormal in several degenerative Parkinsonian syndromes other than PD, including progressive supranuclear palsy (PSP) and multiple system atrophy (MSA), and does not distinguish PD from these disorders. PET and SPECT techniques are available to measure pre-and post-synaptic neurons in the nigrostriatal pathways. 123-iodine-labeled 2-β-carbomethoxy-3β-(4-iodophenyl) tropane ([^{123}I] β-CIT) SPECT, which assesses the DAT, and [^{18}F] fluorodopa ($_F$-dopa)-PET, which assesses dopamine storage capacity and dopa-decarboxylase activity, have probably been the most widely used tracers in research to measure the integrity of the nigrostriatal system. In addition, the SPECT tracer, ioflupane ^{123}I (DaTscan, GE Healthcare, UK), was approved by the US FDA for the detection of DATs in patients with suspected Parkinsonian syndromes and is available for clinical use. Other tracers that evaluate the vesicular monoamine transporter are available as research tools. These tracers capture much of the same information as DAT or $_F$-dopa imaging. Dopaminergic imaging hasproven to be a useful natural history biomarker, showing consistent declines in binding of approximately 5–10% per year. In addition, a recent study showed that patients with more severe dopaminergic loss at baseline experienced more rapid motor and cognitive decline.

While they are generally accepted as diagnostic and natural history biomarkers, the use of dopaminergic imaging as a marker of therapeutic response is controversial. In three trials where they have been used as biomarkers, the changes observed in the imaging biomarkers were inconsistent with clinical measures. In each of these cases, patients treated with levodopa had deterioration in imaging results that were not correlated with changes in clinical status. The failure of these biomarkers to capture the effect on clinical status has led many experts to question their validity as surrogate end points. The difficulty in interpreting these studies demonstrates the challenges in validating biomarkers for use as surrogate end points in interventional studies.

A number of other imaging tests have been investigated as PD biomarkers. One example is metabolic imaging with ^{18}F-deoxyglucose PET, which is a marker of cerebral metabolism. PD and other Parkinsonian syndromes, such as PSP and MSA, each produce distinctive patterns of abnormal cerebral metabolism that can be detected by ^{18}F-deoxyglucose PET and computer-assisted, voxelbased analysis systems. Using these techniques, PD can be differentiated from other Parkinsonian syndromes, something that is not possible with dopaminergic imaging. A specific metabolic pattern has also been identified in patients with PD dementia that differentiates these individuals from nondemented PD patients.

Conventional MRI shows nonspecific abnormalities in PD and has not been useful as a biomarker. However, newer MRI techniques may have greater value. A study using diffusion tensor imaging of the substantia nigra (SN) showed 100% differentiation between PD patients and controls. Diffusionweighted MRI has been reported to be highly sensitive to changes in striatal structure and can differentiate PD (which is relatively normal) from PSP but not the Parkinsonian form of MSA. In addition, studies using high-field strength (7 T) MRI allow for detailed visualization of the SN and accurate quantification of SN volume. These advanced MRI techniques may prove to be useful biomarkers in the future. However, the results of studies using MRI as a diagnostic need to be replicated in independent groups of patients with early PD and longitudinal studies are needed to test whether MRI is sensitive to disease progression.

Transcranial sonography (TCS) is another structural imaging technique that has been widely used in PD. Approximately 90% of patients with clinically diagnosed PD have been reported to show increased mid-brain echogenicity by TCS. However, TCS does not detect abnormal midbrain signals in either MSA or PSP. Interestingly, midbrain hyperechogenicity has also been reported in asymptomatic carriers at risk for monogenic forms of Parkinsonism. Thus, TCS may be useful as both a diagnostic and a risk marker for PD.

In summary, there are some imaging biomarkers that may be useful in PD. Of these, dopaminergic imaging is the best developed. Dopaminergic imaging modalities have been shown to accurately diagnose dopaminergic degeneration. Their weakness as diagnostic biomarkers is that they do not distinguish PD from other degenerative Parkinsonian syndromes. Dopaminergic imaging is also useful as a natural history biomarker; however, its utility as a measure of treatment response remains uncertain. Other imaging technologies, particularly those based on MRI, are developing rapidly and may prove to be useful in the future. While the field of imaging biomarkers is well developedin comparison with biochemical biomarkers for PD, there is a clear gap in the ability of imaging technology to measure disease mechanisms that are specific to PD. In particular, a tracer that could identify deposits of α-syn *in vivo* would fill several key gaps. As a research tool, for example, it could provide *in vivo* evidence of the pathological spread of PD pathology. It would also be useful in monitoring experimental treatments that target α-syn. In clinical practice, α-syn imaging would probably be fairly comparable to current dopaminergic imaging but would improve the differential diagnosis of PD versus PSP (although not necessarily PD vs. MSA). α-syn imaging would also allow for monitoring of clinically meaningful disease progression from pathology confined to the mid-brain to widespread limbic and neocortical pathology (Wu et al, 2011).

Summary

- PD is a neurodegenerative disorder characterized by motor findings of rest tremor, bradykinesia and rigidity. Non-motor features of PD have received greater attention in the past two decades owing to their recognized contribution to disability in advancing disease. These include hyposmia and other sensory abnormalities, autonomic changes, sleep impairment and neurobehavioral problems including depression and dementia.
- Sensory symptoms, and pain, in particular, are common non-motor features of PD. Indeed, virtually all patients with PD experience at least one sensory symptom as part of their prodrome, and such symptoms increase in prevalence and severity with the progression of the disease.
- Pain is a common NMS of PD and in some severe or intractable pain may be a dominant problem that some patients find more distressing than the motor disability. PD-related pain is heterogeneous and in up to a quarter of patients, chronic pain precedes the onset of motor symptoms or the start of anti-Parkinsonian treatment.
- Akathisia, defined as a subjective inner restlessness associated with an inability to remain still and a constant need to move or change positions, is also a common cause of discomfort in patients with PD.
- Cognitive and behavioral abnormalities are prominent over the course of PD. As the neuropsychiatric disturbances are frequently disabling, often more so than motor aspects of PD, comprehensive management of the patient with PD requires recognition and treatment of these comorbidities.
- Sleep disturbances are common problems in PD patients. Because of depression and/ or hallucination, patients may become restless at night and have difficulty falling asleep. Those at higher risk for pathologic sleep are male patients with advanced disease, cognitive impairment, drug-induced psychosis, and orthostatic hypotension. After falling asleep, patients may still wake up frequently because of stiffness of their bodies or urinary urgency at night. As a result, they have difficulty achieving restful sleep.
- Dysfunction of the autonomic nervous system is almost always present in patients with Parkinson's Disease, but its severity varies. It is important for clinicians to be aware of and recognize autonomic impairment because many of its features can be treated, which can dramatically improve quality of life.
- Biomarkers are objectively measured characteristics that are indicators of either normal physiological function or pathophysiology. Biomarkers have the potential to aid in diagnosis, prognosis and predicting response to therapy. In the case of Parkinson's disease, imaging biomarkers that assess the integrity of the dopaminergic system have been investigated extensively. Development of biomarkers that assess the status of α-synuclein pathology or that address specific disease mechanisms is an area of substantial unmet need. Such biomarkers have the potential to accelerate the discovery of disease-modifying treatments.

References

1. Abbott, R. D., Petrovitch, H., White, L. R., et al. (2001). Frequency of bowel movements and the future risk of Parkinson's disease. *Neurology, 57*(3), 456–462.
2. Beiske, A. G., Loge, J. H., Ronningen, A., et al. (2009). Pain in Parkinson's disease: prevalence and characteristics. *Pain, 141*, 173–177.
3. Braak, H., Del Tredici, K., Rüb, U., et al. (2003). Staging of brain pathology related to sporadic Parkinson's disease. *Neurobiology of Aging, 24*, 197–210.
4. Brefel-Courbon, C., Thalamas, C., Rascol, O., et al. (2000). Lack of autonomic nervous dysfunction in progressive supranuclear palsy, a study of blood pressure variability. *Clinical Autonomic Research, 10*(5), 309–312.
5. Buhmann, C., Kassubek, J., & Jost, W. H. (2020). Management of Pain in Parkinson's Disease. *Journal of Parkinson's Disease, 10*(s1), S37–S48.
6. Chaudhuri, K. R., & Schapira, A. H. (2009). Nonmotor symptoms in Parkinson's disease: dopaminergic pathophysiology and treatment. *The Lancet Neurology, 8*, 464–474.
7. Chaudhuri, K. R., Prieto-Jurcynska, C., Naidu, Y., et al. (2010). The nondeclaration of nonmotor symptoms of Parkinson's disease to healthcare professionals: an international study using the non-motor symptoms questionnaire. *Movement Disorders, 25*, 704–709.
8. Davidsdottir, S., Cronin-Golomb, A., & Lee, A. (2005). Visual and spatial symptoms in Parkinson's disease. *Vision Research, 45*, 1285–1296.
9. Deeb, J., Shah, M., Muhammed, N., et al. (2010). A basic smell test is as sensitive as a dopamine transporter scan: comparison of olfaction, taste and DaTSCAN in the diagnosis of Parkinson's disease. *QJM: An International Journal of Medicine, 103*(12), 941–952.
10. Delenclos, M., Jones, D. R., McLean, P. J., & Uitti, R. J. (2016). Biomarkers in Parkinson's disease: Advances and strategies. *Parkinsonism & Related Disorders, 22*(Suppl 1), S106–S110.
11. Emamzadeh, F. N., & Surguchov, A. (2018). Parkinson's Disease: Biomarkers, Treatment, and Risk Factors. *Frontiers in Neuroscience, 12*, 612.
12. Goldstein, D. S., et al. (2000). Cardiac sympathetic denervation in Parkinson's Disease. *Annals of Internal Medicine, 133*(5), 338–347.
13. Guo, X., Gao, G., Wang, X., et al. (2008). Effects of bilateral deep brain stimulation of the subthalamic nucleus on olfactory function in Parkinson's disease patients. *Stereotactic and Functional Neurosurgery, 86*(4), 237–244.
14. Haehner, A., Boesveldt, S., Berendse, H. W., et al. (2009). Prevalence of smell loss in Parkinson's disease – a multicenter study. *Parkinsonism & Related Disorders, 15*, 490–494.
15. Haehner, A., Hummel, T., & Reichmann, H. (2011). Olfactory loss in Parkinson's disease. *Parkinson's Disease, 2011*, 450939.
16. Hawkes, C. H. (2008). The prodromal phase sporadic Parkinson's disease: does it exist and if so, how long is it? *Movement Disorders, 23*(13), 1799–1807.
17. Izawa, M. O., Miwa, H., Kajimoto, Y., et al. (2012). Combination of transcranial sonography, olfactory testing, and MIBG myocardial scintigraphy as a diagnostic indicator for Parkinson's disease. *European Journal of Neurology, 19*(3), 411–416.

18. Jankovic, J. (n.d.). Parkinson's disease: diagnosis, motor symptoms and non-motor features. *Future Medicine*. DOI: 10.2217/9781780843391.

19. Kaufmann, H., & Biaggioni, I. (2003). Autonomic failure in neurodegenerative disorders. *Seminars in Neurology, 23*(4), 351–363.

20. Kaufmann, H., Malamut, R., Norcliffe-Kaufmann, L., et al. (2012). The Orthostatic Hypotension Questionnaire (OHQ): validation of a novel symptom assessment scale. *Clinical Autonomic Research, 22*(2), 79–90.

21. Kaufmann, H., Nahm, K., Purohit, D., et al. (2004). Autonomic failure as the initial presentation of Parkinson's Disease and dementia with Lewy bodies. *Neurology, 63*(6), 1093–1095.

22. Kinateder, T., Marinho, D., Gruber, D., Hatzler, L., Ebersbach, G., & Gandor, F. (2022). Sexual Dysfunctions in Parkinson's Disease and Their Influence on Partnership-Data of the PRISM Study. *Brain Sciences, 12*(2), 159.

23. Lang, A. E. (2011). A critical appraisal of the premotor symptoms of Parkinson's disease: potential usefulness in early diagnosis and design of neuroprotective trials. *Movement Disorders, 26*(5), 775–783.

24. Muller, B., Larsen, J. P., Wentzel-Larsen, T., et al. (2011). Autonomic and sensory symptoms and signs in incident, untreated Parkinson's disease: frequent but mild. *Movement Disorders, 26*(1), 65–72.

25. Norcliffe-Kaufmann, L., & Kaufmann, H. (2013). Autonomic dysfunction in Parkinson's Disease. DOI: 10.2217/9781780843391.

26. Ondo, W. (2009). Parkinson's disease and restless legs syndrome. In K. R. Chaudhuri, E. Tolosa, A. Schapira, & W. Poewe (Eds.), *Non-Motor Symptoms of Parkinson's disease (1st Edition)* (pp. 195–203). University Press, Oxford, UK.

27. Orimo, S., Takahashi, A., Uchihara, T., et al. (2007). Degeneration of cardiac sympathetic nerve begins in the early disease process of Parkinson's disease. *Brain Pathology, 17*(1), 24–30.

28. Rahayel, S., Frasnelli, J., & Joubert, S. (2012). The effect of Alzheimer's disease and Parkinson's disease on olfaction: A metanalysis. *Behavioral Brain Research, 231*(1), 60–74.

29. Riedel, O., Klotsche, J., Spottke, A., Deuschl, G., Förstl, H., Henn, F., et al. (2010). Frequency of dementia, depression, and other neuropsychiatric symptoms in 1,449 outpatients with Parkinson's disease. *Journal of Neurology, 257*, 1073–1082.

30. Saadat, P., Faramarzi, M., Salimkhani, F., & Khafri, S. (2020). Psychiatric Symptoms in Patients and Caregivers with Parkinson's Disease. *Oman Medical Journal, 35*(6), e205.

31. Trojano, L., & Papagno, C. (2018). Cognitive and behavioral disorders in Parkinson's disease: an update. II: behavioral disorders. *Neurological Sciences, 39*(1), 53–61.

32. Velseboer, D. C., de Haan, R. J., Wieling, W., et al. (2011). Prevalence of orthostatic hypotension in Parkinson's disease: a systematic review and meta-analysis. *Parkinsonism & Related Disorders, 17*(10), 724–729.

33. Visser, M., Marinus, J., Stiggelbout, A. M., et al. (2004). Assessment of autonomic dysfunction in Parkinson's disease: the SCOPA-AUT. *Movement Disorders, 19*(11), 1306–1312.

34. Wattendorf, E., Welge-Lüssen, A., Fiedler, K., et al. (2009). Olfactory impairment predicts brain atrophy in Parkinson's disease. *Journal of Neuroscience, 29*(49), 15410–15413.

35. Westermann, B., Wattendorf, E., Schwerdtfeger, U., et al. (2008). Functional modulation of cortical olfactory pathways in Parkinson's disease: an fMRI study. *Journal of Neurology, Neurosurgery, and Psychiatry, 79*, 19–24.

36. Wu, Y., Le, W., & Jankovic, J. (2011). Preclinical biomarkers of Parkinson's disease. *Archives of Neurology, 68*, 22–30.

Chapter

SURGICAL THERAPY FOR PARKINSON'S DISEASE

6

Contents

Introduction

An estimated one million Americans, both men and women of all ages and races, are thought to be affected by PD, though men are slightly more likely to get it than women. The primary risk factor for Parkinson's disease is getting older, but environmental and genetic factors also play a role. Although there isn't a cure, there are plenty of effective symptomatic interventions. Treatments such as holistic approaches, holistic medicine, nutrition, exercise, and surgery can all help to improve quality of life and lessen symptoms. Tremor, bradykinesia (slowness of movement), rigidity (muscle stiffness), and postural instability (difficulty balancing) are common signs of Parkinson's disease. These are known as PD "motor" symptoms. Numerous non-motor symptoms also exist, the most notable of which are fatigue, apathy, depression, anxiety, and sexual dysfunction.

Early on in PD (i.e., the first few years following a diagnosis), most patients' symptoms are usually under control with medication. However, as the illness worsens, people might need to take higher doses of their medications, take them more frequently, and sometimes even more frequently. People with PD may observe that as the disease progresses, there will be times during the day when their symptoms are adequately controlled (also known as "on time"), times when their symptoms are significantly worse (also known as "off time"), and times when their medication peaks (usually an hour after taking a dose) and causes them to move involuntarily. Dyskinesia is the term used to describe these uncontrollable movements. People are said to have motor fluctuations when they transition between any one of these three states. a kind of surgery that can be used to lessen Parkinson's disease symptoms in a subgroup of people who have been carefully chosen and have a particular symptom or symptoms that may respond to this kind of therapy. Deep brain stimulation is the name of the treatment (DBS). Some, but not all, of the debilitating symptoms of PD can be treated with DBS, a well-researched and successful surgery. Thalamotomy, pallidotomy, and subthalamotomy are a few more surgeries that have been used to treat Parkinson's disease symptoms.

Orientation and Directional Terms:

Term	Definition	Illustration
Globus pallidus internus (GPi)	A specific region of the brain that is involved in motor pathways. It is one target site for DBS therapy.	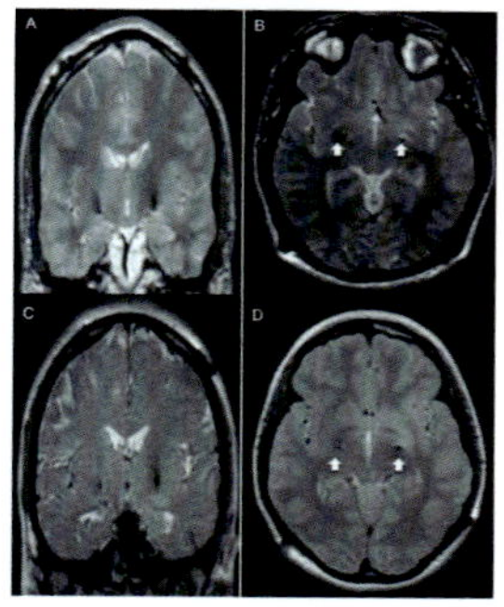
Implantable pulse generator (IPG)	Also called the neurostimulator, the IPG is the battery-powered device that is used to deliver electricity to the brain lead. A similar generator is also used for heart pacemakers. It is most often surgically implanted under the skin of the upper chest just below the collarbone.	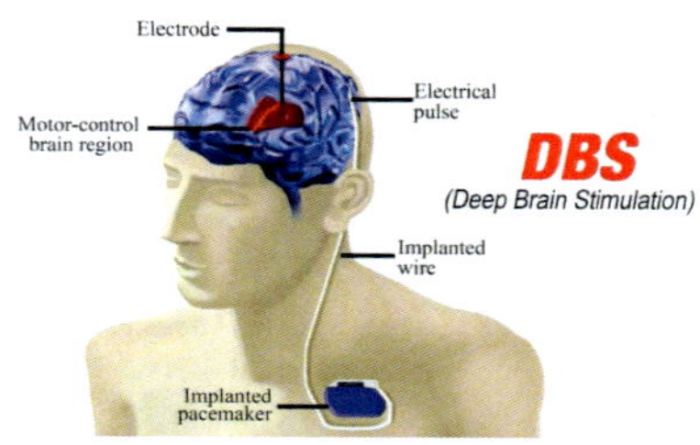
Lead	A thin, metal wire that allows for transmission of electricity. In DBS therapy the lead is surgically implanted into the brain. There are four different electrodes along the tip that deliver electrical pulses to exact locations of the brain.	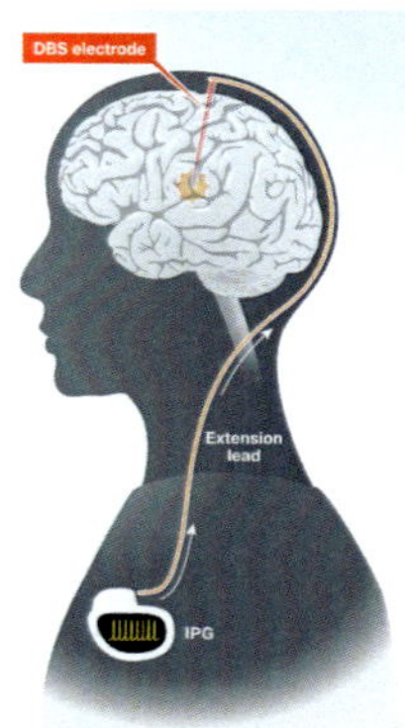
Lewy body disease	A neurological disease in which abnormal protein deposits called Lewy bodies are found in certain areas of the brain. Symptoms can be similar to PD and Alzheimer's disease.	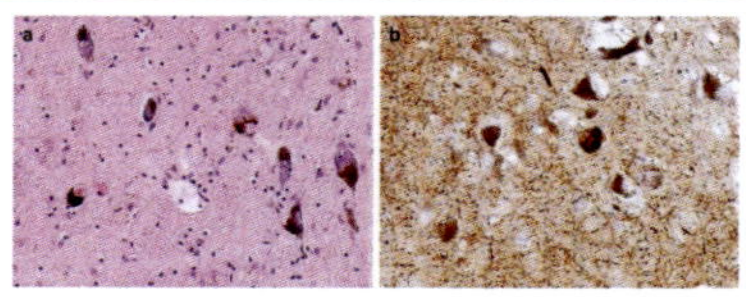
Neurophysiologist	A scientist who specializes in understanding brain cell firing patterns. A neurophysiologist or neurologist may use these patterns to map your brain function during a DBS operation.	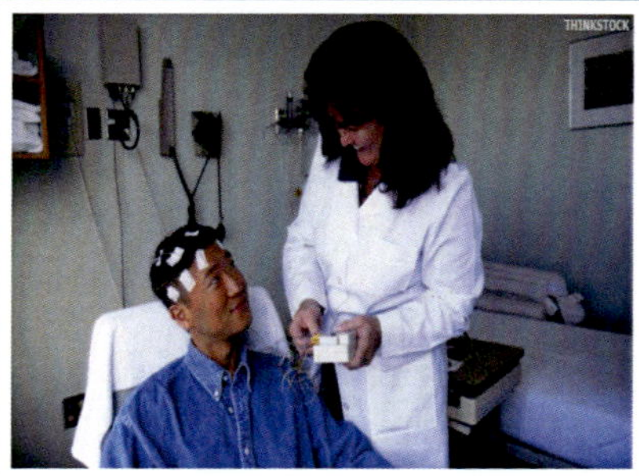

Motor symptoms	Symptoms of PD that affect movement, such as tremor, rigidity, and bradykinesia.	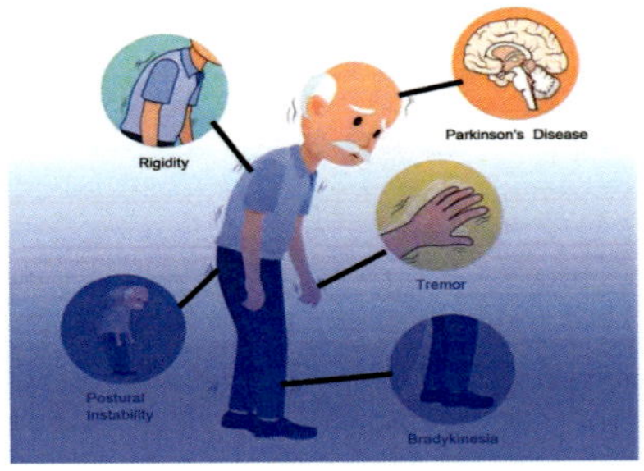
Diathermy	A type of ultrasound therapy that involves applying a heat coil to the skin or body. Most often used by dentists, pain specialists, and physical therapists to help reduce pain. Diathermy should never be used on someone who has DBS therapy as it can heat the brain electrodes, causing serious brain damage and even death.	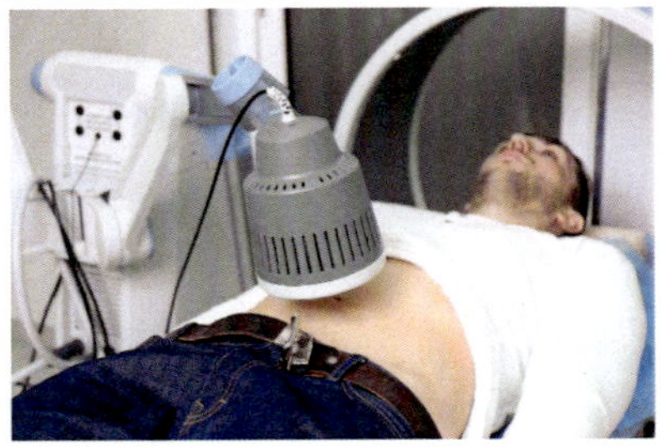

6.1. Pallidotomy, Thalamotomy, and Subthalamotomy

A tiny heated probe is inserted into a specific area of the brain during a thalamotomy, subthalamotomy, or pallidotomy surgical procedure to destroy tissue. Pallidotomy is the term used to describe the process of lesioning the globus pallidus internus. In a similar vein, we refer to the procedure as a thalamotomy when it involves treating the thalamus. And we call the operation a subthalamotomy when the subthalamic nucleus is injured. Among these three techniques, pallidotomy has been used the most frequently to treat Parkinson's disease symptoms over the past few decades. Tremor, rigidity, bradykinesia, motor fluctuations, and, in certain situations, walking and balance, may all be improved by a pallidotomy lesion. Except for tremor and dyskinesia, pallidotomies are only useful for treating Parkinson's disease symptoms that improve when treated with levodopa (Sinemet). Pallidotomy may be able to alleviate tremor and dyskinesia if medication is ineffective. Compared to DBS, pallidotomy offers the advantages of not requiring electronic programming sessions to fine-tune the parameters and of not requiring batteries or wires to be implanted. Furthermore, after the initial surgical procedure is completed, there is no risk of infection from an implanted device, and there are no hardware malfunctions to deal with. Pallidotomy might be a wise option for people who might find it difficult to travel for DBS programming (from another area or nation) or in situations where DBS is too costly or unavailable. In treating PD symptoms, pallidotomy can be just as successful as DBS, but the lesion needs to be positioned precisely. Pallidotomy can have long-lasting benefits, according to recent research. One significant drawback of pallidotomy is that, unlike DBS, it should not be done on both sides of the brain. Two pallidotomies may result in lifelong difficulties with speech, swallowing, and cognition. When a patient needs a second surgery after having an existing pallidotomy, DBS is typically placed on the opposite side of the brain. Because subthalamotomy can offer similar benefits to pallidotomy and can be safely performed on both sides of the brain by numerous medical groups, it is becoming more and more popular. In Cuba, subthalamotomy is the preferred PD procedure, and evidence points to its high efficacy. Hemiballism, or the uncontrollable flinging of one arm or leg, is a side effect that a small number of subthalamotomy patients have experienced. However, in most cases, this side effect is temporary and goes away over time. Since thalamotomy is typically limited to treating tremor, it is an uncommon procedure in Parkinson's disease (Hariz, 2009; Okum, 2012; Fenoy & Simpson, 2014).

6.2. Deep Brain Stimulation (DBS)

A surgical therapy called deep brain stimulation (DBS) is used to treat PD. A lead, a type of special wire, is implanted into a particular part of the brain during DBS surgery. A thin wire with four electrical contacts at its tip is surgically inserted into a very precise and carefully chosen brain region in order to perform DBS. The thalamus, subthalamic nucleus, and globus pallidus internus are the three main regions of the brain where this wire, also known as the DBS lead (pronounced "leed"), can be positioned. Unlike pallidotomy, thalamotomy, and subthalamotomy, DBS does not result in the permanent destruction of brain tissue. Potentially reversible, the procedure typically leaves little to no brain tissue damage behind. For instance, there is nothing you can do to stop slurred speech if you have a pallidotomy. You can tweak the settings with DBS, and most, if not all, slurred speech will get better. While modifying the settings does not always ensure that slurred speech or other side effects will go better, the likelihood of improvement is significantly higher than with permanent procedures like pallidotomies. This is because the DBS lead itself may have a lesioning effect.

The pacemaker-like device that is implanted in the area of the chest beneath the collarbone is connected to the DBS lead. The battery and computer source that power the neurostimulator, also known as the implantable pulse generator (IPG), produce the electrical pulses that are then sent to the brain through a lead. Both the patient and the clinician can turn the system on or off. Furthermore, the clinician has the ability to choose which of the four electrodes on each brain lead to activate to deliver electrical stimulation. This procedure makes it possible to target a very specific area of the brain with electrical stimulation.

A physician assistant, nurse practitioner, doctor, or other qualified staff member can program the DBS and change many electrical parameters or settings to regulate the level of stimulation. The DBS system is being "programmed" by these changes. The clinician can minimize side effects and maximize benefits by making the necessary adjustments. One advantage of DBS that is not possible with pallidotomy, thalamotomy, or subthalamotomy is its adjustability. Many patients give their justifications for selecting DBS over a lesioning procedure: the procedure can be carried out safely on both sides of the brain; it is reversible; and the device can be programmed and reprogrammed for symptoms and symptom changes. The entire procedure is needed for individuals and families thinking about DBS treatment. Everything from the decision to have surgery to the day of the procedure, surgical recovery, and DBS programming is covered in the content. This book's content is meant to help you have DBS discussions with family, friends, and members of your healthcare team; it is not meant to take the place of the advice you receive from the knowledgeable medical professionals who are involved in your care.

6.2.1. How DBS Works?

Even though we still don't fully understand the mechanisms underlying DBS, we have found a lot of significant hints over the past 20 years. A fundamental understanding of brain function is necessary to comprehend DBS and how it might be able to suppress symptoms. The brain is an intricate organ made up of billions of cells connected by synapses. Axons, sometimes known as "pipes," connect these cells to one another and transmit messages back and forth. A network of circuits designed to sort and process information facilitates communication. The electrical wiring in your home or vehicle is comparable to the connections found in brain circuits. A single circuit failure can cause the system as a whole to malfunction. Studies have indicated that PD is caused by abnormal signals in multiple brain circuits. Several symptoms of PD, such as stiffness, tremor, and slowed movement, appear to be caused by these flawed or disrupted signals. By "disrupting the disruption," electricity improves the symptoms of disabling and returns order to the circuit. It is believed that the electric current causes the brain cells known as astrocytes to release calcium, stimulate the axons (the pipes), and inhibit cell firing. Blood flow is stimulated and neurotransmitters are released as a result of a sequence of events that calcium appears to set off. In some unidentified way, this symphony of changes brought about by electrical stimulation helps to mitigate Parkinson's disease symptoms.

The substantia nigra pars compacta (SNc) is a region of the brain that is abnormally affected by PD in terms of electrical signal processing. More than 400,000 brain cells that produce dopamine are located in this area. These brain cells may sustain damage over time and eventually die. This procedure lowers dopamine's natural production, and dopamine loss has a major impact on how PD symptoms manifest. Important brain regions that regulate both motor and non-motor functions are connected to the SNc. The subthalamic nucleus (STN) and the globus pallidus internus (GPi) are two significant interconnections. These are important brain regions that transmit signals that impact your arms, legs, neck, and other body parts in addition to other functions (like mood and thought processes). The transmission of electrical signals through the GPi and STN can be changed by inserting DBS leads into these regions, which typically leads to more fluid and smooth movement. It has been demonstrated that specific regions in the GPi and STN are effective DBS targets, particularly when it comes to treating tremor, rigidity, bradykinesia, motor fluctuations, and dyskinesia symptoms (Okun et al., 2012).

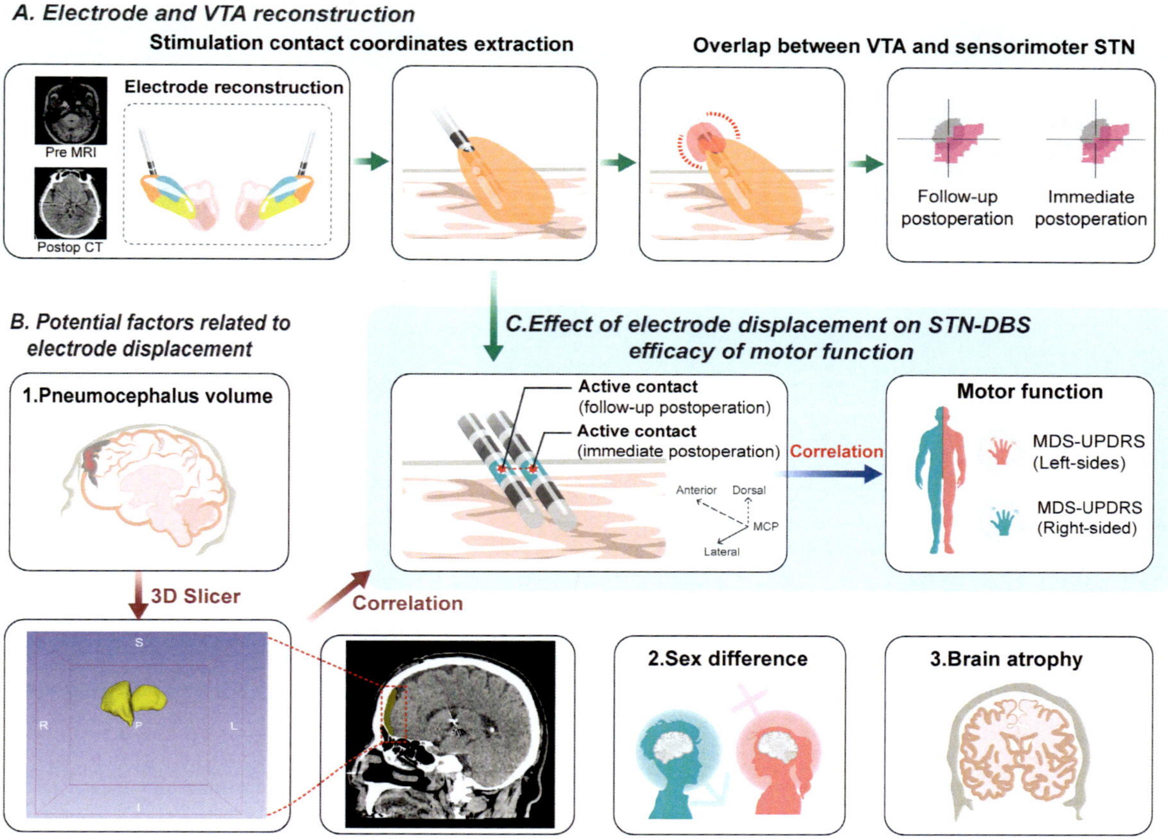

Figure 6.1. *Deep brain stimulation (DBS).*

Source: Yuan T, Chen Y, Zhu G, Zhang J. The Related Factors and Effect of Electrode Displacement on Motor Outcome of Subthalamic Nuclei Deep Brain Stimulation in Parkinson's Disease. Journal of Clinical Medicine. 2023; 12(24):7561. https://doi.org/10.3390/jcm12247561.

6.2.2. Location of DBS Target Areas and Substantia Nigra (SN)

DBS has been used for a variety of neurological disorders and can be positioned in many different parts of the brain. Treatment occasionally also targets the ventralis intermediate nucleus of the thalamus (Vim). Arm tremor can be significantly reduced with a DBS lead in this area. However, in the majority of cases, it does not alleviate rigidity, dyskinesia, bradykinesia, or lower extremity tremor. Thus, Vim is the recommended location for another ailment called essential tremor (Table 6.1).

Table 6.1. *Experiences Shared Over 11 Years of DBS Therapy*

		At Enrollment			At 11-Year Interview				
Patient	**Treatment Group ***	**Medication Duration (Years)**	**Age (Years)**	**PDQ-39 Summary Index**	**DBS Duration (Years)**	**Medication Duration (Years)**	**Age (Years)**	**PDQ-39 Summary Index**	**11-Year Washout Duration (Days)**
1	eDBS	1.0	73.9	7.5	10.4	12.1	85.0	d.n.p.	d.n.p.
2	eODTsDBS	0.9	63.2	19.5	5.2	14.3	76.6	15.2	4
3	eODTsDBS	3.9	55.5	14.6	0.5	16.8	68.3	14.3	5
4	eODT	3.0	59.7	9.6	n.a.	15.6	72.3	15.6	7
5	eODT	1.3	67.9	24.9	n.a.	12.2	78.8	36.8	w.n.a.
6	eDBS	1.7	56.4	19.7	13.0	15.0	69.7	18.1	w.n.a.
7	eDBS	0.6	55.4	14.3	10.9	11.7	66.5	51.8	7
8	eODT	1.4	52.3	14.5	n.a.	14.1	64.9	30.0	7
9	eDBS	1.4	53.6	6.8	13.3	15.2	67.4	15.8	2.5
10	eODTsDBS	3.5	60.8	20.3	7.6	17.1	74.4	35.2	4
Mean ± SD (Range)		1.9 ± 1.2 (0.6–3.9)	59.9 ± 6.8 (52.3–73.9)	15.2 ± 6.0 (6.8–24.9)	8.7 ± 4.6 (0.5–13.3)	14.4 ± 1.9 (11.7–17.1)	72.4 ± 6.3 (64.9–85.0)	25.9 ± 13.3 (14.3–51.8)	5.2 ± 1.7 (0–7)

* eDBS = randomized to early DBS+ODT; eODT = randomized to early ODT and never received DBS; eODTsDBS = randomized to early-ODT and later received standard of care DBS after the trial concluded; d.n.p. = did not participate in 11-year study; w.n.a. = 11-year washout not attempted.

Source: Stoehr K, Pazira K, Bonnet K, Schlundt D, Charles D, Hacker M. Deep Brain Stimulation in Early-Stage Parkinson's Disease: Patient Experience after 11 Years. Brain Sciences. 2022; 12(6):766. https://doi.org/10.3390/brainsci12060766.

Leads, which are wires with tiny electrodes, are inserted into a narrow target region of the brain during DBS surgery. The STN, GPi, or Vim will be the target, depending on the circumstances. The best targets for reducing most PD symptoms are STN or GPi. Leads can be positioned bilaterally (on both sides of the brain) or unilaterally (on one side). After the lead is positioned, it is fastened to a wire that passes beneath the neck's skin and beneath the scalp. Next, a pulse generator, also known as a neurostimulator, is connected to it. The neurostimulator is situated beneath the skin of the chest, directly beneath the collarbone. The pulse generator functions similarly to a pacemaker in that it provides electricity to the lead that is implanted in the brain. Either a single-chamber or dual-chamber pulse generator—which connects two leads—is available. A remote control resembling that of a television is used to turn on and off the pulse generator. The DBS programmer can achieve the best possible symptomatic improvement by adjusting the DBS settings in thousands of combinations.

The affected circuit brain signals will return to normal as a result of DBS activation, the lead, and the electricity it emits. The majority of DBS patients report feeling more "on" time, responding to medication more smoothly, and seeing improvements in their rigidity, tremor, and dyskinesia. Certain side effects are possible when the DBS electrode is activated. The DBS programmer can try to prevent these side effects in different ways, depending on the type of DBS electrode that is implanted.

6.2.3. DBS Devices

The intended brain target area, or as close to it as feasible, is implanted with the DBS lead (thin wire). The diameter of the wire is slightly over a millimeter, making it comparable in size to a thin picture hanging wire. The Medtronic lead can target the GPi or STN and has four electrodes. The eight electrodes on the Abbott and Boston Scientific devices are aimed at the STN. The implantable pulse generator, also known as a neurostimulator or implantable pulse generator (IPG), receives the connecting wire after it has been connected to the brain electrode. The 4–8 electrode contacts on the DBS lead receive power from the IPG via the connecting wire. The IPG is normally positioned in the chest, though it is occasionally positioned in the abdomen (Table 6.2).

Table 6.2. *IPG Devices*

TABLE 3 | Commercially available IPG devices.

Device	Frequency	Pulsewidth	Mode	Ampltiude (Joohi, 2021)	Feature	Application
Medtronic Activa™ PC (Paff et al., 2020)	2–250 Hz	60–450 μs	CC or CV	0–25.5 mA 0–10.5 V	conditionally safe with MRI	Bilateral STN and Gpi Stimulation for PD, Unilateral Thalamic Stimulation for Ets,Unilateral or Bilateral stimulation of the Gpi or STN for treatment of chronic, drug refractory segmental or generalized dystonia
Medtronic Activa™ RC (Paff et al., 2020)					dual channel, rechargeable, conditionally safe with MRI	
Medtronic Activa™ SC (Paff et al., 2020)	3–250 Hz				single channel, conditionally safe with MRI	
Medtronic Percept™ PC (Joohi, 2021)	2–250 Hz	20–450 μs	CC	0–25.5 mA	closed loop feature (using local field potential as biomarker)	
Abbott Infinity 5 (Paff et al., 2020)	2–240 Hz	20–500 μs	CC	0–12.75 mA	dual channel	Bilateral STN and GPi stimulation for PD and for bilateral thalamic stimulation for ETs
AbbottInfinity 7 (Paff et al., 2020)						
Boston Scientific Vercise PC (Paff et al., 2020)	2–255 Hz	20–450—μs	CC	0.1–20 mA	dual channel	Bilateral STN stimulation for PD
Boston Scientific Vercise RC (Paff et al., 2020)			CC		dual channel, rechargeable	
Boston Scientific Gevia (Paff et al., 2020)					dual channel, rechargeable, conditionally safe with MRI	
PINS Medical G102 (Paff et al., 2020)	2–250 Hz	30–450—μs	CC or CV	0–25 mA; 0–10 V	dual channel, remote wireless programming	PD, tremor, dystonia (Joohi, 2021)
PINS Medical G102R (Paff et al., 2020)					dual channel, rechargeable, remote wireless programming	
PINS Medical G101A (Paff et al., 2020)					single channel, remote wireless programming	
SceneRay 1180	1–1600 Hz	60–960 μs	—	—	dual channel remote wireless programming	—
Neuropace (Joohi, 2021)	1–333 Hz	40–1000 μs	CC	0–12.0 mA	closed loop feature (responsive neurostimulation), rechargeable (Shaikhouni, et al., 2015)	Drug-Resistant Epilepsy (DRE)

Source: Silverio AA and Silverio LAA (2022) Developments in Deep Brain Stimulators for Successful Aging Towards Smart Devices—An Overview. Front. Aging 3:848219. doi: 10.3389/fragi.2022.848219.

The N' vision programmer, a radio-transmitting device that can control the amount of electricity delivered to the electrodes, is used to adjust the Medtronic IPGs. Holding the programmer over the IPG—that is, over the chest or abdomen—is how programming is done. During office visits, healthcare providers use an iPad Mini to program the Abbott device leads. Wireless assessments of motor skills can be performed by clinicians. Physicians utilize a Surface Pro 3 and the Patient Remote Control to program the Boston Scientific device. Placing the remote control over the IPG allows you to program it.

The system's final component is one that is not inserted into the body. It is the controller who is patient. The remote for the Activa SC, PC, and RC is the same. The patient controller for the Infinity device is an Apple iPod Touch with Bluetooth wireless connectivity. The IPG can also be wirelessly connected to the Boston Scientific Patient Remote. The patient can check the battery level and turn the IPG on and off with any of the three controllers. Additionally, they enable the patient to self-adjust within the DBS programmer's parameters.

6.2.4. BG-Thalamo-Cortical Circuitry in PD

The BG is made up of the putamen and caudate nucleus of the corpus striatum, the GPi and globus pallidus externus, the STN, the pedunculopontine nucleus (PPN), and the substantia nigra. Through segregated parallel circuits to and from the cortex, the BG are involved in motor, associative-cognitive, and limbic functions. The BG is in charge of "the automatic execution of learned motor plans" when it comes to movement execution, and the GPi is the primary output structure that goes from the thalamus to the cerebral cortex and brain stem nuclei. Thus, the BG's function includes regulating and streamlining movement execution. The balance between glutamatergic excitatory and gaba-ergic inhibitory pathways allows for this. This balance is upset in PD. The absence of dopamine in the striatum causes it to become more inhibitory on the globus pallidus externus. This, in turn, reduces the striatum's inhibition on the STN, enabling the latter to increase its glutamatergic excitation on the GPi, which in turn increases its inhibitory activity on the thalamus.

Concurrently, there is a reduction in the striatum's direct inhibitory projection to the GPi, enabling the GPi's inhibitory activity on the thalamus to be further enhanced. Ultimately, this leads to an overactivity of the STN and GPi, which in turn inhibits the thalamo-cortical projections, causing PD patients to become rigid and akinesic. Akinesia, rigidity, and tremors are reduced by "silencing" the pathologically increased neuronal activity of the GPi or the STN through lesioning or high-frequency DBS of these nuclei, which results in the restoration of a roughly normal movement pattern. This is the rationale behind the use of high-frequency DBS of either the GPi or the STN in the surgical treatment of patients with advanced PD (Marwan Hariz, & Patric Blomstedt, 2022) (Figure 6.2).

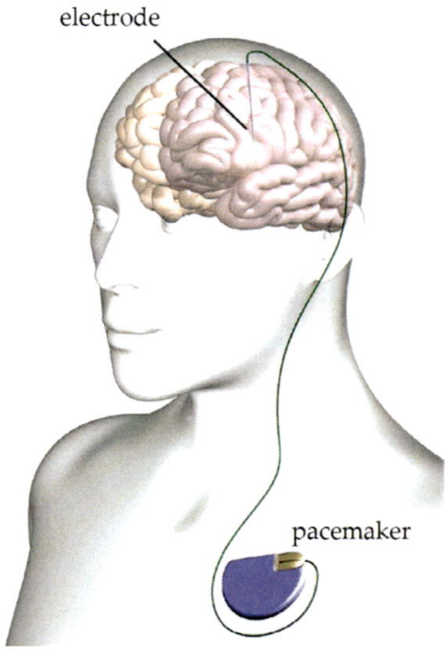

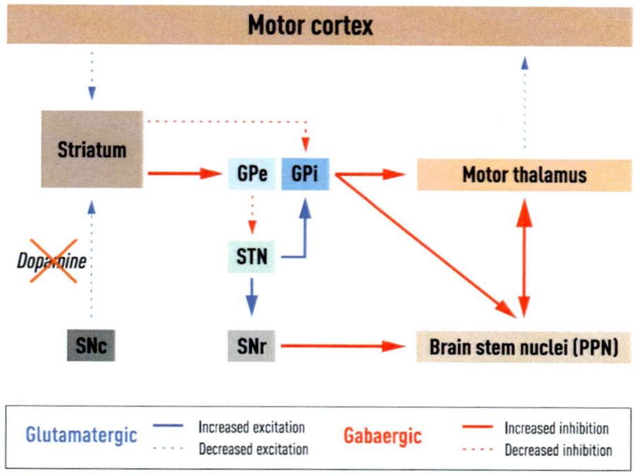

Figure 6.2. *DBSPD*

Source: Auxiliadora de Paula Vasconcelos, L. (2020). Parkinson's Disease Rehabilitation: Effectiveness Approaches and New Perspectives. IntechOpen. doi: 10.5772/intechopen.89360.

6.2.5. DBS Hardware, Surgical Procedure and Mechanism of Action of DBS

The components of contemporary DBS hardware are as follows: an electrode with a diameter of 1.3 mm and 4–8 1.5 mm contacts at the tip, spaced 0.5 or 1.5 mm apart. By using three-dimensional magnetic resonance imaging (MRI), the desired brain target is located and these electrodes are inserted stereotactically. Thanks to advancements in imaging technology, patients can now undergo surgery while unconscious, maintaining the same level of clinical outcome as before. The electrodes are affixed to the skull's burrhole and linked to an implanted neuropacemaker via cables that pass beneath the skin and into a pocket typically formed beneath the collarbone. MRI or computed tomography imaging, either intra- or postoperative, is used to confirm the precise location of the brain electrodes. A few days following surgery, the neurosurgeon, neurologist, or specialized DBS nurse will apply electrostimulation by screening the lead's various contacts with an external computer that is remotely connected to the neuropacemaker in an attempt to detect any effects on the patient's symptoms or potential side effects. The stimulation is typically programmed with a current of 130 Hz, a pulse width of 60 ms, and an amplitude that can be adjusted between 1 and 4 milliampere based on the patient's response.

The different electrode contacts can be turned on individually or in combination, depending on what the clinical context dictates. Monopolar or bipolar stimulation can be used (Figure 6.3. Instead of using an omnidirectional electric field, the newest DBS hardware brands use electrodes with directional contacts, which can "direct" the current perpendicular to the lead's axis in order to more precisely focus stimulation on the relevant brain target. The neuropacemaker is composed of primary cells, which require replacement after the battery runs out (usually after 3–5 years of continuous stimulation). Alternatively, the device can be recharged, in which case it can last for an additional 15–25 years. The precise workings of high-frequency DBS remain unclear. High-frequency DBS mimics an ablation in the majority of targets (STN, GPi, VIM) used in PD treatment, as previously mentioned. High-frequency stimulation is supposed to produce noise that jams the pathological neuronal firing pattern of the stimulated structure's cells. But the stimulation also affects axons in the orthodromic and antidromic directions. Therefore, DBS may disrupt pathological oscillatory neuronal activity in the BG-thalamus circuitry at different nodes in the network through a number of nonexclusive mechanisms. In any case, the overall clinical effect of high-frequency DBS is comparable to that of a lesion, albeit reversible; that is, symptoms are suppressed while stimulation is applied, and symptoms reappear when stimulation is removed (Holewijn & Verbaan, 2021).

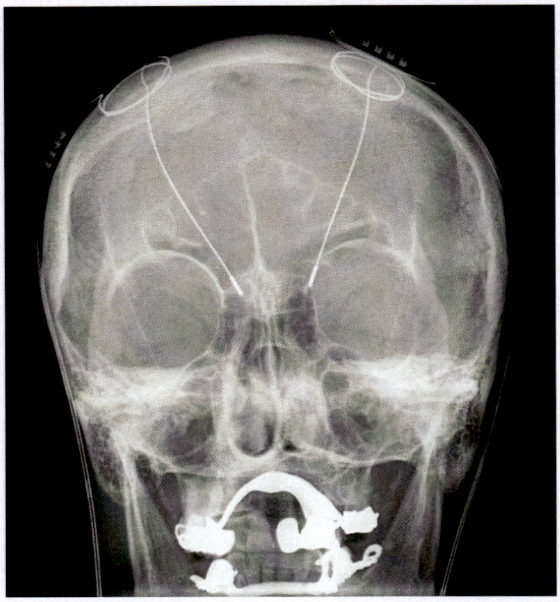

Figure 6.3. *DPS probes.*

Source: By Hellerhoff – Own work, CC BY-SA 3.0, https://commons.wikimedia.org/w/index.php?curid=13785677.

6.2.6. Current Practices of DBS for PD

A specialized multidisciplinary team comprising a functional neurosurgeon, a neurologist specializing in movement disorders, a neuropsychologist, and a DBS nurse is necessary for DBS for Parkinson's disease.

This is required to allow for an appropriate lifetime follow-up of patients who have had surgery as well as a proper selection of patients who are suitable for DBS.

Deep-seated electrode placement in the brain is now a relatively safe, routine neurosurgical procedure that, in skilled, multidisciplinary centers, has almost no surgical morbidity and almost no mortality.

The primary surgical complication is the potential for infection of the extracranially implanted hardware, which is uncommon, and the possibility of mistargeting electrodes if appropriate imaging verification of targeting accuracy is not carried out during the procedure or afterward. While DBS is now being studied for the treatment of various other neurological and neuropsychiatric conditions, it is still primarily used to treat PD.

However, DBS has also been used to treat other movement disorders, such as essential tremor and dystonia.

According to a recently published review of the literature, nearly half of the papers on DBS over the previous 35 years dealt with DBS for PD, with the STN, GPi, and VIM nucleus of the thalamus being the most frequently published brain regions targeted by DBS. The following will provide specifics on each of the most popular DBS procedures used on patients with Parkinson's disease, including indications, contraindications, clinical outcomes, and possible side effects (Tables 6.3 and 6.4).

Table 6.3. *DBS in Various Brain Targets*

Subthalamic nucleus	Disabling motor symptoms
	Dyskinesia
	Motor fluctuations
Globus pallidus internus	Improvement of motor symptoms in general
Ventral intermediate thalamic nucleus	Tremor
Pedunculopontine nucleus	Gait instability
	Gait freezing phenomenon

Source: Auxiliadora de Paula Vasconcelos, L. (2020). Parkinson's Disease Rehabilitation: Effectiveness Approaches and New Perspectives. IntechOpen. doi: 10.5772/intechopen.89360.

Table 6.4. *Summary of Different Mechanistic Pathways by Which DBS Affects AD And PD, as well as Their Consequent Physiological Outcomes*

Disease	Action of DBS	Physiological Effects	Year	Author
AD	Neuronal activation through fornix DBS.	Increased hippocampal volume.	2020, 2012, 2019, 2015	Jakobs, Smith, Aldehri, Sankar
	Increased acetylcholine levels using NBM DBS.	Increased glucose uptake in amygdalo-hippocampal, temporal, and superior lingual gyrus.	2021, 2014	Maltête, Kuhn
	Increased prefrontal glucose uptake.	Decreased clinical decline.	2021	Lam
PD	Neuronal inhibition.	Depletion of glutamate and release of GABA and adenosine.	2012, 2001, 2001	Lozano, Contreras, Wu
	Neuronal activation.	Increased glutamate and dopamine levels.	2013, 2005, 1992	Lozano, Stefani, Benazzouz
	Neuronal activation and inhibition.	Decoupling of the soma and axons.	2013	Lozano
	Disrupt pathologic oscillatory patterns.	Neurotrophin release and generation of new neurons.	2013, 2010	Lozano, McIntyre

Source: Senevirathne DKL, Mahboob A, Zhai K, Paul P, Kammen A, Lee DJ, Yousef MS, Chaari A. Deep Brain Stimulation beyond the Clinic: Navigating the Future of Parkinson's and Alzheimer's Disease Therapy. Cells. 2023; 12(11):1478. https://doi.org/10.3390/cells12111478.

6.2.7. VIM DBS for Tremors

In the modern era of DBS, tremor (both Parkinsonian and essential) was the first application. The tremor reacts less well to dopaminergic treatment, despite the fact that it effectively relieves akinesia and stiffness. Therefore, VIM DBS offers a stable and long-lasting control of tremor in patients with PD whose other PD symptoms are well managed with medication, who do not show signs of dopa-induced dyskinesias, and in whom tremor is the only symptom that causes them distress. If the patient is in otherwise good health and the MRI results do not demonstrate significant brain atrophy, there is no upper age limit for this procedure. If necessary, bilateral VIM DBS can be carried out; however, it is advisable to stage the two procedures at least six months apart in elderly patients. Usually, stimulation of the VIM is initiated in the waking hours and ought to be discontinued when the patient retires for the night. Dysarthria and imbalance disorders are potential side effects of stimulation in the VIM, particularly if bilateral, but these can occasionally be controlled by adjusting the electric parameters of the stimulation. Over time, certain patients may develop a tolerance or habituation to stimulation, necessitating higher stimulation amplitudes to control their tremors. Occasionally, ataxia may arise, in which case a temporary cessation of stimulation (a "stimulation vacation") will be necessary to eliminate the ataxia. Not turning off the DBS at night increases the risk for both ataxia and tolerance in patients. VIM DBS is not as common in practice as DBS in the GPi or STN because most patients referred for surgery are in a more advanced stage of the disease and have symptoms other than tremors.

6.2.8. GPi DBS for Advanced PD and Dopa-Induced Dyskinesias

Pallidotomy has essentially been superseded by DBS in the posteroventral GPi. This procedure treats akinesia, rigidity, and dyskinesias, three of the main motor symptoms of Parkinson's disease. Bilateral-GPi DBS is more tolerable than bilateral VIM DBS or bilateral STN DBS, despite being performed bilaterally in patients with more advanced disease (see below). With GPi DBS, there is no upper age limit, and there is a lower chance of dysarthria and negative affect on balance than with VIM DBS. The primary effects of GPi DBS are dopa-induced dyskinesias, such as painful dystonia, rigidity, akinesia, and tremors; gait disturbances, such as freezing of gait, are least affected. The patient can keep taking their dopaminergic medications at the same doses or even raise them if necessary because GPi DBS has a great effect on dyskinesias and reduces the risk of dopa-induced dyskinesias. In most countries, DBS in the STN has overshadowed GPi DBS, despite the latter's leniency towards patients with advanced Parkinson's disease and positive effects on symptoms.

6.2.9. STN DBS for PD

No surgical technique for Parkinson's disease has received as much praise and publicity as STN DBS. This procedure is very popular for the following reasons: STN DBS is the most effective surgical treatment for PD; it is the only surgery that allows patients with advanced PD to drastically reduce their daily doses of dopaminergic medications, and in some cases, stop them completely; it has undergone the most stringent scrutiny with multiple multicenter randomized blinded studies and outcome meta-analyses; and it has the longest documented follow-up. However, in contrast to DBS in other brain targets, STN DBS has the strictest selection criteria for PD patients, and it necessitates careful postoperative patient management by skilled neurologists specializing in movement disorders.

There have been constant efforts to refine the indications of STN DBS since its inception in the mid-1990s, as well as to establish clinical standards for eligibility. The goal is to optimize patient benefits and minimize unintended side effects of stimulation. Levodopa response was determined to be the primary eligibility criterion for STN DBS: good motor outcome was obtained with STN DBS in patients who responded well to levodopa in terms of symptoms. Since then, every PD patient who is referred for DBS has to go through a procedure known as the "L-dopa challenge," which measures motor symptoms by first having the patient not take any medication and then giving them a sizable dose of levodopa. The patient will gain more from STN DBS if their symptoms improve more following this L-dopa challenge. The second criterion was age: although there was still a meaningful benefit from surgery, it was discovered that the older the patient was at the time of the procedure, the less improvement from STN DBS and the more side effects from stimulation. In certain locations, 69–70 years old was determined to be the cutoff age for this procedure. The third requirement for a favorable outcome was having good cognitive function since it has been suggested that STN DBS may worsen cognitive decline. As a result, all patients who are referred for DBS take a neuropsychologic exam to assess their cognitive abilities, including memory and executive function. The patient's mood is the final criterion, and it should be formally assessed in order to prevent STN DBS from being performed on patients who have relevant or untreated depression. The following selection criteria have been established by an expert consensus to ensure the best outcomes after STN DBS in patients with advanced PD: excellent levodopa response, younger age, no or very mild cognitive impairment, and absence of, or well controlled, psychiatric disease. Strict contra-indications for STN DBS include: severe axial symptoms not alleviated by levodopa; so-called nondopaminergic symptoms (poor balance, falls, advanced freezing of gait, severe dysarthria), relevant cognitive decline, and severe depression. Levodopa inresponsiveness of cardinal symptoms of PD, especially rigidity and akinesia (which would question the diagnosis of idiopathic PD in the first place).

Given the safety and effectiveness of STN DBS, along with its stringent inclusion criteria, particularly for younger patients, some eminent neurologists suggested that patients might benefit from it at an earlier stage of their progressive disease. The younger patients would be able to continue living their regular lives, avoid retiring too soon, lessen their family's burden, prevent marital problems, and help to preserve their opportunities in life. Therefore, patients with early on/off motor complications who received STN DBS after a mean of 7 years after diagnosis (instead of the usual 11 years or more) participated in a randomized trial named the EARLYSTIM trial, which compared best medical management strategies to STN DBS. It was demonstrated that, in terms of both motor symptoms and quality of life measures, patients who had received STN DBS fared considerably better at the 2-year follow-up than those who had received the best medical care alone. Other aspects of the disease, such as anxiety, pain, and difficulties sleeping, show improvement following STN DBS. These are nonmotor symptoms of Parkinson's disease.

6.2.10. STN DBS versus GPi DBS

Movement disorders clinicians generally agree that stimulating the thalamic VIM is a useful surgical treatment for PD patients whose primary symptom, or sometimes only symptom, is tremor. However, opinions differ regarding the superiority of STN DBS versus GPi DBS in patients with advanced PD who experience motor fluctuations and dyskinesias. Numerous trials have been conducted to compare the results of these two procedures. In terms of motor improvement, some trials demonstrated that STN DBS was superior to GPi DBS, while other trials revealed no differences. Furthermore, it is critical that patients, particularly those with STN DBS, receive care from highly skilled neurologists who specialize in movement disorders. This is because it allows them to carefully adjust medication dosages and stimulation amplitude in the months and years following surgery, maintaining improvement and reducing the risk of developing a hypodopaminergic syndrome (apathy, depression, suicide) or a hyperdopaminergic syndrome (dyskinesias, impulsivity, hypersexuality, mania).

6.2.11. Side Effects of DBS

Any brain target for DBS carries some risk of adverse effect induction. These vary slightly depending on the target brain and are caused by the electric current diffusing outside of the intended area, particularly when the electrodes are not positioned precisely. Furthermore, the majority of side effects brought on by stimulation can be partially reversed and controlled by varying the intensity of the stimulation, including its frequency, amplitude, pulse width, and/or polarity. Stimulation-induced dysarthria is a common potential side effect of bilateral DBS to any brain target, albeit to varying degrees. Diffusion of the current to the adjacent motor internal capsule is the primary cause of dysarthria and balance disturbance in VIM thalamic DBS, especially when bilateral. Dysarthria may worsen with GPi DBS as well, though not as much as with bilateral VIM DBS. Apart from the possibility of dysarthria, the STN also carries the risk of eyelid opening dyspraxia, which can be managed with injections of botulinum toxin. Additionally, if the electrode is placed too ventral–anterior–medial, there is a chance of behavioral abnormalities as this region of the STN is linked to limbic cortical structures. Furthermore, STN DBS will intensify the effects of dopaminergic drugs, particularly dopamine agonists, if dosages are not lowered following surgery, resulting in heightened impulsivity and manic episodes. However, patients will experience apathy and even depression if their dopa medication is reduced excessively, even though STN DBS alone can give them a very good motor improvement. In rare cases, this can even result in suicide. All of this clarifies why a movement disorders neurologist with expertise in Parkinson's disease management is necessary to oversee this most effective surgical procedure, STN DBS. This also explains why GPi DBS is regarded as more lenient for older patients and preferred by some clinicians even for younger patients, despite not being as effective on motor symptoms as STN DBS. Unlike STN DBS, GPi DBS is less time-consuming, labor-intensive, and difficult to manage, and it does not require adjusting medication doses. However, it might be advisable to offer STN DBS rather than GPi DBS to patients with advanced PD who have relevant dopaminergic medication-induced impulse control disorders. This is because only STN DBS would permit a reduction in dopaminergic medication dosages, helping to treat the medication-induced impulse control disorder.

6.2.12. Limits and Issues in DBS for PD

While DBS, particularly STN DBS, may be the greatest thing for Parkinson's disease patients since levodopa was developed, it's important to keep in mind that not everything that seems perfect is. Initially, as with levodopa therapy, DBS is not a treatment for the disease; rather, the illness will continue to progress, albeit at a different and unique rate. As previously mentioned, DBS treats some of the primary symptoms of the illness symptomatically. A number of patients experience dopaminergic symptoms that become resistant to DBS as their disease worsens and they stop responding to dopa. These dopaminergic symptoms primarily impact axial aspects like speech, gait abnormalities like freezing, postural instability, and cognitive decline. They continue to be resistant to both medical and surgical interventions. But after years of STN DBS, a new phenotype of the illness may emerge, as with any PD treatment: while the effect on appendicular symptoms, such as hand tremors, rigidity, and dyskinesias, is still good, and quality of life measures are still better than they were prior to surgery, the axial symptoms worsen and the patient may experience walking difficulties, falls, dysarthria, and cognitive decline.

Another problem with DBS is that it can be hard to predict who will continue to benefit from it and who won't, particularly in cases of certain genetic forms of Parkinson's disease. Individuals who possess mutations in either the Parkin or leucine-rich repeat kinase 2 (LRRK2) genes exhibit superior dopa responsiveness and long-lasting positive results from dopaminergic stimulation. Conversely, individuals with glucocerebrosidase mutations tend to be older, exhibit an akinetic–rigid phenotype, and may experience cognitive decline earlier in life. As a result, both the beneficial effects of dopa and DBS are not long-lasting in these patients. Therefore, even though the majority of idiopathic PD cases are sporadic, it may be useful to know whether there is a genetic predisposition for the disease when providing counseling to PD patients and their families prior to DBS surgery. For some patients with unusual presentations or whose disease onset occurs before the age of 40, a genetic screening may be advised.

For PD patients, DBS is a lifelong treatment—"once DBS, always DBS." This reiterates the need for clinicians who are knowledgeable about DBS to provide care for patients with the condition. A sudden stop of stimulation owing to a neuropacemaker malfunction or low battery may cause a severe rebound of Parkinson's disease symptoms, particularly in patients with STN DBS. This may call for immediate medical attention, including emergency surgery to replace the neuropacemaker. Patients who were unable to pay for a neuropacemaker replacement or who had to have the implanted hardware removed due to infection, sometimes with fatal results, have been reported to have a status of therapy-resistant malignant Parkinsonian crisis.

Other problems with DBS are more widespread: research has demonstrated that, independent of the disease's gender prevalence, DBS is significantly more common in male PD patients than in female patients worldwide. This could be related to social issues and referral patterns. Furthermore, because DBS requires regular neuropacemaker replacements, it is only available to patients with the means to pay for it in nations without universal healthcare.

6.2.13. Other Investigated Brain Targets for DBS in PD

There are continuous efforts to explore DBS in alternative brain targets, with the goal of either improving nonmotor symptoms of PD like dementia or addressing some motor symptoms that would not respond well to DBS in conventional brain targets. A densely packed region of sensory and motor tracts lies beneath the thalamus and is called the posterior subthalamic area (PSA). The dentato-rubro-thalamic tract is one such tract that is involved in mediating the tremor symptom. Research on DBS directed at this region of the PSA, including a randomized trial, has demonstrated a good impact on essential and Parkinsonian tremor, with potentially fewer adverse effects than DBS in the VIM.

DBS has been studied as a potential target for treating therapy-resistant gait and balance disorders. The PPN, which is a portion of the brain stem locomotor area, and the substantia nigra reticulata, which is a part of the output structures of the BG, are shown in Figure 6.3. These studies haven't included nearly enough patients, followed them up for too little time, and produced inconsistent findings thus far. The primary source of cholinergic innervation of the cortex, the nucleus basalis of Meynert (NBM), atrophy in PD dementia patients. The hypothesis was that slowing down the cognitive decline might be helped by using low-frequency DBS to stimulate that nucleus rather than high frequency DBS to inhibit it. In a PD patient experiencing cognitive decline, apraxia was lessened by DBS in the NBM, according to a prior single-case report. Later, six PD patients with cognitive decline participated in a randomized controlled trial that compared the effects of six weeks of DBS on versus six weeks off. The results revealed no differences in the cognitive outcome.

6.2.14. Future Prospects of DBS in PD

DBS is still the most popular and effective surgical treatment for certain cardinal symptoms of PD after thirty years of use. Research into the new brain targets indicated above as well as potentially other brain regions will persist with the goal of enhancing results even more. This will be made easier by advancements in brain imaging, such as connectivity and functional MRI. Furthermore, since DBS was once the sole domain of a single company, there are now at least three major DBS companies.

This has led to a number of technical DBS innovations that are either being tested or implemented, such as MRI-compatible DBS hardware; neuropacemakers with rechargeable batteries and a 25-year lifespan; neuropacemakers with sensing technology that records the depth electroencephalogram, particularly beta activity, and adjusts stimulation accordingly, a feature known as closed loop stimulation, which may reduce side effects and battery drain; directional DBS electrodes that allow the electric current to be precisely focused on the region of interest, potentially reducing side effects like dysarthria and improving results; remote web-based follow-up. Notwithstanding all of the aforementioned characteristics, DBS for PD is still a successful symptomatic treatment; however, over time, the degree of improvement tends to diminish, and DBS may cause some late-stage disability milestones to be delayed.

This therapy will place even more pressure on clinicians to stay up to date due to the growing technological advancements and sophistication of DBS. As a result, they will need to specialize more in the complex modern treatments of PD and take advantage of the increased potential that DBS technology offers to further improve patient outcomes.

6.3. Risks and Complications of DBS

Deep brain stimulation (DBS) is a highly effective treatment for movement disorders like Parkinson's disease, essential tremor, and dystonia, but it does come with inherent risks and potential complications. Surgical risks include infection, bleeding, and damage to surrounding brain structures during electrode placement. Complications can arise post-surgery, such as device malfunction or migration, leading to inadequate symptom control or the need for additional surgeries. There's also a risk of cognitive and psychiatric side effects, including mood swings, depression, or impulsivity, though these are often manageable with adjustments to stimulation settings or medication. Long-term concerns revolve around device battery life and the potential for lead breakage or infection over time. Additionally, while rare, there's a risk of intracranial hemorrhage during the procedure, which can have serious consequences. Overall, while DBS can significantly improve quality of life for many patients, it's crucial to weigh these potential risks against the benefits and carefully consider candidacy with a healthcare team specialized in movement disorders and neurosurgery. Like any surgery, deep brain stimulation (DBS) carries with it a risk of complications. Problems that may occur as a result of the procedure can be serious and permanent, or alternatively temporary and reversible. In addition, malfunctioning DBS devices can result in post-operative problems (Fenoy & Simpson, 2014).

6.3.1. Serious or Permanent Complications

The possibility of major or long-lasting side effects from DBS treatment is extremely minimal. There is a 1% or less chance of dying. About 2 to 3% of strokes occur as a result of brain hemorrhage during surgery. While the majority of complications are asymptomatic, some people may have persistent symptoms akin to a stroke, including numbness, weakness, blurred vision, or slurred speech. A stroke during DBS surgery is more likely in those who have a history of bleeding issues. A rare but potential side effect of DBS is hydrocephalus, which is typically brought on by an accumulation of fluid in the brain that raises intracranial pressure. A neurosurgeon might have to place a shunt to reroute the fluid and release pressure if hydrocephalus occurs.

6.3.2. Temporary or Reversible Complications

Temporary or reversible complications may result as a side effect of the surgery or electrical stimulation. These potential complications include the following:

- ***Changes in Mood, Memory, and Thinking*:** DBS may make thinking and memory worse. Additional alterations may comprise of anxiety, depression, disorientation, delusions, or becoming excessively enthusiastic. After the procedure, these so-called psychiatric symptoms usually get better over the course of a few days or weeks and eventually go away entirely. Medication or stimulation modifications may be necessary to address these symptoms if they continue. Individuals who are known to have cognitive or psychiatric issues, like dementia or severe depression, are generally ineligible for DBS therapy and are far more likely to experience these complications. There have also been reports of suicidal thoughts and actual suicide after DBS therapy.
- ***Seizures*:** A small percentage of DBS patients will experience seizures. If a seizure does happen, it usually happens during the procedure or in the first week following it. Surgery-related seizures typically go away. If the seizures persist, there's a greater chance that they're caused by a brain infection, stroke, or DBS lead irritation. Medication for seizures may be recommended in these circumstances.
- ***Infection*:** At the surgical sites in the chest, scalp, or brain, there is a 5–20% chance of infection. Antibiotics are given during surgery in order to prevent infection. It might be necessary to remove the electrode, connecting wire, and/or neurostimulator if a serious infection occurs.
- ***Problems with Movement and Speech*:** It is possible to experience dyskinesia, a transient worsening of movement, balance issues, and slurred speech after DBS. Expert DBS programming can occasionally alleviate these symptoms. In certain situations, these signs are irreversible.
- ***Headache, Dizziness, Tingling of the Face or Limbs, and an Electrical Jolting Sensation*:** The stimulator settings can be changed to help with these issues as well as worsening dyskinesia. By using the patient controller or the hand-held magnet to turn off the stimulator, these unpleasant effects can often be improved almost instantly. These side effects can usually be resolved by adjusting the stimulation settings.

1. ***Other Risks of Surgery***

a. Pain, inflammation, or swelling at the surgery sites.

b. A very small risk of swelling or an allergic response to implanted materials.

6.3.3. Malfunctioning DBS Devices

Finally, there are some technical problems that can be associated with the DBS lead, connecting wire, and neurostimulator. These types of difficulties include the following:

- Lead migration, when the electrode has moved away from the optimal target site.
- Fracture, disconnection, or damage of the connecting wire.
- Malfunction or injury to the neurostimulator.
- Misplacement of the brain electrode.

Many of these issues are unpredictable and unavoidable. Avoid doing anything that directly applies pressure to the implanted devices. The lead may not always be positioned in the ideal part of the brain, even with the best tools, expertise, and technique. Electrodes can occasionally be misplaced by even the most skilled professionals employed by DBS centers. Sometimes a second surgery is required to correct a malfunctioning device or to realign the implant. Steer clear of twisting or pushing the implanted DBS system components, like the neurostimulator (battery). Surgery may be necessary if manipulations cause skin erosion or system damage.

6.4. Preparing for Surgery

The next stage, should you choose to proceed with deep brain stimulation (DBS) therapy, will be to schedule and get ready for your surgery and recuperation. Recognize that choosing a facility with a staff of professionals with expertise in DBS therapy for PD treatment is crucial. Once you have been referred to a DBS center, schedule your appointments so that a family member or friend can accompany you. Make sure you schedule appointments with the nurses, neuropsychologist, neurosurgeon, movement disorders neurologist, and psychiatrist who will be involved in your care. A physical therapist, occupational therapist, and speech therapist are frequently required team members. Make sure you have all the answers you need to ask about DBS before the procedure happens. Be ready to ask questions. If there are other patients who have undergone the surgery, ask the staff if you can talk to them about their experiences, both good and bad.

6.4.1. Pre-Surgery Tests and Evaluations

There might need to be multiple trips to the DBS center. Undertake a baseline Unified Parkinson's Disease Rating Scale (UPDRS) assessment by the movement disorders neurologist. This scale will assist the neurologist in assessing your Parkinson's disease. Both when you are taking medication and when you are not, the neurologist will probably administer the UPDRS. Your neurologist will use the UPDRS to determine which symptoms DBS has the best chance of curing (i.e., symptoms that improve with medication usually do so with DBS).

A battery of memory and cognitive tests known as a neuropsychological battery will also be administered to you. These tests are done to make sure you don't have depression, untreated mood disorders, memory problems, or confusion. A neuropsychologist with experience treating PD patients should administer these tests. Before being placed on DBS, you might also need to see a psychiatrist for treatment of anxiety, depression, or other mental health issues. To make sure you have support both before and after surgery, a social worker may evaluate your network of friends and family. If you are undergoing DBS, it is imperative that you have a spouse or full-time caregiver. Other standard, pre-operative tests may be performed by your local physician or the DBS staff. The specific tests will depend on your age and other health conditions. You may have one or more of the following:

- Magnetic resonance imaging (MRI) of the brain to make sure there are no other important issues such as brain shrinkage, strokes, or tumors
- Chest X-ray
- EKG, which measures heart rhythm
- Blood tests for blood counts, bleeding times, kidney function, and liver function
- Blood pregnancy test if female and of childbearing age
- Possible type and cross-match of blood, or donation of patient's own blood

6.4.2. Preparing for the Surgery

It's common to feel anxious or nervous as the surgery day draws near. Patients are frequently initially thrilled about the possibility of receiving DBS therapy. However, following the review and approval procedure, some people start to worry about the real event. Being anxious, afraid, or apprehensive is a typical and expected behavior. Speaking with others who have undergone the procedure could allay your worries. You can better prepare for the surgery by keeping yourself organized, making plans in advance, and understanding what to expect. It can be comforting to have a friend or family member make plans to stay by your side prior to, during, and following the procedure. This checklist will assist you in maintaining organization while you get ready for DBS.

A few weeks before surgery:

- Make sure you know where to go the day of surgery. This may be a different location from where you were evaluated. Write down the address, phone numbers, and parking instructions of the center. You may wish to practice in a rehearsal trip.
- If traveling from out of town, make arrangements to arrive a day early. Be sure to stay near the hospital. Check with the DBS center for recommended lodging and potential discounts.
- Get instructions from the DBS staff about when to take your PD medication the night prior to and the day of surgery. Most doctors will instruct you to not take PD medication the day of surgery. Therefore, your last dose will likely have to be taken the night before.

It's likely that you will be awake during the procedure, so being able to relax can make it go more smoothly. Practicing mindfulness, meditation, or music listening could be beneficial. Certain surgical centers permit their patients to take a light anesthetic and fall asleep during the procedure. This is generally not recommended as it may alter your brain's cell firing patterns and complicate brain mapping.

6.5. The Surgery

Plan to arrive at the center one hour prior to your scheduled surgery time on the day of the procedure. You'll be taken from the admitting area to a preoperative room, where you'll change into surgical clothes and have your breathing, blood pressure, and pulse assessed. You will have the chance to attend to any toilet requirements. At this point, an intravenous line (IV) might be inserted. The neurosurgeon will attach the head frame to your skull in the operating room. To precisely guide the neurosurgeon to the target, the frame resembling a box is essential. Due to the potential discomfort associated with applying the head frame, the areas where the screws that will secure the head frame to the skull are numbed by injection of local anesthetic. Additionally, mild painkillers might be provided. Throughout the entire procedure, the head frame will not be removed. An MRI or CAT scan (computed axial tomography) will be performed following the attachment of the head frame. The neurosurgeon uses this scan to pinpoint the precise location in the brain where the lead will be inserted. A specific shampoo or shaving cream will be applied to the area where the skull will be opened. It is no longer required in many operating rooms to shave the head entirely (Figure 6.4).

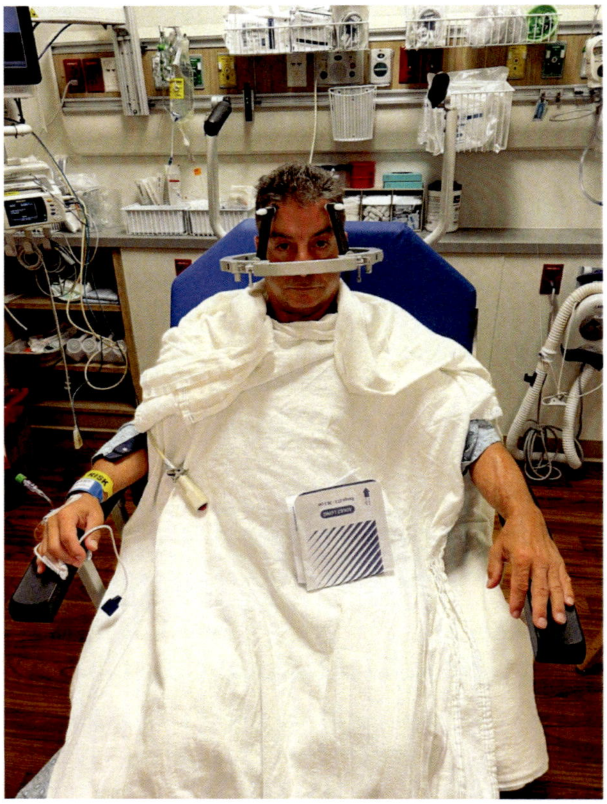

Figure 6.4. *Pre-operative head frame placement.*

Source: By Whoisjohngalt – Own work, CC BY-SA 4.0, https://commons.wikimedia.org/w/index.php?curid=131942246.

Some surgical practices will make use of a DBS system that is "frameless." You will see the neurosurgeon for this procedure at least one day prior to the operation. To hold the frameless system in place, he or she will insert a number of screws and plates into your skull. He or she will perform the surgery in the operating room, essentially in the same way as the frame-based system, after attaching the recording equipment to the plates. Neurosurgeons will select one approach over the other according to their personal preferences and experience. Be it a frame or not, the most crucial thing is that your surgeon is at ease performing the surgery.

You will be taken to the operating room following the brain scan. In addition to the neurosurgeon, the brain activity will be recorded by nurses, a movement disorders neurologist, or a neurophysiologist. After administering additional anesthesia to your scalp, the neurosurgeon will use a drill to make a hole in your skull the size of a dime, through which a microelectrode will be inserted (Figures 6.5 and 6.6).

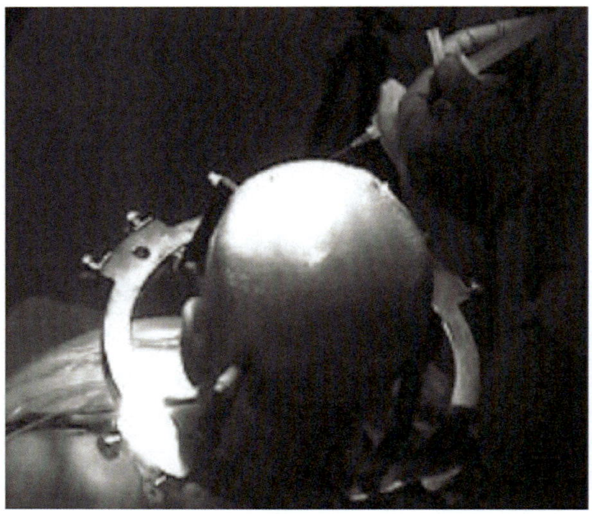

Figure 6.5. *Numbing of surgical site.*

Source: https://www.med.upenn.edu/pdmdc/assets/user-content/deep-brain-stimulation-guide-Parkinsons.pdf.

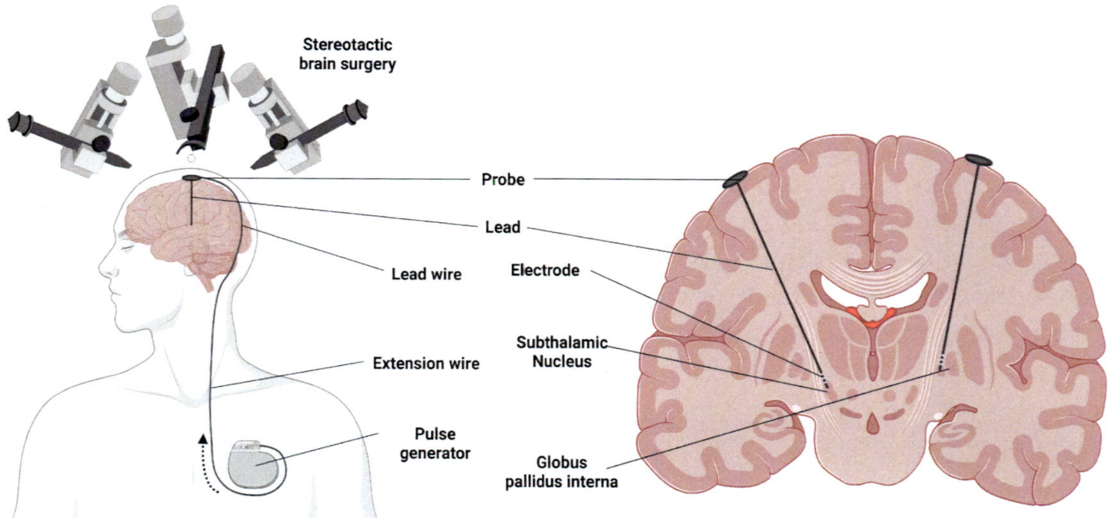

Figure 6.6. *The process.*

Source: Senevirathne DKL, Mahboob A, Zhai K, Paul P, Kammen A, Lee DJ, Yousef MS, Chaari A. Deep Brain Stimulation beyond the Clinic: Navigating the Future of Parkinson's and Alzheimer's Disease Therapy. Cells. 2023; 12(11):1478. https://doi.org/10.3390/cells12111478.

An essential component of the procedure is the microelectrode recording. The neurosurgeon will use this specialized procedure as guidance to precisely place the lead where it will produce the best results. Depending on how many microelectrode passes are needed to identify the target site and whether or not both sides of the brain are being operated on in a single session, this portion of the surgery may take several hours.

You might be asked to move your arm, leg, or face during the microelectrode recording, or the examiner might move them themselves. While the microelectrode is receiving electrical current, you might experience twitches, pulling, or tingling. All of these feelings are typical and to be expected. During the recording, you will be asked to remain silent so that the neurologist can move your arm, leg, or face to identify the specific areas of your brain that respond to touch or movement. To guarantee the best outcomes, you will need to be cooperative, quiet, and patient. The permanent DBS lead will be inserted after the neurosurgeon and neurologist have determined the optimal location based on the microelectrode recording's ability to pinpoint the exact target.

The neurologist or neurosurgeon will attach the lead to an external generator after it has been inserted and give you brief electrical stimulation to see if it helps your Parkinson's disease symptoms. The amount of improvement that is seen in the operating room, however, may not be the same as the amount that is eventually achieved. The neurologist and neurosurgeon will intentionally cause side effects, like tingling or pulling sensations or seeing spots. Measuring side effects aids in determining the DBS lead's location. The neurosurgeon will use a capping device to secure the permanent lead into place and run the connecting wire beneath the scalp's skin, outside the brain, once it has been verified that the lead is in the intended area. The skull's opening is closed with stitches and a plastic cap. In certain facilities, the pulse generator will then be inserted while you are unconscious under general anesthesia. This is usually done in the area of your chest beneath your collarbone. This second procedure will be carried out on a different day in other centers.

Patient will be brought to a post-operative area after the procedure and kept under close observation for at least an hour. After the surgery, it's critical to monitor for complications, such as disorientation or seizures, for the first 24 hours. You might occasionally be admitted to a specialized unit for intensive observation. The majority of patients leave the hospital the following day. On the other hand, if you experience weakness or confusion, infection symptoms, or an unanticipated consequence like stroke-like symptoms, you might need to stay longer. 10 to 20% of patients will stay in the hospital more than once after surgery.

It is possible to implant the implantable pulse generator (IPG) on the same day as the brain lead implantation, though this is usually done as a separate procedure several weeks later. The connecting wire will then be fastened to the IPG and brain lead at that point. This requires general anesthesia and takes about forty minutes. While some surgeons may need an overnight stay, the majority of surgeons will implant the IPG and release the patient that same day. Make sure you enquire with your DBS personnel about whether the IPG will be implanted concurrently with the brain leads or if it will be placed afterwards. Medication for PD should be taken as prescribed by your neurologist or as previously prescribed. Medication adjustments are typically made following the DBS system's programming.

6.6. After Surgery Care

The deep brain stimulation (DBS) staff will give you discharge instructions at the conclusion of your hospital stay so you can take care of yourself at home. These instructions include specifics on when to schedule follow-up appointments, how to take care of your surgical cuts, and how much medication to take for PD. In the event of an emergency, these instructions should also include phone numbers to call. To check the battery life of your device and turn on and off the DBS system, you might be given a patient controller or hand-held magnet of your own. These supplies are sometimes given out at the time of hospital discharge, but they could also be given out during follow-up clinic visits, particularly in cases where the DBS system is delayed. Make sure you understand how to operate the remote devices once you have these items. A wallet-sized card containing details about the DBS device and the name and phone number of your doctor will also be mailed to you. The information card and the magnet/patient controller should be carried at all times.

Be sure to schedule appointments for the following:

- Removal of sutures or staples
- Placement of the neurostimulator, if it has not been implanted at the time of the brain surgery
- Your first stimulator programming session

Complications can develop during the first few weeks or even months after surgery. You should know the signs and symptoms of infection, and you should be on the look-out for changes in mood, stroke-like symptoms and seizures.

1. **Infection:** Around the time of surgery, your doctor may prescribe antibiotics to reduce the chances of an infection at the incision sites. Other precautions that you can take to prevent an infection include the following:

- Carefully follow any instructions that were given by the DBS staff about caring for your incision.

- Wash hands frequently.
- Keep the stitches clean and dry. Clean stitches with a small amount of antibacterial soap and water, then pat dry with a clean towel or gauze. Keep stitches covered with a dry bandage or piece of gauze, especially while bathing.
- Do not go swimming or bathe in a hot tub while you have stitches.
- Never scratch, touch, or put any pressure on the incision.
- Be sure pillows, sheets, and bedding are clean.
- Make sure that hats and wigs are clean.
- Wash hands after handling pets.
- Return to have sutures and/or staples removed at the scheduled time. Most centers will remove sutures 7 to 10 days after surgery. Some surgeons may use stitches that dissolve on their own.
- Look for the signs of infection:
- Redness, swelling, or warmth at the incision or around the stitches
- A fever of 100 degrees or higher
- Pain or tenderness at the incision
- Puss, blood, or oozing at the incision

You should notify your doctor of any infection symptoms as soon as possible; they will probably prescribe antibiotics. While an infection may necessitate the removal of some or all system components, this can occasionally be avoided with early detection and antibiotic treatment.

2. **Mood Changes:** Notifying your neurologist of any mood changes is advised, particularly for depression and anxiety. Patients with DBS have reportedly experienced severe depression and even suicidal thoughts. Inform your doctor right away if you're feeling down. Inform a friend or family member if you are contemplating suicide. Either call 911 or have someone drive you to the closest emergency room. With the right care, depression that may be connected to DBS can be reversed. Here are some of the signs of depression:

- Saddened mood
- Excessive tearfulness or crying episodes
- Not feeling like doing your normal daily activities
- Wanting to be alone
- A sudden change in your sleeping habits—either sleeping too much or not enough
- Change in appetite, along with weight gain or loss
- Loss of libido, or sex drive
- Feeling irritable, anxious, or having feelings of panic
- Thinking and talking negatively
- Extreme loss of energy, tiredness, or fatigue

It has recently come to light that dopamine dysregulation syndrome, which is characterized by a patient's craving for dopamine, and impulse control disorders—such as improper eating, gambling, shopping, and/or sexual behaviors—can both be made worse by DBS. Furthermore, there have been multiple documented instances where DBS surgery can result in these kinds of behavioral side effects. Get in touch with your doctors right away if you encounter any of these behaviors so they can treat you.

3. **Stroke-like Symptoms:** Signs and symptoms of a stroke or brain bleed include the following:

- Sudden severe headache, nausea, and vomiting
- Suddenly becoming confused
- Numbness and weakness on one side of the body
- Difficulty talking
- Worsening of balance, or falling to one side
- Thinking and memory problems
- Loss of vision

If you experience these symptoms, seek medical attention immediately. A brain scan can determine if there is bleeding or a stroke. The brain scan can also be used to check DBS lead placement.

4. **Seizure:** Brain cells can become inflamed by head trauma, infection, blood, or, in the case of DBS, the actual placement of the electrodes, which can result in seizures. Rarely, seizures brought on by DBS therapy happen during surgery or in the first 24 hours after the procedure. Loss of consciousness and uncontrollably jerking the arms, legs, and face are the most common symptoms of seizures. They may also cause abrupt numbness or confusion. You should contact your doctor and get medical attention right away if you think you may have had a seizure. You might be prescribed anti-seizure medication, which will probably help you manage your symptoms. The majority of patients who have a seizure during or soon after surgery won't require medication for longer than six months, and the seizures typically don't come back.

6.7. Adjustment of Stimulation

The stimulator system is typically programmed as an outpatient procedure, though in certain deep brain stimulation (DBS) facilities, the system might be turned on prior to hospital discharge. In addition, activation can take place in a rehabilitation facility that offers alternative therapy. Typically, programming begins a few weeks after the DBS procedure. The majority of centers choose to wait for brain swelling around the DBS lead to subside for two to four weeks following surgery. The DBS programmer will use a tiny device to change the DBS system's settings while it is being programmed. He or she will test the effects of different electrode and stimulation settings by holding a tiny wand over the neurostimulator. You will be assessed and asked about your feelings during this process. Your tremor, stiffness, bradykinesia, dyskinesia/dystonia, and side effects like tingling, numbness, pulling, cramping, or electrical shock-like sensations will all be monitored by the programmer. It's also possible that your PD symptoms will worsen. Some Parkinson's disease symptoms frequently improve right away, but they can also reappear in a few hours or days. After a programming session, some programmers may ask you to remain close to the clinic for a few hours or may ask you to come back on a regular basis for the first six months. It is also possible for you to be admitted to a rehabilitation center, where your response to DBS programming and medication modifications can be closely monitored.

For best symptom control, most PD patients receiving DBS therapy will need multiple programming sessions. In DBS centers across the US, the typical number of programming sessions reported in the first half-year is approximately six. In the initial few months after DBS surgery, some patients might be able to reduce their PD medication dosages. Following the determination of the optimal settings and medication adjustments, you will be required to attend routine follow-up appointments. The precise timetable will change based on your health and the advice of your neurologist.

It is advisable that you inquire as to whether you need to take your regular prescription before the visit. When your last medication dose is taken the night before the programming session, your symptoms will be more noticeable and will not be confused with the side effects of your medication. This makes programming generally more successful. Later that day, or after you've taken your PD meds, more programming might be done. If you are asked to take your medications during or after programming, always have them with you.

Due to the numerous setting combinations and the possibility of multiple DBS leads being activated, determining the best setting for a patient can take some time. Every DBS electrode contains four leads. Not every one of the four electrodes is in use. Typically, one or two electrodes are activated based on the response. Three electrodes are rarely activated. Furthermore, the stimulation field's form is dictated by the manner in which these electrodes are triggered. Other parameters that can be changed are the voltage, pulse width, and frequency. Interleaving in more recent neurostimulators, like the Activa SC, enables even more sophisticated programming choices. Patients frequently request "higher" settings, but higher does not always mean better. Slurred speech is one example of a side effect of stimulation that can occasionally be caused by an excessive setting. Finding the ideal configuration for each unique person takes time. Similar to how a combination lock can be opened with low or high numbers, the DBS device needs to have the correct settings in order to give the patient the best results. The objective is to modify the settings to influence the targeted brain region (STN or GPi) when the DBS electrode is activated. Speech slurring, tingling, pulling sensations, nausea, and other side effects may occur as the settings are increased and the stimulation field expands to surrounding brain regions. The leads of conventional DBS electrodes can be turned on to try to prevent these side effects. But as the benefits of the stimulation diminish, so too might the side effects. In the clinic, it's possible that certain DBS settings won't immediately reveal their advantages or disadvantages. A patient may not fully understand and value a side effect, like tingling or slurred speech, in comparison to the advantages of DBS for several days to a few weeks. This is an additional explanation for why determining the ideal setting may require multiple DBS programming visits.

Patients with the Medtronic neurostimulators Activa SC, PC, and RC have "group" setting options. This is at the discretion of the DBS programmer. Patients can have up to 4 groups that are lettered: Group A, Group B, Group C, and Group D. Patients can be provided a different combination of settings in each group and can switch to a different group with their patient controller. This allows the patient to try alternative settings between programming visits.

When patients need higher voltage settings to control their tremor but the high-voltage setting causes slurred speech, there is another way to use the group settings. One group that has more precise tremor control but slurred speech could be used. Then, if you want to talk to someone without slurring your words, you can move to another group where there may be less slurring of speech but still only partial control over tremors. The DBS programmer can also try other kinds of advanced programming. Giving the patient the option to change the voltage, pulse width, or frequency within predetermined limits is another choice available with the more recent neurostimulators.

After selecting the best settings, you will be urged not to switch off your DBS system. You can use your patient controller device or a hand-held magnet to turn the device back on if it has been turned off for any reason. The neurostimulator's battery life should last two to five years, depending on the settings. Low battery life may make your PD motor symptoms worse. Your neurologist or neurosurgeon will want to arrange for you to have the old neurostimulator replaced as soon as its battery life is almost out. An incision is made to expose the area where the neurostimulator is implanted, the DBS extensions are disconnected, and a new neurostimulator is inserted and connected during this straightforward outpatient procedure. After being implanted, the new neurostimulator can be turned on right away.

It is crucial that the programmer checks the battery life and has a replacement strategy in place before beginning any programming session. There are situations when the battery life indicators can be deceiving, necessitating a replacement.

Your DBS programmer can use web-based DBS estimators that take into consideration your clinical symptoms. Estimators will give a ballpark estimate of how long the DBS battery should last. The DBS battery might need to be changed before the projected period ends, or it might last for a few more months after that. To prevent battery failure and loss of therapy efficacy, it is crucial that a DBS programmer inspect the device on a regular basis. This will help determine when the DBS battery needs to be changed.

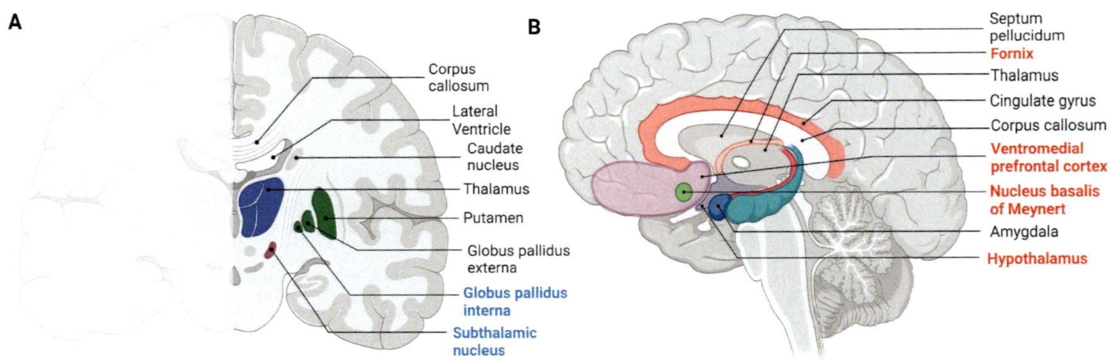

Figure 6.7. *Targets of DBS.*

Source: Senevirathne DKL, Mahboob A, Zhai K, Paul P, Kammen A, Lee DJ, Yousef MS, Chaari A. Deep Brain Stimulation beyond the Clinic: Navigating the Future of Parkinson's and Alzheimer's Disease Therapy. Cells. 2023; 12(11):1478. https://doi.org/10.3390/cells12111478.

- **Magnetic Fields and Household Appliances:** Any electromagnetic or magnetic field, such as that produced by theft detection devices in department stores or security equipment at airports and public buildings, has the potential to inadvertently turn off the neurostimulator. The neurostimulator can also be impacted by common magnets like those in wireless phones and radios, cabinet door closers, and refrigerator magnets. If the device is unintentionally turned off, symptom control will be compromised, but it is not dangerous. Using the patient controller or the hand-held magnet, the neurostimulator can be turned back on. The sensitivity of neurostimulators to magnetic fields and unintentional device deactivations is increased. Both the Infinity and the more recent Activa SC/PC/RC neurostimulators are less susceptible to magnetic fields and have a lower rate of unintentional device deactivations (Oliveira & Marta Ruiz-Lopez, 2021) (Figure 6.7).

6.7.1. Special Information and Warnings

There are tight guidelines you must adhere to when using other electrical devices after these electrical wires, or leads, have been inserted into the brain.

The deep brain stimulation (DBS) system may malfunction and pose a risk due to magnetic and electrical currents in the surrounding environment.

- **MRI and X-rays:** Radio waves and magnetic fields are used in MRI scanning to create images of the brain and other organs. After receiving DBS, you can have an MRI, but only under the strict supervision of medical professionals experienced in treating DBS patients. For instance, only a head coil MRI with a strength of 1 point 5 Tesla or less should be used for brain MRIs. This kind of head MRI is safe for people with DBS and has not been associated with any problems or injuries. Certain DBS systems are able to be turned on and off by the magnetic field of the head coil MRI. It is necessary to turn off the device and set the voltage to zero volts for the Soletra and Kinetra systems. Turning off the Activa SC/PC/RC is all that is required. While the Activa SC 37603 is safe for full-body MRI with certain precautions, the Activa SC 37602 is only safe for head MRIs. (Full-body MRI is not safe if the DBS batteries are positioned in the abdomen. The kind of MRI that is safe for each individual depends on additional factors. You should always confirm with the personnel at your DBS center that the type of MRI is safe for your specific DBS system before having any MRIs. People with DBS can safely undergo fluoroscopy, CAT scans, DAT/SPECT scans, standard X-rays, and PET (positron emission tomography) scans. Nevertheless, the quality of the image may be harmed in brain or head scans due to some distortion from the DBS leads.
- **Diathermy:** Physical therapists and dentists occasionally employ diathermy, a deep heat treatment, to relieve pain. When someone has DBS leads, they should never use diathermy because it can cause the leads to heat up too quickly and cause a stroke or even death. Additionally, it may harm the neurostimulator system.
- **Electrocautery:** Most surgeons use electrocautery, a form of electrical heat, to stop minor bleeding during surgery. Electrocautery can be used on people with DBS, but only with the following safeguards to minimize

any flow of the electrical current toward the DBS device:

i. Inform the surgeon that you have DBS therapy well before the surgery; contact your neurologist to let him or her know that you are having surgery.

ii. Just before surgery, the leads should be turned off, and the amplitude settings turned to zero.

iii. Bipolar electrocautery should be used to lessen transfer of electricity. Do not use a unipolar device.

iv. A ground lead should be placed on one of your legs. Any electrical charges that might transmit from the electrocautery device will be directed to the ground lead on your leg instead of the neurostimulator system.

- **Ultrasound:** It is safe to carry out ultrasound procedures like abdominal ultrasound and carotid doppler. Once more, before beginning any procedures, the DBS system's amplitude and voltage should be set to zero and the device turned off. Additionally, the ultrasonic microphone needs to be at least six inches away from the chest wall neurostimulator. A person should not have an echocardiogram, or ultrasound of the heart, if they have a DBS neurostimulator inserted in their left chest, unless the microphone is more than 6 inches away from the device. It is a good idea to visit your DBS center to ensure that your device is functioning properly following any ultrasound procedure. The primary issue with ultrasound procedures is that the quality of the ultrasound may be impacted by the neurostimulator, potentially leading to inaccurate test results. Otherwise, having these procedures done carries no significant risk.

- **Cardiac Pacemakers:** Cardiac pacemakers can usually be placed in persons who have had DBS therapy as long as the neurostimulator and cardiac pacemaker are 10 inches apart.

- **Miscellaneous Procedures:**

i. Any type of medical procedure that will be performed directly over the neurostimulator device or connecting wire is not recommended. It could damage the device. Most X-rays can be performed safely.

ii. Do not allow your dentist to place electric drills or cleaning tools near the neurostimulator, connecting wire, or implant site on the scalp. Dental X-rays are okay.

iii. If you have a mammogram, be sure that the pressure of the machine on the breast does not directly compress the neurostimulator or connecting wires.

iv. Radiation therapy for the treatment of cancer can be performed as long as it is not performed too close to the neurostimulator and a protective shield is placed over it.

v. Lithotripsy, a procedure to break up kidney stones, is not recommended unless it is the only medical option, as the treatment can damage the neurostimulator. If it is the only medical option, then protective shielding should be placed over the neurostimulator, which should be turned off and amplitude/voltage set to zero.

6.8. Emerging Changes and Future Directions in Deep Brain Stimulation for Parkinson's Disease

For some patients with PD, deep brain stimulation (DBS) is a potent tool that can help improve their quality of life. Researchers are constantly looking into DBS in an effort to improve and secure DBS management for patients. New insights from research will help scientists come up with innovative ways to improve the surgery.

Actually, the primary motivation behind scientists' ongoing research into DBS is the initial groundbreaking, life-altering success of DBS surgery—now regarded as the gold standard.

Even though there have been many positive developments, including better batteries, programming and targeting that enables DBS devices to operate longer on the same batteries, and electrodes that provide the best stimulation possible, scientists' work is still far from being finished.

Following are some innovations that will put you in the driver's seat, letting you make more choices about your Parkinson's therapy.

6.8.1. A New DBS Approach to Surgery

Patients undergoing deep brain stimulation surgery have the choice between being awake or asleep during the procedure. Originally, this surgery was performed with patients awake in order to receive feedback from them during the surgery. Many medical teams still prefer this method as it has been linked to successful treatment outcomes. Patients who are awake can actively participate in the procedure by helping the neurologist and neurosurgeon map the brain and find the relevant cells. Furthermore, being awake and off Parkinson's medications for a certain period of time allows neurologists to accurately identify the signals indicating Parkinson's disease, aiding in the precise placement of the electrode. Some medical teams have recently begun using anesthesia to put patients to sleep during the surgery, as this can alleviate the anxiety many patients feel about the procedure. However, this makes it more difficult for the surgeon to determine the exact placement of the electrode. While experienced surgeons can usually place the electrode correctly, verifying the placement using microelectrode recording can provide additional reassurance. Unfortunately, this method is less effective when the patient is asleep. There is ongoing debate among doctors about whether the benefits of microelectrode recording outweigh the challenges of managing patient anxiety.

6.8.2. MRI- or CT-Guided DBS versus Traditional Microelectrode Recording

There are two approaches your neurosurgeon can use to place your DBS electrode:

- *Microelectrode recording (MER-guided)*: This "gold standard" approach involves the surgeon using MRI or CT scans to plan the surgery, but using microelectrode recording to listen to your brain cells' signals, the surgeon confirms that the electrode is positioned correctly.
- *MRI or CT scans in the operating room (imaging-guided)*: With this new method, the surgeon uses MRI or CT scans to plan the surgery as

usual, but during the procedure, a scanner is used to monitor the electrode's placement into the brain and ensure that it is correctly placed within the intended target region. The patient can undergo this procedure while sedated (under anesthesia).

With imaging-guided surgery, the neurosurgeon can see the targeted area while performing the procedure and can react fast to any changes in the brain's movement. But when it comes to pinpointing the exact location of an electrode, MER is superior at identifying the brain cells. Cells are invisible in a scan. It is far more difficult for the neurologist to program the electrode appropriately to treat your Parkinson's disease if it is not positioned correctly. Rarely, patients have needed to have additional surgery to correct the placement. Many patients want a faster DBS procedure that allows them to stay asleep, so research is being done to better understand and achieve better results with this approach. Whatever instruments your surgeon employs, the most crucial aspect of treating Parkinson's disease is placing the electrodes correctly.

6.8.3. On the Horizon

Even though DBS therapy has brought about some significant advancements, there are still many areas that could be improved upon and a number of significant issues that need to be investigated. The effects of Parkinson's disease on the brain are extremely complex, and our understanding of the most effective methods and strategies for treating this illness with stimulation is still limited. DBS stimulates a "target"—a region of the brain impacted by Parkinson's disease. However, there are a number of novel targets to take into account, including the motor cortex, the pedunculopontine nucleus, the zona incerta, and the centromedian thalamus. Additionally, it's possible that activating one of these will alleviate symptoms (such as walking, balance, talking, and thinking) that don't currently respond well to standard DBS targets.

DBS devices these days pulse on a clocklike schedule. These "adaptive DBS" devices, which pulse only when your brain needed stimulation, are almost a reality. Imagine if a computer could listen for warning indications of trouble and then respond by pulsing to bring it back to normal, similar to a heart pacemaker. Electrodes with precise targeting capabilities, meaning they can be precisely positioned to stimulate the right cells rather than the wrong ones, may help your doctor minimize side effects and maximize your benefits. We may soon be able to monitor brain signals from PD and even remotely program multiple leads that have been implanted into different brain regions. Better DBS devices will allow us to treat specific symptoms in real-time, giving you the ability to combat Parkinson's wherever and whenever it suits you (Hariz, 2009; Okum et al, 2012; Fenoy & Simpson, 2014).

A Closer Look

Pedunculopontine Nucleus

The pedunculopontine nucleus (PPN), situated in the brainstem's rostral pons, has garnered increasing attention for its potential therapeutic role in movement disorders, particularly PD. Despite its intricate neural connections and multifunctional properties, the precise role of the PPN remains elusive. Functionally, the PPN serves as a crucial node in the neural circuitry governing motor control, integrating inputs from the basal ganglia, cerebellum, and cortex to regulate locomotion, posture, and balance. In PD, characterized by the degeneration of dopaminergic neurons within the substantia nigra and dysfunction in basal ganglia circuits, the PPN's role becomes pivotal. Emerging evidence suggests that PD pathology extends beyond the classical basal ganglia model, implicating brainstem structures like the PPN in motor symptomatology. Studies using animal models and neuroimaging in PD patients have highlighted alterations in PPN activity and connectivity, correlating with gait disturbances and postural instability. Consequently, PPN stimulation has emerged as a potential therapeutic strategy to ameliorate these symptoms. By delivering targeted electrical impulses to the PPN via deep brain stimulation (DBS), this intervention aims to modulate aberrant neural activity and restore motor function. Clinical trials evaluating PPN-DBS in PD have shown promising results, with improvements observed in gait velocity, freezing of gait, and postural stability. However, challenges persist in optimizing stimulation parameters and patient selection, given the its complex and heterogeneous connectivity. Moreover, the precise mechanisms underlying the therapeutic effects of PPN stimulation remain incompletely understood. Proposed mechanisms include modulation of basal ganglia output, enhancement of locomotor rhythm generation, and restoration of cortico-cerebellar interactions. Furthermore, PPN stimulation may exert non-motor effects, such as improving cognitive function and sleep disturbances, underscoring its potential utility beyond motor symptom management. Despite these advances, controversies persist regarding the ideal target within the PPN and the long-term sustainability of therapeutic benefits. Future research endeavors aim to elucidate the neurophysiological underpinnings of PPN function in health and disease, refine surgical techniques and stimulation protocols, and explore adjunctive therapies to augment its therapeutic efficacy. In conclusion, while the therapeutic potential of PPN stimulation in PD holds promise, further investigations are warranted to unlock its full clinical utility and address existing challenges, ultimately enhancing the quality of life for individuals living with PD and related movement disorders.

Summary

- Pallidotomy, thalamotomy, and subthalamotomy are types of surgical procedures in which a tiny heated probe is inserted into a precise region of the brain to destroy tissue. When the region known as the globus pallidus internus is lesioned, we refer to the procedure as a pallidotomy.
- Deep brain stimulation (DBS) is a surgical therapy used for the treatment of PD.
- DBS for PD requires a dedicated multidisciplinary team including a functional neurosurgeon, movement disorders neurologist, neuropsychologist and a specialist DBS nurse. This is necessary to enable a proper selection of patients suitable for DBS and an adequate life-long follow-up of operated patients.
- Deep brain stimulation (DBS) is a highly effective treatment for movement disorders like Parkinson's disease, essential tremor, and dystonia, but it does come with inherent risks and potential complications.
- Programming of the stimulator system is usually performed on an outpatient basis, although in some deep brain stimulation (DBS) centers the system may be activated before discharge from the hospital.
- MRI scanning uses magnetic fields and radio waves to view images of organs and other structures, including the brain. While you can have an MRI after you have DBS, it should only be done under close supervision by physicians who are familiar with procedures for DBS patients.
- A person with DBS leads should never have a total-body or full-body radio frequency coil MRI, or a head transmit coil MRI that extends over the chest. MRI should only be performed on the head region, not the neck or body. Some DBS systems are full-body MRI-compatible, while other systems are not. Always check with your implanting institution for the type of MRIs that are safe with your DBS system.
- The DBS system consists of the lead, connecting wire, implantable pulse generator (IPG), programmer, patient controller, and/or magnet.

References

1. Andy, O., Jurko, M., & Sias, F. (1963). Sub thalamotomy in treatment of parkinsonian tremor. *Journal of Neurosurgery, 20*, 860–870.
2. Benabid, A. L., Pollak, P., Louveau, A., Henry, S., & de Rougemont, J. (1987). Combined (thalamotomy and stimulation) stereotactic surgery of the VIM thalamic nucleus for bilateral Parkinson's Disease. *Applied Neurophysiology, 50*, 344–346.
3. Benazzouz, A., Gross, C., Féger, J., Boraud, T., & Bioulac, B. (1993). Reversal of rigidity and improvement in motor performance by subthalamic high-frequency stimulation in MPTP-treated monkeys. *European Journal of Neuroscience, 5*, 382–389.
4. Blomstedt, P., & Hariz, M. I. (2010). Deep brain stimulation for movement disorders before DBS for movement disorders. *Parkinsonism & Related Disorders, 16*, 42–33.

5. Cif, L., & Hariz, M. (2017). Seventy years with the globus pallidus: pallidal surgery for movement disorders between 1947 and 2017. *Movement Disorders, 32*, 972–982.

6. Coffey, R. J. (2009). Deep brain stimulation devices: A brief technical history and review. *Artificial Organs, 33*, 208–220.

7. De Bie, R. M., Schuurman, P. R., Esselink, R. A., Bosch, D. A., & Speelman, J. D. (2002). Bilateral pallidotomy in Parkinson's disease: A retrospective study. *Movement Disorders, 17*, 533–538.

8. Dietrichs, E., & Odin, P. (2017). Algorithms for the treatment of motor problems in Parkinson's disease. *Acta Neurologica Scandinavica, 136*, 378–385.

9. Fahn, S., Elton, R. L., & UPDRS Development Committee. (1987). Unified Parkinsons Disease Rating Scale. In S. Fahn, C. D. Marsden, D. B. Calne, & M. Goldstein (Eds.), *Recent Developments in Parkinsons Disease* (pp. 153–163). Florham Park: Macmillan Healthcare Information.

10. Fan, S., Liu, D., Shi, L., Meng, F., Fang, H., Liu, H., et al. (2022). Differential effects of subthalamic nucleus and globus pallidus internus deep brain stimulation on motor subtypes in Parkinson's disease. *World Neurosurgery, 77*(4), 710–719.

11. Fenoy, A. J., & Simpson, R. K. Jr. (2014). Risks of common complications in deep brain stimulation surgery: management and avoidance. *Journal of Neurosurgery, 120*(1), 132–139.

12. Fox, S. H., Katzenschlager, R., Lim, S. Y., Ravina, B., Seppi, K., Coelho, M., et al. (2011). The movement disorder society evidence-based medicine review update: treatments for the motor symptoms of Parkinson's disease. *Movement Disorders, 26*(Suppl 3), S2–S41.

13. Gildenberg, P. L. (1985). Surgical therapy of movement disorders. In R. H. Wilkins & S. S. Rengachary (Eds.), *Neurosurgery* (pp. 2507–2516). New York: McGraw-Hill.

14. Gildenberg, P. L. (2006). Evolution of basal ganglia surgery for movement disorders. *Stereotactic and Functional Neurosurgery, 84*, 131–135.

15. Hariz, M. I. (2009). Pallidotomy for Parkinson's disease. In *Textbook of Stereotactic and Functional Neurosurgery* (pp. 1540–1541).

16. Hariz, M. I., Blomstedt, P., & Zrinzo, L. (2010). Deep brain stimulation between 1947 and 1987: the untold story. *Neurosurgical Focus, 29*(2), E1.

17. Hariz, M., & Blomstedt, P. (2022). Deep brain stimulation for Parkinson's disease. *Journal of Internal Medicine, 292*, 764–778.

18. Hassler, R. (1955). The influence of stimulations and coagulations in the human thalamus on the tremor at rest and its physiopathology mechanism. In J. Greenfield Godwin & D. Russell (Eds.), *Proceedings of the Second International Congress of Neuropathology, London* (pp. 195–203). Amsterdam: Excerpta Medica.

19. Heath, R. G. (1977). Modulation of emotion with a brain pacemaker. Treatment for intractable psychiatric illness. *Journal of Nervous and Mental Disease, 165*, 300–317.

20. Hoehn, M. M., & Yahr, M. D. (1967). Parkinsonism: onset, progression and mortality. *Neurology, 17*, 427–442.

21. Holewijn, R. A., Verbaan, D., van den Munckhof, P. M., Bot, M., Geurtsen, G. J., Dijk, J. M., et al. (2021). General anesthesia vs local anesthesia in microelectrode recording-guided deep-brain stimulation for Parkinson's Disease: The galaxy randomized clinical trial. *JAMA Neurology, 78*, 1212–1219.

22. Jankovic, J., & Tolosa, E. (2007). *Parkinson's Disease and Movement Disorders* (5th ed.). Philadelphia: Lippincott Williams & Wilkins.

23. Katz, M., Luciano, M. S., Carlson, K., Luo, P., Marks Jr., W. J., Larson, P. S., et al. (2015). Differential effects of deep brain stimulation target on motor subtypes in Parkinson's disease. *Annals of Neurology, 77*, 710–719.

24. Krauss, J. K., & Fernandes, F. W. (2021). Svennilson's publication on pallidotomy for Parkinsonism in 1960: a most influential paper in the field. *Movement Disorders Clinical Practice, 9*, 173–177.

25. Laitinen, L. V., & Hariz, M. I. (1996). Movement disorders. In J. R. Youmans (Ed.), *Neurological Surgery* (4th ed., pp. 3575–3609). Philadelphia: Saunders.

26. Laitinen, L. V., Bergenheim, A. T., & Hariz, M. I. (1992). Leksell's posteroventral pallidotomy in the treatment of Parkinson's disease. *Journal of Neurosurgery, 76*, 53–61.

27. Lees, A. J., Hardy, J., & Revesz, T. (2009). Parkinson's disease. *The Lancet, 373*, 2055–2066.

28. Limousin, P., Krack, P., Pollak, P., Benazzouz, A., Ardouin, C., Hoffmann, D., et al. (1998). Electrical stimulation of the subthalamic nucleus in advanced Parkinson's disease. *New England Journal of Medicine, 339*, 1105–1111.

29. Limousin, P., Pollak, P., Benazzouz, A., Hoffmann, D., Le Bas, J. F., Broussolle, E., et al. (1995). Effect of Parkinsonian signs and symptoms of bilateral subthalamic nucleus stimulation. *The Lancet, 345*, 91–95.

30. Lindvall, O. (2016). Clinical translation of stem cell transplantation in Parkinson's disease (review). *Journal of Internal Medicine, 279*, 30–40.

31. Okun, M. S., & Zeilman, P. R. (2012). *Parkinson's Disease: Deep Brain Stimulation a Practical Guide for Patients and Families.* National Parkinson Foundation (U.S.).

32. Oliveira, L. M., Ruiz-Lopez, M., Boutet, A., Elias, G. J. B., Kalia, S. K., Hodaie, M., et al. (2021). Self-adjustment of deep brain stimulation delays optimization in Parkinson's disease. *May–June, 2021*, 676–681.

33. Pollak, P., & Krack, P. (2007). Deep-brain stimulation for movement disorders. In J. Jankovic & E. Tolosa (Eds.), *Parkinson's Disease and Movement Disorders* (5th ed., pp. 653–691). Philadelphia: Lippincott Williams & Wilkins.

34. Pollak, P., Benabid, A. L., Gross, C., Gao, D. M., Laurent, A., Benazzouz, A., et al. (1993). Effects of the stimulation of the subthalamic nucleus in Parkinson's Disease. *Revue Neurologique, 149*, 175–176.

35. Rehncrona, S., Johnels, B., Widner, H., Törnqvist, A. L., Hariz, M., & Sydow, O. (2003). Long-term efficacy of thalamic deep brain stimulation for tremor: Double-blind assessments. *Movement Disorders, 18*, 163–170.

36. Siegfried, J., & Lippitz, B. (1994). Bilateral chronic electrostimulation of ventroposterolateral pallidum: A new therapeutic approach for alleviating all Parkinsonian symptoms. *Neurosurgery, 35*, 1126–1129.

37. Strutt, A. M., Lai, E. C., Jankovic, J., Atassi, F., Soety, E. M., Levin, H. S., et al. (2009). Five-year follow-up of unilateral posteroventral pallidotomy in Parkinson's disease. *Surgical Neurology, 71*, 551–558.

38. Svennilson, E., Torvik, A., Lowe, R., & Leksell, L. (1960). Treatment of Parkinsonism by stereotactic thermolesions in the pallidal region. A clinical evaluation of 81 cases. *Acta Psychiatrica Scandinavica, 35*, 358–377.

39. The Deep-Brain Stimulation for Parkinson's disease Study Group. (2001). Deep brain stimulation of the subthalamic nucleus or the pars interna of the globus pallidus in Parkinson's disease. *New England Journal of Medicine, 345*, 956–963.

Chapter

7

THE ROLE OF THE NURSE PRACTITIONER/PHYSICIAN ASSISTANT

Contents

Introduction

Specialist practitioners, clinical leadership, case management, education, and care evaluation are the fundamental competencies of Parkinson's nurses. This could occur on a regular or emergency basis, and it could take place in clinics, hospitals, health centers, the individual's home, or a care facility. When necessary, they communicate with professional and volunteer groups in order to offer a full range of Parkinson's services that guarantee continuous, integrated care. Parkinson's nurses are in a unique position to educate patients, caregivers, and families as well as a variety of medical professionals who might only occasionally encounter Parkinson's patients.

Partially in response to mounting demands on consultant-led services and the realization that patient's value their opinions, the nurse specialist role emerged. In response to service demands and observations that patients in trials preferred the frequent, longer appointments with research nurses over the brief, infrequent reviews by their physician, Leeds General Infirmary created a rheumatology nurse specialist role in the early 1980s. Many disease areas, such as diabetes, multiple sclerosis, and chronic rheumatological conditions, now incorporate nurse-led care.

The development of guidelines with multidisciplinary actions that address the complexity of care is currently being observed as part of the remodeling of the health system. By providing health professionals with specialized knowledge, it is possible to standardize behaviors and reduce the obstacles to interprofessional collaboration.

In order to promote health, prevent complications, treat patients, and facilitate their rehabilitation, nursing care for patients with PD must be centered around the biopsychosocial context and grounded in the ethical, legal, operational, and theoretical presumptions of the profession.

Orientation and Directional Terms:

Term	Definition	Illustration
Health system	A health system consists of all organizations, people and actions whose primary intent is to promote, restore or maintain health. This includes efforts to influence determinants of health as well as more direct health-improving activities.	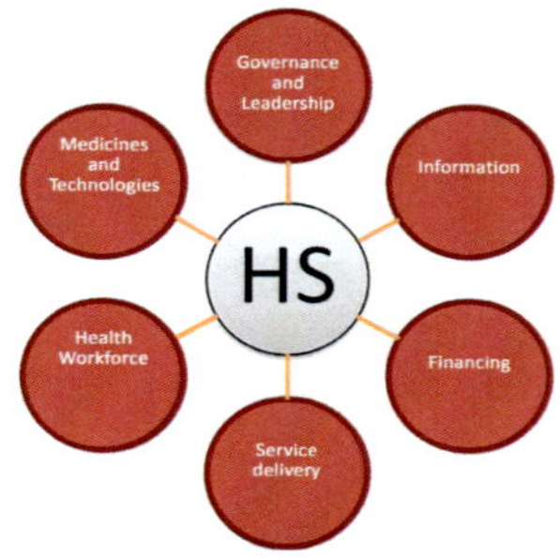
Hypoxemia	Hypoxemia is a low level of oxygen in the blood. It starts in blood vessels called arteries. Hypoxemia isn't an illness or a condition. It's a sign of a problem tied to breathing or blood flow.	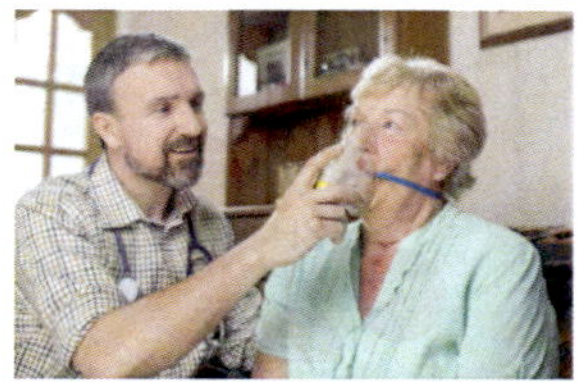
Dysarthria	Dysarthria is a speech disorder caused by muscle weakness. It can make it hard for you to talk. People may have trouble understanding what you say.	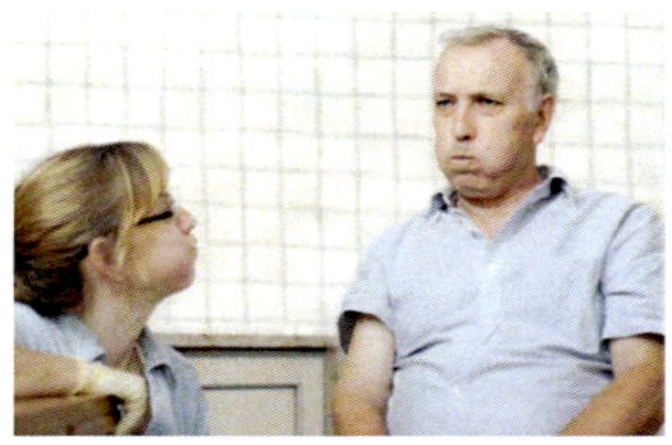
Lee Silverman Voice Treatment	The Lee Silverman Voice Treatment – LOUD (LSVT LOUD) is a treatment for speech disorders associated with PD. It focuses on increasing vocal loudness and is delivered by a speech therapist in sixteen one-hour sessions spread over **four** weeks. A derivative of this treatment, known as LSVT BIG, is used in treating movement aspects of Parkinson's disease.	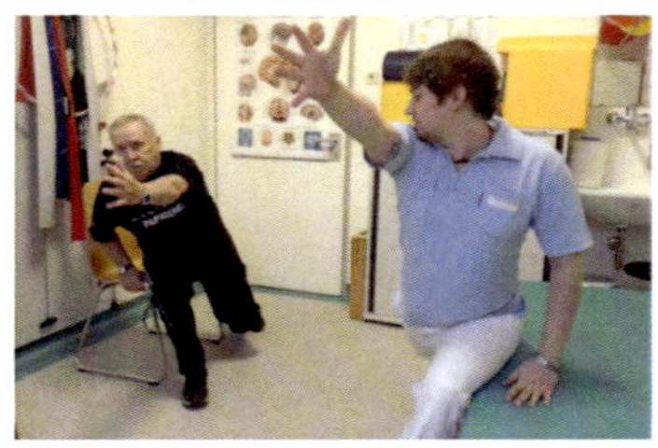
Bradykinesia	Bradykinesia means slowness of movement and speed (or progressive hesitations/ halts) as movements are continued. It is one of the cardinal symptoms of PD.	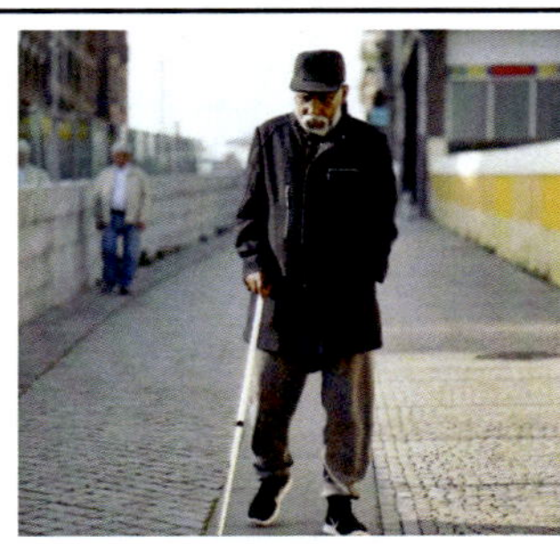

7.1. Improving Respiratory Function

Parkinson's disease is a neurodegenerative condition that mainly affects movement, but it can also significantly impair breathing and other body systems. Parkinson's disease patients frequently experience respiratory issues, which can lower their quality of life. Nonetheless, there exist multiple approaches and measures that can be implemented to enhance respiratory performance in patients suffering from Parkinson's disease (Jennifer Schlette, 2024).

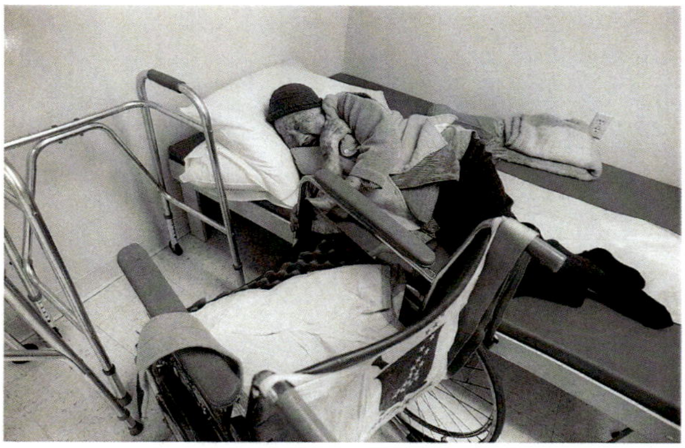

Figure 7.1. *Providing care to patients who are suffering from conditions that affect their breathing.*

Source: By Nancy Wong – Own work, CC BY-SA 4.0, https://commons.wikimedia.org/w/index.php?curid=81990587.

1. ***Observe the patient and assess energy level and endurance, and how these affects respiratory status:*** Age and chronic conditions such as Parkinson's disease reduce energy ability. The most prevalent form of Parkinsonism, PD, has been studied for its impairment of pulmonary function; however, the cause of PD is unknown. As an autonomic disorder, pulmonary dysfunction has been linked to non-motor symptoms of PD abnormalities, such as obstructive, restrictive, and mixed-type pulmonary dysfunction, which worsen disability in PD patients (Figure 7.1).
2. ***Assess respiratory status for rate, depth, ease, use of accessory muscles, and work of breathing:*** A study found that compared to age-matched healthy controls, patients with early idiopathic PD had significantly lower respiratory muscle strength and higher central respiratory drive. Peak expiratory and inspiratory flow abnormalities were discovered in patients with relatively severe PD who did not exhibit any clinical indications of respiratory issues. These alterations can be accounted for by "muscle weakness" and hypokinesia, two hallmark symptoms of Parkinson's disease. The primary causes of the restrictive pattern and dysfunction of the upper airways may be respiratory muscle rigidity or poor coordination.
3. ***Auscultate the lung fields for the presence of wheezes, crackles, rhonchi, or decreased breath sounds:*** Squeezing air past the constricted airways during expiration—a condition brought on by bronchospasms, edema, and obstructive secretions—causes wheezing. An infection or fluid buildup in the lungs is the cause of crackles, which are caused by the consolidation of leukocytes and fibrin in the lung. Reduced breath sounds typically indicate inadequate ventilation and may be a sign of

alveolar collapse with little to no air exchange in the auscultated lung area.

4. ***Assess the patient for pallor or cyanosis in nail beds and/or around the mouth:*** This could be a sign of hypoxemia. According to a number of studies, patients with Parkinson's disease are more likely to have upper airway obstruction. This leads to chronic airflow limitation, which in turn causes weakness, bradykinesia, or dysfunctional contraction of the striated musculature in the upper airway region. These factors have been identified as major risk factors for the development of aspiration pneumonia, atelectasis, and secretion retention.
5. ***Monitor the patient for cough and production of sputum, noting the amount, color, character, and Patient's ability to expectorate secretions and the patient's ability to cough:*** An infection may be present if mucus turns green or yellow in color. Tough, viscous secretions are harder to cough up and clear, and they can obstruct airways and cause stasis, which can result in infection. Pneumonia kills a disproportionately high proportion of Parkinson's Disease patients when compared to the overall population.
6. ***Position the patient in a high Fowler's or semi-Fowler's position, if possible:*** This encourages lung expansion to its maximum. According to a study, dyspnea is a common symptom in the progression of Parkinson's disease, accounting for about 40% of patients' symptomatology. The degree of the illness, reduced ventilatory function, motor fluctuations, dysphagia, and even neuropsychological symptoms like anxiety and depression are all correlated with the presence of dyspnea.
7. ***Turn the patient in every two hours:*** In order to reduce the risk of atelectasis, repositioning encourages the drainage of pulmonary secretions and improves ventilation. Autonomic dysfunction is thought to manifest as dyspnea and subsequent ventilatory dysfunctions. Partially to blame for ventilatory dysfunction in Parkinson's Disease patients are the obstructive and restrictive features, possible drug side effects, and abnormal central control of ventilation.
8. ***Encourage an increase in intake of fluids up to 3 to 4 L/day:*** This provides hydration and helps to thin secretions for easier mobilization and removal. Drinking enough water can aid in swallowing by moistening the throat and making it easier to swallow food and medications. Parkinson's Disease can also cause dysphagia.
9. ***Perform postural drainage and percussion as ordered:*** Gravity is used by postural drainage to help raise secretions and facilitate sputum clearance. With the help of percussion, secretions may be moved away from the bronchial walls, allowing the patient to cough them up and exhale more forcefully.

Certain positions might not be suitable for patients who are older adults. Breathing exercises, incentive spirometry, postural drainage, and airway clearance techniques could all be beneficial.

10. ***Encourage deep breathing and coughing exercises every two hours:*** This promotes lung expansion and facilitates easier expectoration by loosening secretions. Through the relaxation of accessory muscles and the reduction of respiratory rate, deep breathing exercises can lessen the effort required to breathe. By relaxing the diaphragm, diaphragmatic breathing helps to lessen breathing difficulties by lowering the activity of accessory muscles. Breathing at the apical, costal, and basal levels enhances different lung segments.
11. ***Suction patient if warranted:*** It's possible that the patient is too weak or worn out to clear their own secretions. One of the most dangerous side effects and a leading cause of death in patients with PD is respiratory complications. If the patient is unable to effectively expel secretions, the nurse must evacuate the area.
12. ***Administer oxygen as ordered. Monitor oxygen saturation by pulse oximetry:*** This helps the patient by giving them extra oxygen. Furthermore, hyperbaric oxygen therapy (HBOT) has been proposed as an additional treatment option for Parkinson's disease. Hyperbaric oxygen therapy (HBOT) has been found to have neuroprotective effects by reducing hypoxia, inhibiting inflammation, and enhancing nervous system microcirculation.
13. ***Administer bronchodilators as ordered:*** This opens up airways to improve ventilation, encourages bronchial smooth muscle relaxation to reduce spasms, and optimizes air exchange. Once the use of care was taken into account, there was a decreased risk of PD associated with the use of salbutamol and inhaled corticosteroids for both COPd and asthma.
14. ***Instruct the patient to seek help and stop smoking if the patient is a smoker:*** Smoking raises blood pressure, mucus production, and vasoconstriction. The risk of PD is inversely correlated with cigarette smoking, according to a meta-analysis of observational studies. Additionally, nicotine may function as a stimulant to block the striatal dopamine transporter's activity, raising dopamine levels in the synaptic gap. Furthermore, there's a chance that smoking cigarettes will impair cognitive function.
15. ***Assist the patient in respiratory muscle training:*** Exercise of the respiratory muscles may be able to increase peak cough flow, since decreased cough function is linked to decreased respiratory muscle strength. Programs for strengthening the respiratory muscles have been used to enhance swallowing and lung function in patients with PD and other neurodegenerative diseases. Studies on patients with

PD have shown improvements in the strength and endurance of their inspiratory muscles.

16. ***Provide information about chest PNF:*** When it comes to respiratory disorders like COPD, chest PNF is a proven treatment option. It enhances the depth and rate of breathing by giving the respiratory muscles proprioceptive feedback, which triggers reflex respiratory movement responses. Additionally, this makes the diaphragm and abdominal muscles more active. By autogenic inhibition, the inflexible muscles of the chest wall may be inhibited, allowing the wall to become more mobile (Hellqvist & Bertero, 2015; Vlaanderen et al., 2019; Bhidayasiri et al., 2020).

7.2. Enhancing Sensory and Cognitive Function

In patients with Parkinson's disease, sensory impairments and cognitive decline—including issues with attention, memory, and executive functions—are frequently seen. To improve these patients' sensory and cognitive functioning, a number of tactics and interventions can be used.

1. ***Assess the patient for depressive behaviors and causative events, and orient the patient to reality as warranted:*** Patients with PD frequently experience depression; however, it is unclear if this is a result of the disorder or a biochemical abnormality. Identify particular issues and make it possible to create a care plan. The patient's awareness of oneself and environment is aided by reality orientation. But evaluating depression in PD patients is made more difficult by the fact that some PD symptoms—like mask-like facial expressions, sleeplessness, psychomotor slowing, fatigue, and difficulty concentrating—share similarities with depression symptoms.
2. ***Identify the patient's medications currently being taken:*** This helps in identifying drug abuse and side effects that might exacerbate depression symptoms. Anticholinergic medications used to treat Parkinson's disease motor symptoms may make memory loss worse. These drugs should be stayed away from whenever possible.
3. ***Assess the Patient for the potential for suicide and suicidal ideation:*** Individuals who are seriously depressed and have considered suicide already require immediate medical attention. The physical restrictions brought on by PD and the well-known elevated risk of suicide in older adults, in addition to the long-established links between mental disorders and suicide, highlight the possibility of suicide in PD patients.
4. ***Monitor vital signs every four hours and PRN:*** Cardiovascular and cerebrovascular insufficiency can be caused by antidepressants and other psychoactive medications. Amantadine may result in mood swings, hallucinations, and psychiatric problems. In PD patients, autonomic dysfunction is prevalent. Orthostatic hypotension frequently arises as a late-stage concern.

5. ***Use a nonjudgmental attitude toward the patient and actively listen to his feelings and concerns:*** This builds a rapport of trust and gives the patient permission to talk about issues that they can handle in healthy ways. Individuals with PD may experience feelings of embarrassment, apathy, boredom, and loneliness due to their physical slowness and the significant effort even simple tasks require. Encourage and support the patient to do all the tasks necessary to take care of their own everyday needs in order to maintain their independence.
6. ***Prepare the patient for deep brain stimulation (DBS):*** For PD patients, DBS surgery has emerged as the preferred method. It's a type of surgery called stereotactic. It is reversible, does not result in the death of brain tissue, can be modified as the condition worsens or unfavorable outcomes arise, and allows for the completion of bilateral operations without noticeably increasing the risk of unfavorable outcomes.
7. ***Refer the patient to a psychiatrist:*** To rule out active mental illness and screen for pertinent past mental history that may be a contraindication to surgery, such as major depression and suicidality, a psychiatrist with experience in the psychiatric complications of movement disorders may be consulted.
8. ***Administer levodopa and carbidopa:*** The usual course of treatment for Parkinson's disease symptoms is still levodopa plus carbidopa. With the fewest short-term side effects, it offers the strongest anti-Parkinsonian effect. A low dose of levodopa/carbidopa is started and increased gradually. Greater levodopa delivery to the central nervous system is made possible by carbadoxopa, which prevents levodopa from being converted to dopamine in the systemic circulation.
9. ***Administer selective serotonin reuptake inhibitors (SSRIs):*** For the treatment of depression in PD, SSRIs are the most often prescribed drugs. Nonetheless, a number of systematic reviews, meta-analyses, and randomized controlled trials have revealed that SSRIs might not work any better in this circumstance than a placebo. Paroxetine has been shown to produce positive outcomes in randomized clinical trials; it was well-tolerated and did not impair motor function.
10. ***Administer selective serotonin inverse agonists (SSIA):*** In April 2016, pimavanserin received approval for the treatment of delusions and hallucinations connected to PD psychosis. It is the first medication authorized for this particular ailment. It avoids activation at dopamine and other receptors that antipsychotics frequently target in addition to preferentially targeting 5-HT2A receptors.
11. ***Provide information about cognitive behavioral therapy***

(CBT): In PD, CBT can aid in impulse control. CBT dramatically reduced the severity of symptoms, neuropsychiatric disturbances, and levels of anxiety and depression in a study involving 45 patients with idiopathic PD and related impulse control behaviors that had not responded to conventional treatment (Hellqvist and Bertero, 2015; Vlaanderen et al, 2019; Bhidayasiri et al, 2020).

7.3. Improving Speech and Communication

Parkinson's disease patients frequently experience impaired verbal communication as a result of the disease's effects on the muscles involved in speaking and swallowing as well as cognitive impairments that may have an impact on language processing and expression. This can show up as reduced vocal inflection, articulation and pronunciation difficulties, or soft or monotonous speech. It can be challenging for people with Parkinson's disease to be understood by others due to changes in their voice, articulation, and general speech clarity. Nonetheless, a range of tactics and measures can be implemented to enhance speech and communication abilities in these individuals.

1. ***Assess the patient's ability to speak, language deficit, cognitive or sensory impairment, and presence of aphasia, dysarthria, aphonia, dyslalia, or apraxia:*** The majority of Parkinson's Disease patients have speech disorders; this aids in identifying problem areas and speech patterns to help create a treatment plan. Between 45 and 89% of patients experience speech difficulties at some point during the illness, and over 30% of patients consider speech problems to be the most crippling aspect of their condition.
2. ***Monitor the patient for nonverbal communication, such as facial grimacing, smiling, pointing, crying, and so forth; encourage the use of speech when possible:*** When speech is impaired, this suggests that needs or feelings are being communicated. The patient may have to rely on nonverbal cues, excessive mumbling, or striking out as their only means of expressing discomfort. Compared to healthy adults, patients with PD have been found to be less likely to engage in conversations due to a lack of confidence in their ability to communicate.
3. ***Assess vocal loudness, intonation, and quality:*** Assessing the vocal quality, loudness, intonation, and fluidity of speech and articulation should be done while the patient is speaking. Reasonable speech samples can be obtained by counting to fifty, reading a passage that assesses articulation, and maintaining vowel phonation for the maximum amount of time.
4. ***Instruct patients to make a conscious effort to speak slowly, with deliberate attention to what they're speaking:*** This facilitates the establishment of a clear channel of communication with the patient. Speech impairment is one of the early signs of PD, especially hypophonia. Reduced absolute speech volume and pitch fluctuation,

breathiness, tremor, rough or hoarse voice quality, irregular speech rates, and imprecise articulation are all examples of voice and speech problems. Parkinsonian dysarthria, sometimes referred to as hypokinetic dysarthria, is the collective term for these PD-related speech abnormalities.

5. ***Attempt to anticipate the patient's needs:*** Anxiety and frustration are lessened as a result. A small number of research have looked at PD patients' voice-related quality of life. According to one study, people with dysphonia experience psychological distress as a result of their condition. According to a different study, depression and dysphonia in people with Parkinson's disease are strongly associated.
6. ***When communicating with the patient, face the patient and maintain eye contact, speaking slowly and enunciating clearly in a moderate or low-pitched tone:*** Clear, concise communication and giving adequate time for responses are important for ensuring a successful speech. Research has shown that speech and language difficulties in Parkinson's disease can impact both the individual and their family, even before noticeable speech issues arise. These communication challenges can hinder social interactions, leading to feelings of anxiety and isolation.
7. ***Remove competing stimuli, and provide a calm, unhurried atmosphere for communication:*** This lessens needless noise and distraction and gives the patient more time to feel less irritated. Patients with PD who experience speech difficulties such as soft voice, slurred speech, or reduced articulation must work harder and pay closer attention in order to communicate effectively. Patients are better able to concentrate on speaking in a quiet, distraction-free atmosphere, which enhances their ability to pronounce words clearly and speak steadily.
8. ***Use simple, direct questions requiring one-word answers, as well as simple directions:*** When a patient can speak or communicate to some extent, this helps them feel more confident. The results of communicative participation were substantially correlated with the perceived presence of cognitive symptoms. Significantly lower levels of communicative participation were reported by patients who reported cognitive symptoms, such as trouble remembering where things were placed, trouble reading and following complex instructions, or trouble making and keeping appointments. Language ability should be taken into account during assessment and treatment planning because of the connection between cognitive symptoms and severe language impairments in Parkinson's disease.
9. ***Provide a small electronic amplifier if necessary:*** If the patient finds it difficult to be heard, this is beneficial. The main purpose of amplification devices is to make voices louder and more intense,

which improves perceived speech intelligibility. Additionally, using an amplification device can help patients with PD communicate more successfully and with fewer requests for their messages to be repeated.

10. ***Encourage the patient to control the length and rate of phrases, over-articulate words, and separate syllables, emphasizing consonants:*** This facilitates speech when dysarthria is present. Participation in communication was also correlated with speech usage. All things considered, increased speech usage was linked to a better sense of communicative participation. Greater communicative participation was reported by patients who spoke more. For those over 65, social participation has been linked to a higher quality of life.
11. ***Avoid rushing the patient when struggling to express feelings and thoughts:*** A patient experiencing impaired verbal communication may experience feelings of frustration, despair, and isolation. A therapeutic alliance and a feeling of trust are fostered by compassion, which is also necessary for ongoing communication. Hearing someone with PD can be extremely difficult for listeners due to hypophonia, especially when there is background noise. The understanding of PD speech is also affected by the blurring of speech components caused by inaccurate articulation and abnormal speech rate.
12. ***Instruct the patient and/or SO regarding the need to use glasses, hearing aids, and dentures:*** With sensory impairments or other disabilities, this facilitates communication. Treatment options for speech impairments associated with Parkinson's disease are numerous. The use of instrumentally based biofeedback therapy, prosthetic or assistive speech devices, and perceptually based behavioral speech therapy are the three approaches that garner the most attention. The goals of these treatment methods are to decrease rapid speech, enhance articulatory precision and mobility, enhance speech intensity, and improve speech prosody (Figure 7.2).

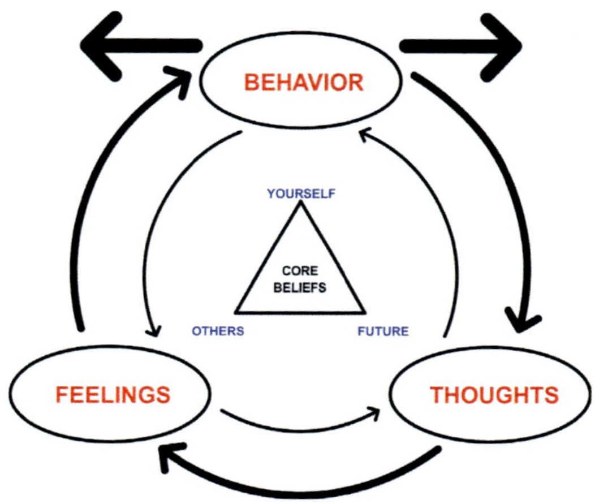

Figure 7.2. *Speech therapy for Parkinson's disease.*

Source: By Urstadt at English Wikipedia, CC BY-SA 3.0, https://commons.wikimedia.org/w/index.php?curid=101734066.

13. ***Instruct the patient and/or SO in the performance of facial muscle exercises:*** By improving muscle tone and coordination, this encourages the use of facial expressions in communication. A common PD-related facial expression loss is

a masked face, also known as hypomimia. It implies a true loss of motor control as opposed to a physical sign of emotional blunting. It matters how you express yourself facially. Studies have indicated that individuals with PD who have received regular facial exercise and therapy to enhance their facial control have a higher quality of life than those who have not.

14. ***Refer the patient to the Lee Silverman Voice Treatment (LSVT):*** A program called LSVT is intended to help PD patients speak louder. The goal of the four-week treatment plan is to maximize respiratory and phonatory functions through the rigorous practice of a small set of tasks four times a week. Without interval intervention, the aim of LSVT is to improve vocal performance in 6 to 24 months. Despite the need to "think loud, think shout," patients with PD speak normally and with a healthy voice quality after LSVT.
15. ***Arrange for the patient's participation in speech and language therapy:*** Conventional speech and language therapy incorporates exercises that target diaphragmatic breathing, pacing, and articulation, among other areas, and is customized to meet the needs of each patient. Although speech therapy is useful in treating the laryngeal manifestations of PD, only 3–4% of patients with the disease receive speech therapy, even though a considerable number of patients experience vocal symptoms.
16. ***Prepare the patient for and assist in surgical treatment methods:*** Although there is no clear-cut evidence linking posteroventral pallidotomy to Parkinsonian dysarthria, a few pilot studies have found improvements in articulatory and/or phonatory measures after the procedure. Vocal fold injection (VFI) augmentation is a transient, minimally invasive procedure that can be safely performed in an office setting. It permits the repeated application of modifications to the vocal fold configuration. The symptoms of glottic insufficiency that are effectively treated by VFI augmentation include trouble swallowing thin liquids, weariness or pain after speaking, and difficulty speaking (Hellqvist & Bertero, 2015; Vlaanderen et al., 2019; Bhidayasiri et al., 2020).

7.4. Enhancing Physical Mobility

Parkinson's disease frequently manifests as impaired physical mobility because the disease causes the neurons that regulate movement to degenerate.

Bradykinesia, tremors, rigidity, and postural instability can result from this, which can make it challenging for patients to carry out daily tasks, keep their balance, and walk unassisted. It is commonly known that a sedentary lifestyle lowers quality of life, raises the risk of falls, and deteriorates the clinical and functional domains of Parkinson's disease. Nonetheless, a range of tactics and measures can be implemented to improve these patients' physical mobility (Figure 7.3).

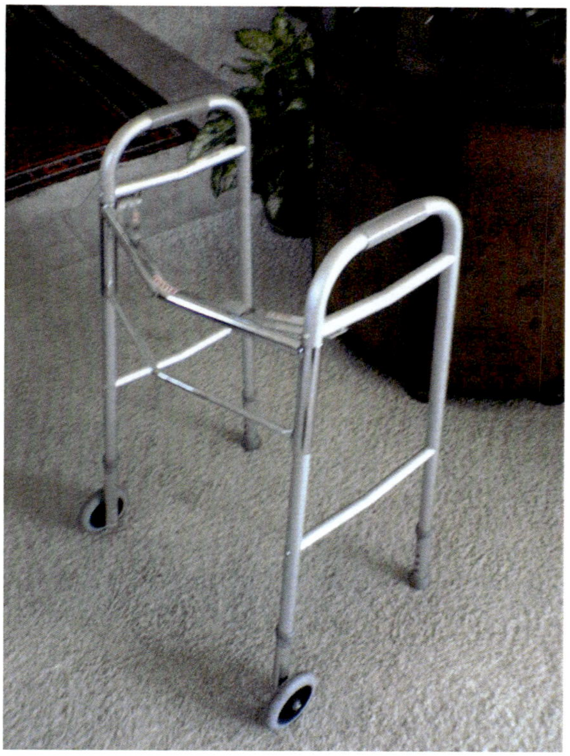

Figure 7.3. *Enhancing mobility and physical health.*

Source: By The original uploader was High Plains Drifter at English Wikipedia. – Transferred from en.wikipedia to Commons., Public Domain, https://commons.wikimedia.org/w/index.php?curid=4353655https://www.countrymeadows.com/blog/therapeutic-modalities-enhancing-mobility-and-physical-health.

1. ***Assess for the presence of rigidity and bradykinesia:*** Flexing and extending the patient's relaxed wrist is a common test for rigidity. It can also be used to highlight rigidity by having the patient use the contralateral limb to make voluntary movements like tapping. One way to evaluate bradykinesia in a patient is to have them tap their toes as quickly and forcefully as they can. To evaluate the patient's ability to get out of a chair, have them stand up from a seated position with their arms crossed.
2. ***Observe for gait abnormalities:*** In the initial phase of Parkinson's disease, patients experience a slowing of their walking pace and shorter steps than healthy individuals of the same age. Decreased arm swing, less smooth movement, and increased differences in movement between limbs are characteristic symptoms of PD and often present as the first signs of motor impairment. The Unified Parkinson's disease Rating Scale is a commonly utilized tool for evaluating symptoms of PD, including a detailed analysis of various aspects of walking that may contribute to functional limitations.
3. ***Assess the patient for postural stability:*** Patients are usually asked to stand with their eyes open and then pull their shoulders back toward the examiner in order to assess postural stability. The patient is instructed to quickly regain their balance and to be prepared for the displacement. It's normal to take one or two steps backward to regain equilibrium. In the event that the patient is unable to regain equilibrium, the examiner should be prepared to intervene.
4. ***Monitor the patient's blood pressure, especially, before and after staying in a prolonged sitting or lying position:*** By monitoring blood pressure and heart rate while the patient is supine and then standing for three minutes,

orthostatic hypotension should be actively screened for at the bedside. A diagnosis of orthostatic hypotension is made when the diastolic or systolic blood pressure falls by more than 10 mm Hg or more.

5. ***Instruct the patient with techniques that initiate movement:*** It's helpful to rock back and forth to initiate the leg movement. Bradykinesia is the term for slowness of movement, but it also describes a decrease in amplitude and spontaneous movement. Furthermore, the patient may also experience postural instability, which is characterized by imbalance and loss of reflexive responses.
6. ***Instruct the patient to get out of the chair by moving to the edge of the seat, placing hands on arm supports, bending forward, and then rocking to a standing position:*** Parkinson's disease can result in bradykinesia, rigidity tremors, and difficulty rising from a chair. An increase in resistance to passive movement about a joint is referred to as rigidity. There are two types of resistance: oscillating and smooth. Additionally, if the patient stands up right away from a seated position, orthostatic hypotension may increase the patient's risk of falling.
7. ***Teach the patient to concentrate on walking erect and use a wide-based gait:*** The inflexibility of the arms, which inhibits them from swinging when walking normally, may negatively impact balance. To counteract the shuffling gait and the inclination to lean forward, a unique walking technique needs to be mastered. Walking with long strides requires a deliberate effort to raise the feet, swing the arms, and place the feet heel-toe.
8. ***Instruct the patient to perform a daily exercise that will increase muscle strength: walking, riding a stationary bike, swimming, and gardening are helpful:*** Exercise lessens muscular rigidity, enhances coordination and dexterity, and prevents contractures that happen when muscles are not used. Walking and exercise regimen adherence slows the disease's progression. Additionally, exercise can enhance gait through a variety of indirect mechanisms, such as increased strength, balance, and fitness, and some that are specific to the central aspects of gait control.
9. ***Teach the patient to sit in chairs with backs and armrests; use elevated toilet seats or sidebars in the bathroom:*** This lessens the risk of falls and facilitates getting up from a sitting position. A straightforward, first-line solution for patients who have trouble transferring or standing for extended periods of time is to add seats, either fixed or free-standing, and boards to showers and bathtubs. Either with or without frames and handles, elevated toilet seats can be helpful for people who have trouble getting off the toilet. When positioned correctly, these facilitate standing, and they are simple to take off and put back on.

10. ***Provide warm baths and massages:*** This aids in releasing tense, painful muscle spasms that come with rigidity. Some patients may report having stiff limbs, but this is more likely to be bradykinesia than stiffness. Sometimes people describe a sensation of stiffness that feels like a ratchet when they move a limb. This could be a sign of cogwheel rigidity.
11. ***Instruct the patient to raise the head of the bed and make position changes slowly:*** These measures reduce orthostatic hypotension. Syncope, inexplicable falls, dizziness, headaches, blurred vision, exhaustion, dyspnea, and pain in the shoulders, neck, or low back that worsens when standing but goes away when lying down are symptoms of orthostatic hypotension. Particularly after spending a prolonged amount of time resting supine, advise the patient to stand up gradually; in this scenario, the patient may hesitate to stand up and resume their sitting position.
12. ***Refer the patient to a physical therapist:*** This could be useful in creating a personalized fitness regimen and teaching the patient and caregiver safe exercise techniques. A comprehensive analysis of 33 randomized studies with 1515 patients assessed a range of physiotherapy interventions, such as exercise, cueing, martial arts, general physiotherapy, and treadmill training. Mobility, balance, step length, walking endurance, and walking speed all showed notable gains.
13. ***Promote increased fluid intake and maintain adequate dietary salt:*** Enhancing hydration (to 2.5 L/day) and salt consumption (6 to 10 g/day) is a crucial non-pharmacological approach to address orthostatic hypotension. Within the next 30 to 90 minutes, consuming a 500 mL bolus of water causes a significant increase in blood pressure. Patients who have a history of heart, kidney, or liver failure should use caution when consuming salt and water.
14. ***Promote the use of mobility aids and other assistive devices:*** Walking sticks and frames are useful tools to help patients with their balance, especially if they are afraid of falling. Wheel-free fixed frames are the most stable and aid in keeping an appropriate erect posture. For use outdoors and over longer distances, a wheeled walker is more convenient. Additionally, many of them come with a storage bag or tray, which allows the patient to transfer items without having to carry them. The safest option are wheeled walkers with brakes because they can lessen the chance of falling in the event that the frame moves too far forward.
15. ***Ensure that the patient's bed height is adjusted to the most optimal position:*** Those with PD frequently experience stiffness and difficulty turning, which can make getting in and out of bed extremely difficult. The height of the bed

should be taken into account first. Similar to a chair, a bed that is the right height enables the patient to position their legs at a 90-degree angle before attempting to stand.

16. ***Encourage the patient to participate in dance practice exercises:*** Several studies have recently shown that dancing exercises combined with musical stimuli appear to activate the reward system by releasing dopamine through the ventral tegmental area. Thai suggests that patients' mood and cognitive states will improve, which will enhance their quality of life. Research findings indicate that dancing improves motor symptoms and functional mobility in people with Parkinson's disease (Hellqvist and Bertero, 2015; Vlaanderen et al, 2019; Bhidayasiri et al, 2020).

7.5. Maintaining Adequate Nutritional Balance

Parkinson's disease patients frequently experience nutritional imbalances because of the disease's effects on the digestive system and decreased levels of physical activity. This may result in weight loss, constipation, decreased appetite, trouble swallowing, and other symptoms that raise the risk of malnutrition and other health issues. As a result, Parkinson's disease patients require adequate nutritional support. For people with Parkinson's disease, maintaining a proper nutritional balance is crucial to promoting their general health and wellbeing. Appropriate nutrition can be ensured by employing techniques like selecting nutrient-dense foods, encouraging hydration, controlling drug interactions, addressing swallowing issues, and keeping a balanced diet.

1. ***Assess the patient's ability to eat:*** This is to give information about factors related to lower nutrient intake. Meal preparation and consumption can be particularly challenging for PD patients due to their decreased grip and dexterity.
2. ***Weigh the patient daily, on the same scale, and same time if possible:*** This gives information on gaining or losing weight. Older adult patients with poor nutritional status have been found to have a lower quality of life; since patients with PD are susceptible to malnutrition, this could be a contributing factor to a lower quality of life. Furthermore, it has been shown that PD patients with poor nutritional status experience higher levels of anxiety and depression. This may result in less appetite and, as a result, weight loss.
3. ***Use assessment tools to identify the presence of malnutrition:*** A quick and easy way to determine the risk of malnutrition is to use the Mini Nutritional Assessment tool. It can be applied as a dual-purpose screening and assessment instrument. Body mass index, weight loss, arm and calf circumference, appetite, mediation, general and cognitive health, dietary concerns, feeding autonomy, and self-perception of nutrition and health are all included in the MNA scale.
4. ***Provide an unhurried environment during mealtime:*** Due to a dry mouth from medication and difficulty chewing and swallowing, eating becomes a very slow process

for patients with PD, making it difficult for them to maintain their weight. Upper extremity bradykinesia can make it difficult to use the hand for fine dexterous tasks like using kitchen utensils.

5. ***Provide the patient with the proper utensils during mealtimes:*** For a patient with PD, large-grip cutlery may be helpful, or the existing cutlery may be modified by adding foam tubing to facilitate gripping. In situations where there is decreased arm strength, lightweight cutlery can be beneficial. Alternatively, if the patient has Parkinson's tremors, heavier, weighted cutlery may be beneficial. Sponks and deep plates with elevated edges, along with non-slip mats, can be helpful for patients who experience food spills.
6. ***Assist the patient when drinking fluids:*** An angled or two-handled beaker or cup with a weighted base should be taken into consideration for patients who have trouble drinking, as these can offer stability and prevent spills in the event of tremors or diminished muscle control. Kettle tippers also reduce the risk of people scalding themselves by enabling the patient to pour boiling water without having to lift the weight of a full kettle.
7. ***Provide a low-protein meal as indicated:*** The total daily protein intake in a low-protein diet is distributed fairly throughout the day. Levodopa competes with dietary proteins for absorption because it is absorbed through a large neutral amino acid active carrier system; however, this effect is usually negligible. Patients who follow a protein-redistributed diet only eat very low-protein foods during the day and a high-protein dinner in the evening.
8. ***Allow the patient to consume moderate amounts of caffeine:*** A methylxanthine class CNS stimulant, caffeine works by reversibly blocking adenosine receptors. There has been prior research suggesting that caffeine may have a neuroprotective effect on the onset of Parkinson's disease. Higher caffeine intake from various sources, such as caffeinated coffee, black and green tea, and other caffeinated beverages, was linked to a significantly lower incidence of PD, according to a follow-up study.
9. ***Promote an increased intake of dietary fiber:*** In patients with PD, autonomic dysfunction results in impaired motility, which impairs absorption and occasionally causes constipation. Sufficient dietary fiber is necessary to avoid the prevalent issue of constipation (Hellqvist & Bertero, 2015; Vlaanderen et al., 2019; Bhidayasiri et al., 2020).

7.6. Managing Dysphagia and Swallowing Difficulties

Parkinson's disease patients frequently experience impaired swallowing as a result of the degeneration of the muscles and nerves involved in swallowing. This may result in dysphagia, which can seriously impair the patient's quality of life and raise the risk of aspiration pneumonia, malnourishment, and dehydration. At the beginning of the disease, up to 80% of patients will experience oropharyngeal dysphagia. Dysphagia can become up to 95% more common in people with PD in its advanced stages. Therefore, treating dysphagia may be a key component in keeping PD patients from developing pneumonia.

1. ***Evaluate the patient's ability to swallow, the extent of paralysis, and the ability to maintain the airway:*** Choking and difficulty swallowing are common in PD, and evaluation offers baseline data from which care interventions can be planned. The O'Neil Dysphagia Outcome and Severity Scale, a visual analog scale, the Dysphagia Severity Scale, and the Functional Dysphagia Scale are a few of the scales and measures that can be used to assess dysphagia. The safest way to swallow can be determined using the Penetration/Aspiration Scale, and the parameters of voluntarily coughing can be measured using Expiratory Muscle Strength Training.
2. ***Assist in the evaluation of swallowing:*** A speech-language pathologist can assess swallowing, and their assessment may involve a fiberoptic endoscope evaluation of swallowing (FEES) and a modified barium swallow. To conduct the modified barium swallow study, the patient is asked to consume barium in varying consistencies. Moving X-rays are then obtained. A very thin, flexible fiberoptic tube with a camera is inserted through the nasal passage for FEES, and swallowing is then monitored.
3. ***Maintain head position and support, with the head of the bed elevated at least 30 degrees or more immediately after feeding:*** This makes swallowing easier and reduces the risk of aspiration. PD can impair the swallowing muscles, resulting in dysphagia. Raising the head of the bed, particularly during eating or drinking, makes it easier for food to pass down the esophagus and lowers the risk of aspiration pneumonia or choking.
4. ***Instruct the patient to chew sugarless chewing gum or suck on hard candy:*** This helps prevent dry mouth, a side effect of PD medications and keeps the mouth moisturised. The medications used to treat PD, especially anticholinergics, may make xerostomia or dry mouth worse. Saliva not only helps with speech, swallowing, and food breakdown, but it's also critical for maintaining dental health.
5. ***Place food on the unaffected side of the patient's mouth:*** This permits taste and sensory stimulation, and it might help set off the swallowing reflex. Swallowing is a multifaceted process that starts in the mouth, moves through the pharynx, and ends in the esophagus. This also entails chewing, moving the food bolus to the back of the throat with the tongue, and coordinating the muscles that protect the trachea or airway from food penetration as well as push the food into the esophagus. A patient with Parkinson's disease may find these tasks challenging.

6. ***Provide foods that are soft and require little chewing; provide thickened liquids if possible:*** These foods are less likely to cause aspiration or choking and are simpler to manage. Moderately textured bread, moistened dry cereals or oatmeal, well-cooked, tender chicken or turkey, well-cooked fish without bones, chopped and ground meats, soft casseroles and pasta, soft, well-cooked vegetables or pureed/mashed fruits, and soft desserts like custard, yogurt, or ice cream are other examples of good food choices.
7. ***Administer tube feedings or enteral alimentation as warranted/ordered:*** This may be required if oral intake is not sufficient. A variety of artificial feeding tubes can be used to deliver medications, guarantee optimal nutrition and fluid intake, and both. While some patients may gain weight through tube feeding, nurses should be aware that frequent adverse events may result from tube insertion and feeding.
8. ***Instruct the patient and/or family to use a straw for drinking liquids:*** This lessens the chance of choking by strengthening the facial and oral muscles. By using a straw, the patient can control and maintain a more steady grip during the drinking process. By delivering liquids in a more focused and controlled manner, straws reduce the possibility of unintentional spills. Additionally, it makes it easier to swallow and lowers the chance of choking or aspiration by facilitating the process of moving the liquid toward the back of the mouth.
9. ***Teach the patient to place food on the tongue, close the lips and teeth, lift the tongue up and then back, and swallow:*** It may be possible to prevent aspiration in patients by teaching them proper chewing and swallowing techniques. It is important to take tiny bites of food or tiny sips of liquid and chew them well. Wait to add more food until you've swallowed the entire first bite before doing so. If the food does not go down completely on the first swallow, the patient should "double swallow," or swallow again.
10. ***Instruct the patient to make a conscious effort to swallow:*** This is to prevent saliva from accumulating. Sialorrhea is the term used to describe poor control of saliva. Because the muscles in the mouth, face, and neck may not be as controlled as they should be and because the patient may take longer to initiate a swallow, people with PD often struggle to control their saliva. Because PD patients generally have slower movements, there may occasionally be an overabundance of saliva in the mouth as a result of their decreased frequency of swallowing.
11. ***Massage the facial and neck muscles before meals:*** Throughout the world, therapeutic massage is a widely used complementary and alternative medical practice. A study revealed that massage improved muscles' ability to move. Five massage techniques

have been shown in a literature review to improve the treatment of both motor and non-motor symptoms; however, a systematic, quantitative review or meta-analysis summarizing the efficacious manual therapy modalities is still lacking.

12. ***Instruct the patient in performing swallow exercises:*** Following a formal swallow assessment, the patient can participate in exercises designed specifically for the mouth and throat regions causing dysphagia as part of swallowing therapy. During sessions, participants may practice compensatory swallowing techniques on a variety of foods to optimize swallowing efficiency and safety.
13. ***Educate the patient on how to perform lip seal exercises:*** Lip seal exercises assist in reducing or controlling excessive saliva. Give the patient instructions to hold their lips in place for four counts, then to relax and do it at least five more times. The patient's lips should be sealed as tightly as possible. Next, tell them to maintain a big smile. After that, allow the patient to hold their lips like they're puffing on a pipe or blowing a whistle. Encourage the patient to firmly swallow their saliva all day long.
14. ***Administer botulinum toxin to the patient as prescribed:*** To decrease the production of saliva, the salivary glands can be injected with botulinum toxin, also known as Botox. Not every patient will respond to this treatment, and it might be necessary to repeat the injections every three to six months. However, Botox injections are not advised and might not be appropriate for certain patients.

(Hellqvist and Bertero, 2015; Vlaanderen et al, 2019; Bhidayasiri et al, 2020)

7.7. Promoting Safety and Preventing Injuries

Due to their decreased reaction times, postural instability, and limited physical mobility, patients with Parkinson's disease are more likely to sustain injuries. Additionally, they run the risk of falling, which can lead to head injuries, fractures, and other complications, especially when the disease is more advanced. Along with decreased step length and gait speed, patients also exhibit increased axial rigidity and poor rhythmicity. As the illness worsens, gait issues become more common and significantly impact quality of life and independence.

1. ***Assess ambulation and movement:*** This facilitates intervention planning. Patients experience stiffness, gait problems, and progressive bradykinesia over time. When walking, the foot on the same side may scrape the floor and the first afflicted arm may not swing fully. Axial posture gradually flexes and strides get shorter with time.
2. ***Assess for bradykinesia and rigidity:*** In addition to reduced spontaneous movement and amplitude, bradykinesia is characterized by slowness of movement. An increase in resistance to passive movement about a joint is referred to as rigidity. To evaluate these, have the patient tap each foot as quickly and widely as they can.

Next, have them stand up from a seated position while crossing their arms to gauge their ability to get out of a chair. After that, the patient is watched as they walk in order to measure their arm swing, stride length, and pace.

3. ***Instruct the patient to swing arms and lift heels during ambulation:*** These exercises improve gait and guard against falls. Reduced forward limb propulsion is likely caused by impaired muscle contraction, rigidity, and postural instability. This can have a detrimental impact on spatiotemporal gait parameters like step length and speed.
4. ***Teach the patient to turn in wide arcs:*** This is to avoid the possibility of a fall resulting from crossing one leg over the other. Freezing of gait, a sudden and transient inability to start or maintain walking, is a common symptom of PD in patients. This can leave them feeling "stuck" or unable to move forward. Patients can gain more momentum by rotating in broad arcs. The bigger steps offer more stability and balance when turning, and the extra momentum can help get past the freezing moments.
5. ***Remind the Patient to maintain an upright posture and look up when walking:*** The patient may bump into objects if they are hunched over. PD impairs postural stability, which results in a bent or stooped posture. Fall risk is decreased when walking erect because it increases stability and balance. It makes it possible for the body's center to align more properly, which lessens the forward inclination that can lead to instability.
6. ***Instruct a wide-based gait:*** A broad base of support is offered by a wide-based gait, which can improve stability and lessen the chance of losing balance. The patient is more stable in their wider stance, which facilitates maintaining an upright posture and navigating uneven surfaces or obstacles. In addition to offering a more stable base during turns, a wide-based gait lowers the chance of losing balance or experiencing freezing of the gait.
7. ***Teach a range of motion exercises and stretching to be performed daily:*** Strength, balance, and flexibility are all improved by exercise. After starting a systematic activity program, balance-related activities showed some improvement, according to multiple meta-analyses of randomized controlled clinical trials. The authors emphasized that improvements are greater in programs that are more difficult. Adapted physical activity programs improve people's quality of life.
8. ***Promote the use of cueing together with exercise training:*** For patients whose freezing of gait is unresponsive to medicine or surgery, cueing may be a helpful tactic. Patients can focus their attention on gait with the aid of sensory cueing. External cues can take the form of visual cues, where the patient steps over lines or other regular patterns on the ground, a laser beam, or a

stick attached to a cane. Auditory cues include counting, using a metronome, listening to rhythmic music, and so on. Cueing increases step length for visual cues and cadence for auditory cues, which in turn causes an increase in gait velocity.

9. ***Provide safety equipment and environmental alterations for the patient's safety:*** In order to help patients get out of bed or stand up to get dressed or perform exercises, handrails are the most commonly installed adaptation that promote independence. They can be installed practically anywhere in the patient's home, including entrances, stairways, bathrooms, and bedrooms. In addition, bath and shower boards can help the patient prevent injuries during bathing or showering; wetroom installations and housing modifications may also be taken into consideration.

10. ***Encourage the patient to use assistive devices and use them properly:*** Walking frames and sticks can help with balance. These are beneficial in cases where there is a risk of the patient falling. Wheel-free fixed frames are the most stable and aid in keeping an appropriate erect posture. When traveling longer distances or outside, a wheeled walker is recommended. The safest option are wheeled walkers with brakes because they can lessen the chance of falling in the event that the frame moves too far forward.

11. ***Promote the use of a treadmill for exercise training:*** A standard treadmill walk improved the freezing gait, as measured by the user, and raised the comfortable gait speed—that is, the speed at which walking does not require effort. The stride length, cadence, walking speed, step length, and walking distance were all increased when walking on a treadmill. When walking at their preferred speed for a longer period of time and distance rather than at their maximal speed on a short distance, patients with PD became faster and increased their step cadence (Hellqvist and Bertero, 2015; Vlaanderen et al., 2019; Bhidayasiri et al., 2020).

7.8. Promoting Positive Coping and Providing Emotional Support

Due to the chronic and progressive nature of Parkinson's disease, patients may find it difficult to cope, which can result in feelings of anxiety, depression, and a loss of independence. This can be made worse by the difficulties in managing symptoms and the social stigma attached to the illness, which can exacerbate feelings of helplessness and frustration. Consequently, "the experience of living with and managing unpredictability" combined with the awareness of one's eventual loss of independence characterizes life with PD.

1. ***Identify expectations from patients for behavior and what consequences will occur if limits are not honed:*** This aids in establishing limits for deceptive conduct. Patient manipulation increases one's sense of power and decreases feelings of insecurity. A person's ability to adjust to

a chronic illness is a dynamic, intricate process that is influenced by a wide range of elements, including personality, coping strategies, and social support.

2. ***Identify successful and ineffective coping strategies that the patient and the family members have previously used:*** Because coping mechanisms are linked to both mental and health-related quality of life, research on them is crucial. Males deal with stress by problem-focused or avoidant coping, whereas females use a combination of coping strategies and seek out social support. Men often repress or ignore their feelings. Compared to men, women seem to employ more emotion-focused coping mechanisms.
3. ***Provide care for patients using the same staff whenever possible:*** This provides for continuity of care and the establishment of a trusting relationship. Individuals differ greatly in the rate at which their symptoms progress, and not everyone experiences the same set of symptoms. Furthermore, the intensity of the symptoms varies over the short term and is readily influenced by variables such as stress. Consequently, in order to assist the patient and family in monitoring the patient's progress and identifying any deviations, a continuous care provider is required.
4. ***Provide uninterrupted time to be spent with the patient, and encourage him to express feelings and concerns:*** This gives the patient the opportunity to express strong, intense emotions. Through dialogue, the patient can also start to understand the significance that recent events have for them personally and form a fair assessment of the circumstances in order to come up with a strategy for handling the situation in a positive way.

Participants in a study felt that accepting the disease required more cognitive work and that patients did not always succeed in doing so. Not every person with Parkinson's disease admitted to accepting their circumstances. Having someone to talk to and communicating their struggles with the illness may help the patient manage their chronic illness.

5. ***Assist the patient only when necessary. offer positive feedback for independent behavior:*** Reliance on the nurse lowers one's sense of worth. Facilitating desired behaviors leads to more efficient coping. Self-tracking devices can be very helpful in assisting PD patients in managing changes to their condition. Self-tracking is beneficial for more than just managing one's own health. Patients perceived tracking technologies as useful resources to assist them in making short- and long-term plans for changes in their health.
6. ***Encourage the patient to make choices about his care:*** This improves self-esteem and lessens helplessness. In one study, PD patients requested tools that would enable them to collaborate with their doctors on medication adjustments in between

appointments. Self-tracking systems were instruments that the patient could use to address problems as they arose. Patients fear that if they only depend on clinicians to solve their problems, they won't be able to solve problems on their own for a long time.

7. ***Assist the patient in identifying behavior and accepting responsibility for actions:*** A sense of accountability must be established prior to making any changes. According to research participants, accepting and attempting to adjust to the disease and the new circumstances is what it means for a person with PD to cope with the condition. For any individual with PD, adjusting to the disease's changes—the majority of which the sufferer views as losses—is an extremely challenging process.
8. ***Identify the patient's positive qualities and accomplishments and assist the patient to recognize these traits:*** Enhancing patients' self-esteem will reduce their need for manipulative behavior. Since personality can influence coping preferences, perceptions, and stress response, it may be important to assess personality in PD patients. According to earlier studies, patients with higher levels of optimism typically employ problem-focused coping mechanisms, whereas patients with lower levels of optimism typically turn to emotion-coping mechanisms like denial.
9. ***Praise the patient when he or she uses effective coping strategies:*** Giving a patient praise or other forms of positive reinforcement can encourage them to follow their medication schedule, take part in therapy activities, and go to rehabilitation sessions. Positive reinforcement is a technique used to boost motivation and motivate patients to keep up their efforts by rewarding desired behaviors or accomplishments with praise or rewards.
10. ***Encourage the patient to utilize community resources, support systems, counselors, and family and friends:*** In older adults, PD is the second most common long-term neurological condition. The need for health and social care is higher among older adults, primarily because they have more chronic illnesses. It is imperative that healthcare systems incorporate interventions aimed at promoting more holistic care for individuals with PD and their family caregivers. These interventions should foster an active and healthy lifestyle in the affected individuals, potentially mitigating the psychosocial impact they face.
11. ***Instruct the patient/family about appropriate coping strategies:*** This disseminates information and suggests alternatives to improper conduct. For PD patients, learning to cope with their illness is essential as it facilitates their ability to adjust and endure the condition. In one study, most participants named two strategies the patient used to deal with Parkinson's disease. the behavioral effort of "trying to bear

it," which meant looking for ways to lessen the impact of the symptoms and the changes taking place in the patient's life, and the cognitive effort of "assuming," which relates to accepting the disease.

12. ***Instruct the patient and/or family regarding the need for support groups and/or counseling:*** In order to provide the patient with appropriate care and help them effectively maintain their coping skills, this may be necessary. Members of support groups can still benefit from having a personal support system and can use professional support services like counseling to locate support groups. An informal, self-managed group of people with PD and their caregivers, a PD support group, like the Parkinson's Foundation support group, aims to provide information about the disease, foster self-acceptance, and provide mutual support.
13. ***Promote the use of positive/ adaptive coping strategies:*** Problem-solving coping strategies, which involve applying rational problem-solving methods to enhance a circumstance, have been linked to higher levels of wellbeing and better quality of life. These techniques, which include actions like formulating and executing a plan of action and problem-solving, are referred to as positive or adaptive coping strategies.
14. ***Redirect the patient if escape/ avoidance coping strategies:*** Avoiding or denying the situation through coping mechanisms has been linked to a lower quality of life and a worse psychological adjustment to Parkinson's disease in PD patients. Escape-avoidance coping techniques include things like imagining a different scenario and refusing to accept that anything has happened. Negative or maladaptive labels are frequently used to describe coping mechanisms linked to a lower quality of life.
15. ***Educate the patient on how to self-track their symptoms:*** According to a study, self-tracking technologies can support individuals with PD and their caregivers in adopting healthy coping mechanisms and overcoming their own inclinations toward denial as the illness worsens. Tremor-like symptoms can be meaningfully recorded in three different ways. Objective measurements, such as phone accelerometer data or the outcomes of a finger tap test, are one method. Subjective metrics, such as a severity rating ranging from mild to severe, are another approach. Functionalist metrics, on the other hand, involve describing how particular tasks and activities of daily life are affected by the tremor (Hellqvist Bertero, 2015; Vlaanderen et al., 2019; Bhidayasiri et al., 2020)

7.9. Initiating Patient Education and Health Teachings

Parkinson's disease patients frequently lack knowledge because of the disease's complexity, wide range of symptoms, and progressive nature.

Patients may be ill-equipped to effectively manage their symptoms and make decisions regarding their care due to a lack of knowledge about the disease process, how to manage symptoms, and how lifestyle choices affect the disease's progression.

1. ***Assess the patient's understanding of the disease process. Consider the older adult's life experiences:*** This offers a starting point for understanding from which a care plan can be created. The patient's prior life experience and knowledge base can be supplemented with new information. More information about the disease itself may help patients with PD and their caregivers recognize and comprehend it more accurately. Conversely, a lack of knowledge about the disease may negatively impact PD patients' care.
2. ***Assess the patient's or family's culture and beliefs about chronic diseases and long-term care:*** The increased burden experienced by male caregivers and female patients may be attributed to cultural differences in caregiving. A different study's findings indicated that the caregiver burden was higher in cases involving female patients and male caregivers, despite some studies suggesting that the quality of life was slightly lower or the caregiver burden was slightly higher in male patient caregivers.
3. ***Educate the patient and/or significant other (SO) about Parkinson's Disease, signs, and symptoms, treatments, and prevention of complications:*** Reeducating older adult patients about current treatments is necessary because they may not be aware of outdated information or the stigma associated with Parkinson's disease and dementia. Eliminating unnecessary stimuli improves learning and the capacity to absorb new information without being distracted. Brief sessions avoid information overload and let the patient learn at their own pace.
4. ***Prepare the patient for surgery as indicated:*** To treat incapacitating drug-resistant tremors, restore dopamine levels, and improve rigidity and dyskinesias, surgery might be necessary. The patient should be made aware before surgery that there is no known cure for Parkinson's disease and that further decline is normal. Working closely with the neurosurgeon and neurologist facilitates decision-making and reduces uncertainty and anxiety in the patient.
5. ***Advise the patient to take the anti-Parkinsonism drugs on schedule:*** Patients can modify their schedule to maximize the drug's peak effect during periods when mobility is most crucial. The effects of levodopa typically last for approximately two hours after prolonged use. The time when the medication is effective in alleviating bradykinesia, rigidity, and tremors is referred to as "on" time, whereas the period when the medication's effects wear off is known as "off" time.
6. ***Instruct the patient and SO regarding medications and the need for adherence with dosage,***

scheduling, and provider follow-up: This increases understanding and makes it easier to follow the treatment plan. In order to notify the provider after the patient is discharged from the hospital, this also enables the prompt identification of significant side effects from the prescribed medication regimen. Follow-up care should be given at least every three to six months once the patient is stable on a medication regimen. The physician will periodically adjust medication dosages during visits if necessary.

7. Instruct the family regarding the side effects of medications and when to notify the healthcare provider

- **Anticholinergic Drugs (Diphenhydramine, Trihexyphenidyl, Procyclidine):** These drugs may result in drowsiness, disorientation, and retention of urine. Anticholinergics can cause side effects such as confusion, hallucinations, and memory loss; therefore, it is best to start low and increase the dosage gradually. Unfavorable cognitive effects are not uncommon, particularly in elderly individuals.
- **Dopaminergic Drugs (Carbidopa-Levodopa):** These may result in dyskinesia, anorexia, nausea, confusion, psychotic episodes, and nightmares. Higher doses should be avoided as they raise the possibility of developing dyskinesia and should not be used in excess of what is required to effectively control symptoms. The levodopa dosage can be taken right after a meal if nausea develops.
- **Dopamine Agonists (Bromocriptine):** These drugs may result in hypotension, dyskinesia, hallucinations, nausea, vomiting, and confusion. In the early stages of a disease, dopamine agonists offer a symptomatic benefit similar to that of levodopa/carbidopa; however, in more advanced stages of the disease, these agents are not effective enough to control signs and symptoms on their own.
- **MAOIs (Selegiline):** These substances may induce headaches, nausea, dizziness, confusion, and insomnia. On the other hand, these drugs have good adverse effect profiles, offer modest symptomatic benefits, and might enhance long-term results. Another medication may be added if the MAO-B inhibitor by itself is insufficient to effectively control motor symptoms.
- **Amantadine:** The antiviral medication amantadine also exhibits anti-Parkinsonian properties. The two most worrisome possible amantadine side effects are disorientation and hallucinations. Insomnia, headaches, nausea, and dizziness are typical side effects. Ataxia, livedo reticularis, peripheral edema, anxiety and irritability, and orthostatic hypotension are less commonly reported side effects.

8. ***Provide time for questions and concerns to be voiced, and answer questions honestly:*** Correcting errors in written materials and information enables documentation that will help with care after the patient is released from the hospital.

By designing an educational program based on an assessment of the patient's and family's level of disease understanding, education can be given more effectively. Information about expected or ongoing challenges and the patient's disease state should be given to patients and their caregivers.

9. ***Instruct the patient and/or family regarding the need for long-term planning and the potential for end-of-life care decisions:*** The patient will eventually experience severe impairment due to the chronic nature of the disease. Future potential problems (tube feedings, DNR, etc.) should be talked about so that, as long as the patient is able to comprehend the seriousness of the condition, the patient and family can make educated decisions. According to recent studies, combining palliative care with PD improves quality of life and lessens the severity and burden of symptoms. In PD, palliative care entails managing non-motor symptoms like pain, exhaustion, and depression.

10. ***Teach the patient and family members how to self-monitor the progression of PD:*** Self-monitoring is regarded as a crucial life management skill. In self-monitoring, physical symptoms, activities of daily living, and cognitive processes that result in self-awareness are all observed, evaluated, and tracked. Consultations with medical professionals and self-care activities can be based on this information.

11. ***Provide information about educational programs that can assist the patient and their caregivers:*** The National Parkinson School (NPS) and Patient Education for Persons with Parkinson's Disease and Their Caregivers (PEPP) were created in partnership with healthcare professionals, researchers, the pharmaceutical industry, and patient organizations. They draw from the insights and experiences gained from cognitive behavioral therapy. Like PEPP, the goal of the NPS is to give people with PD and their loved ones strategies and tools to help them better manage their daily lives while living with the disease and to encourage a higher quality of life.

12. ***Discuss the prevention of falls with the patient and caregivers:*** For older adults, falls and fall-related injuries are frequent and dangerous issues. Falling has a human cost that includes injury, pain, distress, loss of confidence, and death. A properly qualified healthcare professional should provide a home hazard assessment and safety intervention/ modifications to older adults who were treated in a hospital after a fall. This is typically done as part of discharge planning and is completed within a window of time decided upon by the healthcare provider, the patient, or the caregiver (Hellqvist and Bertero, 2015; Vlaanderen et al, 2019; Bhidayasiri et al, 2020)

7.10. Administer Medications and Provide Pharmacologic Support

Parkinson's disease patients require individua lized treatment plans, exact medication timing and dosage, ongoing medication monitoring and adjustment.

Side effect management, patient education and adherence, and routine follow-up in order to effectively administer medications and provide pharmacologic support.

- **Levodopa/Carbidopa:** When treating Parkinson's disease, this combination drug is regarded as the best available. Carbidopa increases levodopa's effectiveness and lessens its side effects, while levodopa is converted to dopamine in the brain, aiding in the replenishment of dopamine levels. It alleviates tremors, stiffness, and bradykinesia, or slowness of movement, among other motor symptoms.
- **Dopamine Agonists:** These drugs imitate the way dopamine functions in the brain. They can be used alone or in conjunction with levodopa to activate dopamine receptors. Examples consist of rotigotine, ropinirole, and pramipexole.
- **MAO-B Inhibitors:** By blocking the enzyme MAO-B, monoamine oxidase-B (MAO-B) inhibitors like rasagiline and selegiline help stop the breakdown of dopamine in the brain. In order to extend the effectiveness of levodopa and shorten its "off" time, they are frequently used as adjunctive therapy.
- **Catechol-O-Methyltransferase (COMT) Inhibitors:** Entacapone and tolcapone are examples of COMT inhibitors that function by preventing the enzyme COMT from degrading dopamine. Together with levodopa, they are used to extend its effects and lessen fluctuations in motor symptoms.
- **Anticholinergic Medications:** These drugs, which block the action of acetylcholine, a neurotransmitter involved in movement regulation, such as trihexyphenidyl and benztropine, help reduce tremors and stiffness. They are usually applied to younger individuals who exhibit noticeable tremors.
- **Amantadine:** Amantadine was initially developed as an antiviral medication, but it has since been discovered to be effective in treating Parkinson's disease. Long-term levodopa use is linked to dyskinesias, or abnormal involuntary movements. It also helps lessen these movements and may offer some mild symptom relief.
- **Antidepressants and Anxiolytics:** A few people with Parkinson's disease may have anxiety, depression, or mood swings. To treat these symptoms, doctors may prescribe anxiolytics like benzodiazepines and antidepressants like tricyclic antidepressants (TCAs) or selective serotonin reuptake inhibitors (SSRIs) (Hellqvist and Bertero, 2015; Vlaanderen et al, 2019; Bhidayasiri et al, 2020).

7.11. Monitoring Results of Diagnostic and Laboratory Procedure

It is crucial to monitor the results of diagnostic and laboratory procedures when managing Parkinson's disease. These tests offer valuable insights into the disease's progression, help evaluate treatment success, and assist in detecting any other health issues.

- **Neurological Examination:** A thorough neurological examination is frequently the first step toward a Parkinson's disease diagnosis. It evaluates reflexes, balance, coordination, muscle tone, motor function, and other neurological indicators that might point to Parkinson's disease.
- **Medical History Review:** Compiling a thorough medical history is essential for diagnosing Parkinson's disease. The medical professional will ask about medication use, family history, symptom onset and progression, and any other pertinent medical conditions.
- **DaTscan:** A diagnostic imaging technique called a DaTscan aids in distinguishing Parkinson's disease from other illnesses that share its symptoms. A radioactive tracer that attaches to dopamine transporters in the brain is injected during the procedure. Positron emission tomography (PET) or single-photon emission computed tomography (SPECT) scans can be used to visualize the density and distribution of these transporters.
- **Blood Tests:** Blood tests can be performed to evaluate general health or rule out other conditions that could mimic Parkinson's disease. A complete blood count (CBC), metabolic panel, thyroid function tests, vitamin B_{12} level, and inflammatory markers are a few examples of these tests.
- **Genetic Testing:** Genetic testing may be necessary in some circumstances to pinpoint particular genetic mutations linked to Parkinson's disease. Those who have a family history of early-onset or hereditary forms of the disease should pay particular attention to this.
- **Lumbar Puncture (Spinal Tap):** In certain circumstances, a lumbar puncture may be necessary to examine the cerebrospinal fluid (CSF) for particular biomarkers, such as tau or alpha-synuclein proteins, linked to Parkinson's disease. Usually, this process is saved for situations in which the diagnosis is unclear or when looking into unusual characteristics.
- **Brain Imaging:** To rule out other neurological conditions or to look for any structural abnormalities that could be causing the symptoms, doctors may order brain computed tomography (CT) or magnetic resonance imaging (MRI) scans.
- **Electromyography (EMG):** The electrical activity of muscles is measured by electromyography (EMG), which can be used to assess muscle function and identify any anomalies or indications of nerve injury that might be causing symptoms.
- **Neuropsychological Testing:**

Cognitive function, including language, executive function, memory, and attention, is assessed through neuropsychological tests. These assessments can guide treatment decisions by identifying any cognitive abnormalities linked to Parkinson's disease.

- **Movement Disorders Rating Scales:** The intensity and course of Parkinson's disease symptoms are evaluated using a variety of rating scales, including the Hoehn and Yahr Scale and the Unified Parkinson's disease Rating Scale (UPDRS). These measures aid in the measurement of daily living activities, motor function, and other disease-related factors (Hellqvist & Bertero, 2015; Vlaanderen et al., 2019; Bhidayasiri et al., 2020).

7.12. Assessing and Monitoring for Potential Complications

A crucial aspect of providing care for patients with Parkinson's disease is evaluating them and keeping an eye out for any potential complications. Parkinson's Disease is a neurological condition that worsens over time and can lead to a number of complications that impact both motor and non-motor functions.

1. ***Perform regular neurological assessments to monitor changes in motor function, including muscle strength, coordination, balance, and gait:*** Examine for the presence of bradykinesia, or slow movement, dyskinesias, or involuntary movements, stiffness, and tremors. To identify any possible complications, note any new or worsening symptoms.
2. ***Assess cognitive function using appropriate screening tools or neuropsychological assessments:*** As cognitive decline can occur in Parkinson's disease, keep an eye out for changes in memory, attention, executive function, and language skills. Early cognitive change detection enables the provision of suitable support and interventions.
3. ***Conduct regular screenings for dysphagia (difficulty swallowing) as it is a common complication in Parkinson's disease:*** Keep an eye out for symptoms like coughing, choking, or trouble swallowing food or liquids. Inform the medical staff of any concerns as soon as possible so that the proper interventions, like a changed diet or swallowing exercises, can be started.
4. ***Monitor for medication-related side effects, such as nausea, dizziness, hallucinations, or orthostatic hypotension (a drop in blood pressure upon standing):*** Regularly check vital signs, particularly blood pressure in various postures, and record any negative outcomes. It is possible to manage medication-related complications appropriately and modify treatment plans by promptly identifying them.
5. ***Conduct routine skin assessments to identify potential complications, such as pressure ulcers or skin breakdown:*** Pressure injuries are more likely in patients with Parkinson's disease because they may have restricted mobility or

difficulty changing positions on their own. Particular attention should be given to areas that have been under constant pressure and bony prominences. Put preventive measures in place, like routine repositioning, sufficient padding, and skin care regimens (Hellqvist & Bertero, 2015; Vlaanderen et al., 2019; Bhidayasiri et al., 2020).

A Closer Look

Cognitive Decline in Parkinson's Disease

There is a strong correlation between the duration of PD and the occurrence of dementia associated with it. 83% of patients with PD survive for twenty years after diagnosis. Retaining patient comfort and reducing caregiver stress require prompt recognition and intervention.

- **Recognizing cognitive decline in Parkinson's disease**

Cognitive, attentional, and alertness fluctuations occur on a daily, or even hourly, basis in PD and dementia with Lewy bodies (DLB). Confusion sometimes gives way to periods of clarity, which is in contrast to the constant, progressive forgetfulness associated with Alzheimer's disease. Up to 90% of patients with Parkinson's disease experience visual hallucinations, which are common and a risk factor for the development of PD but can also occur in the absence of the disease. Impaired light/shadow discrimination, trouble estimating distance, extracampine hallucinations (such as a presence in the periphery of the visual field), and visual illusions are examples of early warning signs. Many accounts describe lilliputian hallucinations, which are characterized by small animals or people. The frequency of hallucinations increases at night or upon waking. Screening for conditions that impair vision and could cause hallucinations is advised (eg, diabetic retinopathy, macular degeneration or cataracts). A dementing illness that develops either before or concurrently with the development of motor symptoms of Parkinsonism is known as dementia-like behavior (DLB). Relatively slow progression and the order in which symptoms first appear are diagnostically significant in order to differentiate PD from DLB. At every stage of the disease, it is crucial to inquire about cognitive concerns, collateral history, and formal assessment from patients. For Parkinson's disease, the Montreal Cognitive Assessment is a more accurate screening tool than the Mini-Mental State Examination.

- ***Treatment approach to neuropsychiatric manifestations of late-stage Parkinson's disease: Prevention:*** In LSPD, taking proactive steps to prevent known reversible causes of delirium is crucial. These authors recommend avoiding anticholinergics, sedatives, and opiates; taking an aperient on a regular basis to prevent constipation; treating infections quickly; and adhering to a regular medication schedule. Though they may seem apparent, these four variables—either separately or in combination—are among the most frequent causes of avoidable declines and extended hospital stays. Parkinson's disease drugs have the potential to intensify cognitive symptoms and trigger delusions and hallucinations. Such complications are much less likely to occur when levodopa is taken alone. There is another discussion of a medication rationalization strategy elsewhere.
- ***Psychosis and hallucinations in Parkinson's disease:*** Apart from visual hallucinations and illusions, PDD/DLB may also be linked to psychotic symptoms like agitation, paranoia, and complex delusions. Risperidone, olanzapine, and haloperidol are

antipsychotics that have higher levels of dopamine antagonism and ought to be avoided. The best treatment for Parkinson's disease psychosis (PDPsy) is clozapine, which can be taken at low doses (up to 50 mg per day). Agranulocytosis is a rare but serious non-dose related complication that limits its routine use and requires frequent laboratory monitoring. In Australia, a referral from a psychogeriatrician and a registered prescriber is normally necessary. Although there isn't as much proof to support quetiapine's effectiveness, its favorable side effect profile encourages regular use. These authors start with a low dose of quetiapine (e.g., 25 mg at night or 12 mg/day) and gradually increase the dosage based on the patient's response. Sedation, falls, orthostatic hypotension, and QT prolongation are possible adverse effects. Because atypical antipsychotics increase the risk of falls, cardiovascular side effects, stroke, and death, their use should be carefully considered.

Cholinesterase inhibitors, namely donepezil and rivastigmine, have potential benefits for treating cognitive and psychotic issues. Although PD/DLB is only licensed for Alzheimer's disease in Australia, many of these patients also have Lewy bodies and Alzheimer's pathology, and it is not always possible to distinguish the two clinically. Cholinesterase inhibitors are useful in treating cognitive impairment brought on by Parkinson's disease, according to clinical data. Anecdotally, it appears to be most useful in lowering attentional fluctuations because Parkinson's disease-related cholinergic denervation has been linked to issues with memory, attention, and executive function. One more advantage of rivastigmine is its transdermal delivery method. LSPD is linked to various neuropsychiatric issues such as depression, anxiety, apathy, impulsive and compulsive behaviors. Depression affects up to 35% of Parkinson's disease patients in residential care, significantly impacting their quality of life. It is important to regularly screen for these symptoms and be vigilant for signs of anorexia, weight loss, fatigue, sleep disturbances, motor or cognitive decline, irritability, guilt, feelings of inadequacy, and pessimism. Depression and anxiety may come and go, especially during 'off' periods. While no clinical trials have been conducted specifically for LSPD, starting selective serotonin reuptake inhibitors like venlafaxine and paroxetine is recommended by these authors. Sertraline may also be effective, especially for cases with a strong anxiety component. Involving family members, staying socially engaged, and promoting good sleep habits are also important for managing LSPD. In LSPD, apathy is common, associated with executive dysfunction, and a sign of impending dementia. Although it can be difficult, differentiating between depression, apathy, demoralization, and cognitive deficits can help with treatment planning. A diminished emotional response combined with a decrease in zeal and goal-directed behavior is what defines apathy. According to these authors, using dopamine agonists sparingly can be advantageous (e.g., rotigotine patch 4 mg/24 hr). There is some evidence of rivastigmine's efficacy. Under the guidance of a mental health professional, trials may be conducted on stimulants and antidepressants like methylphenidate and the norepinephrine–dopamine reuptake inhibitor bupropion. On the other hand, emotional distress or cognitive impairment are the causes of low motivation linked to depression or dementia, respectively. Anxiety, agitation, and irritability are characteristics of depression that are generally absent in apathy. Demoralization, which is defined as emotions of hopelessness, failure, and helplessness, has been connected to a decline in functioning and quality of life in Parkinson's disease patients. Psychotherapy and behavioral therapies are the mainstays of treatment for demoralization.

Summary

- Parkinson's nurses are specialist practitioners whose essential skills are clinical leadership, case management, education and the evaluation of care.
- Respiratory problems in Parkinson's disease are commonly observed and can lead to reduced quality of life for patients.
- Patients with early idiopathic PD had significantly lower respiratory muscle strength and higher central respiratory drive than those in age-matched healthy controls, according to a study.
- Repositioning promotes drainage of pulmonary secretions and enhances ventilation to decrease the potential for atelectasis.
- Respiratory muscle training programs have been utilized in patient with PD and other similar neurodegenerative disorders to improve pulmonary and swallowing function.
- Sensory impairments and cognitive decline, including difficulties with attention, memory, and executive functions, are commonly observed in individuals with Parkinson's disease.
- Depression is common among PD patients, whether it is a reaction to the disorder or related to biochemical abnormality is uncertain.
- Impaired verbal communication is common in patients with Parkinson's disease due to the effects of the disease on the muscles used for speaking and swallowing, as well as cognitive impairments that may affect language processing and expression.
- Impaired physical mobility is a common symptom of Parkinson's disease due to the degeneration of neurons that control movement.
- Imbalanced nutrition is a common problem in patients with Parkinson's disease due to the effects of the disease on the digestive system and reduced physical activity.
- Impaired swallowing is a common problem in patients with Parkinson's disease due to the degeneration of the muscles and nerves involved in the swallowing process.
- Lack of knowledge is common in patients with Parkinson's disease due to the complex nature of the disease, its varied symptoms, and the progressive nature of the condition.
- Administering medications and providing pharmacologic support in patients with Parkinson's disease involves developing individualized treatment plans, precise timing and dosing of medications, monitoring and adjusting medications as needed, managing side effects, patient education and adherence, and regular follow-up.

References

1. Bhidayasiri, R., Boonpang, K., Jitkritsadakul, O., Calne, S. M., Henriksen, T., Trump, S., & Chaudhuri, K. R. (2016). Understanding the role of the Parkinson's disease nurse specialist in the delivery of apomorphine therapy. *Parkinsonism & Related Disorders, 33*, 49–55.

2. Bhidayasiri, R., Panyakaew, P., Trenkwalder, C., Jeon, B., Hattori, N., Jagota, P., & Chaiwong, S. (2020). Delivering patient-centered care in Parkinson's disease: Challenges and consensus from an international panel. *Parkinsonism & Related Disorders, 72*, 82–87.

3. Bloem, B. R., Henderson, E. J., Dorsey, E. R., Okun, M. S., Okubadejo, N., Chan, P., & Munneke, M. (2020). Integrated and patient-centred management of Parkinson's disease: A network model for reshaping chronic neurological care. *The Lancet Neurology, 19*, 623–634.

4. Dorsey, E. R., Constantinescu, R., Thompson, J. P., Biglan, K. M., Holloway, R. G., Kieburtz, K., & Tanner, C. M. (2007). Projected number of people with Parkinson's Disease in the most populous nations, 2005 through 2030. *Neurology, 68*, 384–386.

5. Eggers, C., Dano, R., Schill, J., Fink, G. R., Hellmich, M., & Timmermann, L.; CPN Study Group. (2018). Patient-centered integrated healthcare improves quality of life in Parkinson's disease patients: A randomized controlled trial. *Journal of Neurology, 265*, 764–773.

6. Greenwell, K., Gray, W. K., van Wersch, A., van Schaik, P., & Walker, R. (2015). Predictors of the psychosocial impact of being a career of people living with Parkinson's disease: A systematic review. *Parkinsonism & Related Disorders, 21*, 1–11.

7. Hellqvist, C., & Bertero, C. (2015). Support supplied by Parkinson's disease specialist nurses to Parkinson's disease patients and their spouses. *Applied Nursing Research, 28*, 86–91.

8. Higgins, J. J., & Altman, D. G. (2019). Analyzing data and undertaking meta-analyses. In J. P. T. Higgins, J. Thomas, J. Chandler, M. Cumpston, T. Li, et al. (Eds.), *Cochrane Handbook for Systematic Reviews of Interventions* (pp. 241–284). John Wiley & Sons Ltd.

9. Htay, M., & Whitehead, D. (2021). The effectiveness of the role of advanced nurse practitioners compared to physician-led or usual care: A systematic review. *International Journal of Nursing Studies Advances, 3*, 100034.

10. Hughes, A. J., Daniel, S. E., Kilford, L., & Lees, A. J. (1992). Accuracy of clinical diagnosis of idiopathic Parkinson's disease: A clinico-pathological study of 100 cases. *Journal of Neurology, Neurosurgery & Psychiatry, 55*, 181–184.

11. Kessler, D., Hauteclocque, J., Grimes, D., Mestre, T., Côté, D., & Liddy, C. (2019). Development of the Integrated Parkinson's Care Network (IPCN): Using co-design to plan collaborative care for people with Parkinson's disease. *Quality of Life Research, 28*, 1355–1364.

12. Lempp, H., Baggott, R., Scott, D. L., Parker, L., Bosworth, A., Georgopoulou, S., & Firth, J. (2020). The value, impact and role of nurses in rheumatology outpatient care: Critical review of the literature. *Musculoskeletal Care, 18*, 245–255.

13. Macchi, Z. A., Koljack, C. E., Miyasaki, J. M., Katz, M., Galifianakis, N., Prizer, N. P., & Kluger, B. M. (2020). Patient and caregiver characteristics associated with caregiver burden in Parkinson's disease: A palliative care approach. *Annals of Palliative Medicine, 9*, 24–33.

14. Martinez-Martin, P., Jeukens-Visser, M., Lyons, K. E., Rodriguez-Blazquez, C., Selai, C., Siderowf, A., & Schrag, A. (2011). Health-related quality-of-life scales in Parkinson's disease: Critique and recommendations. *Movement Disorders, 26*, 2371–2380.

15. Montemuro, M. A. (1987). The evolution of the clinical nurse specialist: Response to the challenge of professional nursing practice. *Clinical Nurse Specialist, 1*, 106–110.

16. Nardini, C., Osmani, V., Cormio, P. G., Frosini, A., Turrini, M., Lionis, C., & D'Errico, G. (2021). The evolution of personalized healthcare and the pivotal role of European regions in its implementation. *Personalized Medicine, 18*, 283–294.

17. Pazzaglia, C., Imbimbo, I., Tranchita, E., Minganti, C., Ricciardi, D., Lo Monaco, R., & Parisi, A. (2020). Comparison of virtual reality rehabilitation and conventional rehabilitation in Parkinson's disease: A randomized controlled trial. *Physiotherapy, 106*, 36–42.

18. Postuma, R. B., Berg, D., Stern, M., Poewe, W., Olanow, C. W., Oertel, W., & Deuschl, G. (2015). MDS clinical diagnostic criteria for Parkinson's disease. *Movement Disorders, 30*, 1591–1601.

19. Rahman, S., Griffin, H. J., Quinn, N. P., & Jahanshahi, M. (2008). Quality of life in Parkinson's disease: The relative importance of the symptoms. *Movement Disorders, 23*, 1428–1434.

20. Rajan, R., Brennan, L., Bloem, B. R., Dahodwala, N., Gardner, J., Goldman, J. G., & Eggers, C. (2020). Integrated care in Parkinson's disease: A systematic review and meta-analysis. *Movement Disorders, 35*, 1509–1531.

21. Schlette, J. (2024). 10 pros and cons of being a respiratory nurse + salary + steps to become. Nursingprocess.org.

22. Schrag, A., Jahanshahi, M., & Quinn, N. (2000). What contributes to quality of life in patients with Parkinson's disease? *Journal of Neurology, Neurosurgery & Psychiatry, 69*, 308–312.

23. Strouwen, C., Molenaar, E. A. L. M., Münks, L., Keus, S. H. J., Zijlmans, J. C. M., Vandenberghe, W., & Nieuwboer, A. (2017). Training dual tasks together or apart in Parkinson's disease: Results from the DUALITY trial. *Movement Disorders, 32*, 1201–1210.

24. Thieken, F., Timmermann, L., Sohrabi, K., Woopen, C., Schmitz-Luhn, B., Janhsen, A., & Eggers, C. (2021). Development of a multidimensional assessment tool for the evaluation of holistic quality of life in Parkinson's disease. *Journal of Parkinson's Disease, 12*, 361–370.

25. van der Kolk, N. M., Vries de, N. M., Kessels, R. P. C., Joosten, H., Zwinderman, A. H., Prost, B., & Bloem, B. R. (2019). Effectiveness of home-based and remotely supervised aerobic exercise in Parkinson's disease: A double-blind, randomized controlled trial. *The Lancet Neurology, 18*, 998–1008.

26. Vlaanderen, F. P., Rompen, L., Munneke, M., Stoffer, M., Bloem, B. R., & Faber, M. J. (2019). The voice of the Parkinson customer. *Journal of Parkinson's Disease, 9*, 197–201.

Chapter

THE ROLE OF THE SPEECH LANGUAGE PATHOLOGIST

8

Contents

Introduction

PD frequently causes difficulties with speech and swallowing, which can make it difficult to engage in essential activities of daily living like eating favorite foods or conversing with loved ones. For speech and swallowing difficulties, working with a speech-language pathologist (SLP) is the primary treatment method.

Speech pathologists assist individuals with Parkinson's in improving their speech clarity, volume, and purpose. They also aid in expressing emotions through facial expressions by implementing specialized exercises. Additionally, SLPs work on enhancing word retrieval skills, managing cognitive abilities, comprehension difficulties, memory issues, and following instructions. These professionals administer oral motor activities to support speech, voice, and swallowing functions. Speech therapy sessions incorporate respiration techniques to enhance breath support for achieving proper speech volume. Individuals with Parkinson's often struggle to perceive the volume of their speech due to internal regulatory challenges. Speech therapists can address resonance by shaping airflow in the oral and nasal cavities and improve prosody, which involves speech rhythm, melody, and intonation.

SLPs can also help with safe swallowing practices, which are necessary when food or liquids "go down the wrong pipe" and cause aspiration. Aspiration pneumonia, the leading cause of death in Parkinson's disease, may result from this.

Orientation and Directional Terms:

Term	Definition	Illustration
Audiologists	Audiologists are health care professionals who test for hearing and balance issues. An audiologist can rule out hearing loss as a medical reason for a child's language an issue.	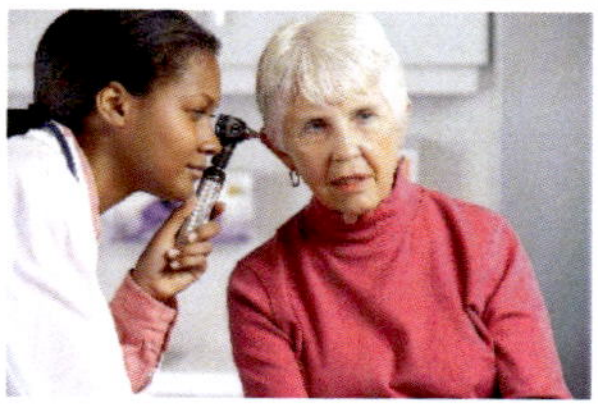
Expressive language	Expressive language allows people to put their thoughts into words, both speaking and writing.	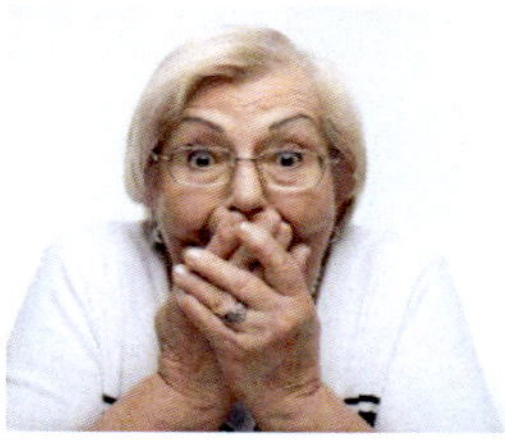
Screening	Screening is often the first step in determining whether a child has a learning difference. It may include observation, interviews, a brief written test, and are view of school and health records.	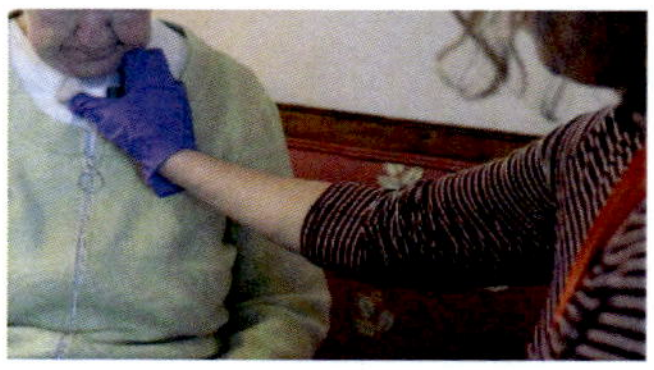
Speech therapy	Speech therapy is treatment that improves your ability to talk and use other language skills. It helps you express your thoughts and understand what other people are saying to you.	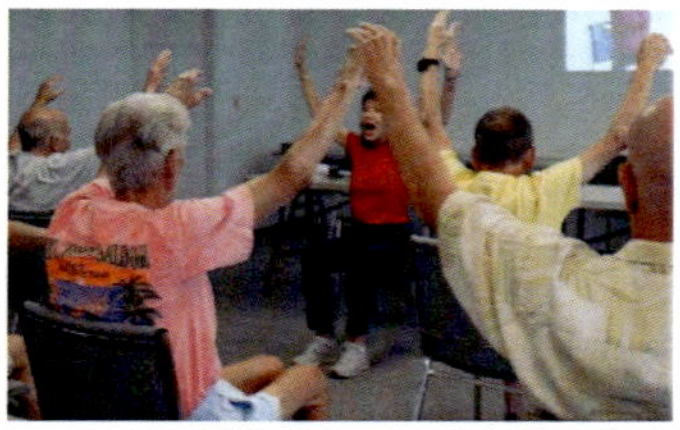

8.1. Communication Disorders in PD

If you have PD, you've probably noticed an increase in the number of times people ask you to repeat what you just said. Additionally, having PD makes it slightly more difficult to speak coherently and clearly. Although the majority of PD patients have some sort of speech issue, very few receive treatment for it. This is regrettable because studies indicate that there are efficient therapies for speech, voice, and language issues associated with Parkinson's disease.

8.1.1. Speech Problems of Parkinson's Disease

The most prevalent speech issues that people with PD face include reduced volume (hypophonia), reduced pitch range (monotone), and dysarthria, or difficulty articulating sounds or syllables. Essentially, you find it harder to express emotion when you do speak, you can't speak as loudly as other people, and you have trouble pronouncing the words you're trying to say. Combining all of these voice issues with PD "masked faces," or the inability to convey emotions through facial expressions, makes it understandable why sometimes it can be difficult for others to understand what you are trying to say. Although it could be tempting to avoid all social interactions, that would be a mistake. No matter how annoying it gets, you must engage with people daily for your mental health, and rest assured that your loved one's desire to do the same. The good news is that PD-related speech issues can be significantly improved with certain treatments, like voice exercises (Lang, 2018).

8.1.2. Language Problems of Parkinson's Disease

Language issues could accompany the annoying speech and voicing issues associated with Parkinson's disease. It is crucial to recognize these language issues as soon as they arise since they most likely make managing the speech issues more challenging.

Speaking is the process of using words to convey ideas. One cognitive ability that can exist even in the absence of speech is language. People with PD may have trouble finding words and with grammar. For instance, they frequently employ more straightforward sentence structures and a higher proportion of open-class (nouns, verbs, and adjectives) to closed-class (determiners, auxiliaries, prepositions, etc) items, as well as a rise in the quantity and length of pauses and hesitations.

People with PD may find it difficult to understand others when they are speaking, especially if they use complex language to convey their ideas. Thus, persons with PD occasionally encounter serious challenges with language comprehension as well as language production.

8.1.3. The Impact of Communication Difficulties on Quality of Life

The foundation of human connection and a high quality of life is effective communication. Our main means of communicating ideas, feelings, and intentions are through spoken and written words. Speech abnormalities and a hoarse voice can cause communication difficulties, social isolation, and a decline in self-esteem in people with Parkinson's disease. For this reason, resolving these problems is essential to maintaining a high standard of living.

- **Communication and Connecting with Others:** Through shared experiences, emotional expression, and the development of strong bonds, spoken communication helps us connect with others. But people with PD may have voice and speech abnormalities that make it difficult for them to express their ideas and emotions clearly, which can cause frustration and social isolation.

- **Social Interaction:** Maintaining relationships and actively participating in social events still depend heavily on effective verbal communication. Unfortunately, speech problems can cause people with PD to retreat from social interactions, which can have a negative effect on their general wellbeing.
- **Self-Confidence:** Speech and voice changes can undermine someone's confidence. Low self-esteem can result from communication anxiety or difficulties being understood.

8.1.4. Causes of Communication Disorders

Parkinson's disease patients experience smaller, less powerful movements than usual due to brain abnormalities. This may result in issues with your communication and speech. Problems could include not speaking loud enough, pronouncing words clearly enough, and using the appropriate tone of voice.

Chewing and safe swallowing can also be impacted by issues producing strong enough movements. As a result, you might find mealtimes more challenging and run the risk of food "going down the wrong way." The way you think affects other aspects of communication in Parkinson's disease patients. You might find it more difficult to process ideas quickly due to changes in your brain. This includes having trouble putting things into words or quickly figuring out what other people are trying to say. It also includes difficulty gathering your ideas fast enough to reply to someone while a conversation is in progress. This is particularly likely to occur when you have to multitask (talk and walk, for instance) (Simms et al. 2020).

8.1.5. Evaluation and Treatment of Communication Disorders

For a diagnosis, the patient should speak with a speech-language pathologist (SLP) who has experience treating individuals with PD if speech abnormalities are suspected. To determine the precise type of speech and voice disturbance, the clinician will review the patient's medical history and complaints. We will also talk about the patient's occupation, routine activities, and social background in relation to how the patient uses their voice in daily life.

The doctor will then go ahead and assess the patient's speech quality. This is accomplished by using the clinician's subjective assessment of particular measures in addition to the aid of tools like a Sound Level Meter to measure speech loudness. Simple speech-related tasks, like pronouncing particular consonants and vowels and reading aloud words, phrases, and brief texts, will be required of the patient. Additionally, the doctor will evaluate the patient's impromptu speech.

Acoustic analysis is another technique used to detect speech abnormalities in patients with Parkinson's disease. This method records the patient while they engage in different speech tasks, providing objective, trustworthy, and highly sensitive information. After that, the voice volume, tone, speech rate, and other acoustic properties are evaluated through analysis of these recordings. Additionally, the speech pathologist will assess the various components of the speech apparatus by assessing the tongue, lips, cheeks, and jaw's range of motion, tone, and movement. For additional assessment, the patient might occasionally be referred to an ENT specialist (ear, nose, and throat).

- **Evaluation:** Healthcare professionals with expertise in speech and language therapy can assess and counsel on all facets of communication, including body language, facial expressions, and speech and communication aids. According to clinical guidelines, if you have Parkinson's in its early stages, your general practitioner, a specialist, or a Parkinson's nurse should think about referring you to a speech and language therapist who has experience with the condition.

This is crucial because small adjustments to your speech and communication may go unnoticed by you. However, a speech-language pathologist can identify any problems, assist you in managing them, and prevent them from getting worse. Regular check-ups might be beneficial for you. This will make it possible for your speech-language pathologist to keep an eye on any alterations to your speech. If so, they can suggest particular workouts or programmes that will be beneficial to you.

- **Treating Speech and Language Problems in Parkinson's Disease:** Medication, behavioral therapy, and surgery are some possible treatments for PD-related speech and language issues. Recent evaluations of these treatments, however, indicate that while surgery—especially deep brain stimulation—may help with some of the more severe motor issues associated with PD, it is not helpful for speech difficulties. Furthermore, there are no drug therapies that work well on their own.

Improving speech issues seems to require treating PD basic motor issues as best as possible (with medication). In other words, behavioral therapies for speech impairments are ineffective if the PD motor issues remain untreated. Therefore, PD medication is required but insufficient. In summary, a combination of PD medication (such as levodopa) and behavioral speech therapy appears to be the most effective treatment approach for the speech and language impairments associated with Parkinson's disease (Zajac et al, 2018).

- **Behavioral Speech Therapy for Parkinson's Disease:** A skilled and certified speech therapist will typically give a series of voice exercises as part of behavioral speech therapy. In order to support the voice, these exercises train the control of speech rate, loudness, articulation, breathing, stress/intonation, or emotional expression. The therapist may occasionally employ assistive technology, like pacing boards, voice amplifiers, or delayed auditory feedback. Using the so-called Lee Silverman Voice Treatment (LSVT), an intensive program of voice exercises that targets vocal intensity, quality, and variation — precisely the areas of difficulty for persons with PD — some investigators have reported significant success with PD patients.

With the LSVT approach, all of the effort is focused on achieving just one therapeutic target at a time. Increasing vocal loudness or improving speech intelligibility could be therapeutic goals. In order to achieve these kinds of therapeutic goals, the patient is trained to self-monitor their voice quality and patterns, as well as to be aware of the sensory feedback that comes from their voice through a series of voice exercises. The voice's enhanced self-awareness enables error correction and expedites progress toward the goal. Behavioral speech therapy regimens seem to be effective based on the evidence that is currently available. Therefore, you shouldn't continue to have frustrating conversations with people who act as though they understand you. Rather, you will relearn how to express yourself loudly and clearly.

8.2. Swallowing Disorders in PD

Parkinson's disease patients frequently experience difficulty swallowing due to a loss of control over their mouth and throat muscles. It can be challenging to manage and chew solid foods as a result. Parkinson's disease patients who have difficulty swallowing are more likely to aspirate, or breathe in liquid or food particles into their lungs, and develop pneumonia. Certain swallowing techniques can alleviate these issues for certain individuals. Some people must alter their diets. (Anna Potulska, Andrzej Friedman, 2003).

8.2.1. Signs and Symptoms

For dysphagia, early intervention is crucial. Early treatment initiation can lower your chance of complications and death. Some dysphagia symptoms, like the following, might not always be evident, but being aware of them can help you catch any early warning signs:

- Weight loss
- Difficulty drinking or keeping liquids and food in your mouth
- Drooling
- Coughing or choking during eating
- A feeling of food stuck in your throat or gumline
- Heartburn or sore throat after eating

8.2.2. Risks Associated with Dysphagia

Dysphagia can be upsetting or embarrassing for a lot of people. In addition to lowering your quality of life, difficulty swallowing can have major consequences.

Malnutrition or dehydration can be brought on by dysphagia. Aspiration, the medical term for "food going down the wrong pipe," can also result from it.

Aspiration can result in aspiration pneumonia, the primary cause of death for Parkinson's disease patients.

This kind of lung infection happens when food particles, liquids, saliva, or vomit enter the lungs through the airways and are inhaled rather than swallowed.

8.2.3. Causes of Dysphagia

Swallowing is a multi-muscled, multi-nerve process. Dysphagia can be brought on by any illness that weakens or damages these muscles and nerves or narrows the esophagus or back of the throat. Generally speaking, dysphagia fits into one of the following groups.

- **Esophageal Dysphagia:** The feeling that food sticks or gets trapped in the base of the throat or in the chest after swallowing is known as esophageal dysphagia. The following are a few reasons of esophageal dysphagia:

a. Achalasia: One condition that causes difficulty swallowing is achalasia. It is difficult for the esophagus to push food and liquids into the stomach when there is damage to the muscles or nerves. Over time, achalasia typically gets worse.

b. Esophageal spasm: This disorder results in irregularly timed, high-pressure esophageal contractions, usually following swallowing. The lower esophageal wall's involuntary muscles are impacted by esophageal spasm.

c. A narrowed esophagus: Large food fragments can become trapped in a narrowed esophagus known as a stricture. Narrowing can be caused by tumors or scar tissue, which are frequently brought on by gastroesophageal reflux disease (GERD).

d. Esophageal tumors: Swallowing difficulties usually worsen over time when esophageal tumors are present. The esophagus gradually narrows due to growing tumors.

e. Foreign bodies: Food or other objects can occasionally obstruct the throat or esophagus, especially in older adults who wear dentures or individuals who have difficulties chewing their food. This can increase the risk of food getting stuck in the throat or esophagus.

f. Esophageal ring: Occasionally, a small area of narrowing in the lower esophagus can make it difficult to swallow solid food.

g. GERD: The tissues lining the esophagus may sustain damage from stomach acid backing up into it. This may result in lower esophageal spasm, scarring, or constriction.

h. Eosinophilic Esophagitis: Immune system illness is known as eosinophilic esophagitis. It is brought on by an accumulation of white blood cells in the esophagus known as eosinophils.

i. Scleroderma: Tissues become stiffer and harder due to the development of scar-like tissue brought on by scleroderma. The lower esophageal sphincter may become weaker as a result. Acid backs up into the esophagus as a result, frequently causing heartburn.

j. Radiation Therapy: This cancer treatment may cause esophageal scarring and inflammation.

- **Oropharyngeal Dysphagia:** When swallowing, food may be difficult to pass from the mouth into the throat and esophagus due to conditions that weaken the throat muscles. When trying to swallow, a person may choke, gag, cough, or feel as though food or liquids are going up their nose or down their trachea, or windpipe. Pneumonia may result from this.

Among the causes of oropharyngeal dysphagia are neurological conditions.

a. Neurological disorders. Dysphagia can be brought on by a number of illnesses, including Parkinson's disease, muscular dystrophy, and multiple sclerosis.

b. Neurological damage. Swallowing can be impacted by sudden neurological damage, such as that caused by a stroke or injury to the brain or spinal cord.

c. Pharyngoesophageal diverticulum, also known as Zenker diverticulum. Food particles get trapped in a little pouch called a diverticulum that forms in the throat, usually right above the esophagus. This can cause gurgling sounds, bad breath, and frequent coughing or clearing of the throat.

d. Cancer. Swallowing problems may result from specific cancers and some cancer treatments, such as radiation.

8.2.4. Diagnosis and Disease Monitoring in PD

The diagnostic process is made more difficult by Parkinson's disease's diverse clinical presentation. The primary basis for diagnosis is the existence of characteristic motor signs, such as i. e. bradykinesia, postural instability, muscle rigidity, resting tremor, reaction to dopamine replacement therapy, and brain imaging. However, a conclusive diagnosis is usually only corroborated after death. As previously mentioned, a number of non-motor and other motor symptoms of PD, such as difficulty swallowing, appear early in the illness and frequently go undiagnosed until much later (Heijmans, 2019).

- ***Disease Severity Rating Scales:*** It is challenging to distinguish between different disease stages clinically, so different measures are employed to assess the severity and course of the illness while diagnosing it. The most widely used instrument for assessing the severity of PD is the Unified Parkinson's Disease Rating Scale (UPDRS). It is divided into three subsections, each containing several separately scored signs on a scale from 0 to 4, where 0 denotes no dysfunction and 4 denotes severe dysfunction. The scale assesses three areas: (1) daily living activities, (2) motor control, and (3) mentation, behavior, and mood. Sadly, the UPDRS only includes two questions—one about salivation and one about swallowing—which does not adequately capture the complexity or severity of dysphagia in Parkinson's disease. Based on the UPDRS, the Hoehn and Yahr Scale (H and Y) evaluates the degree of motor impairments in Parkinson's disease. This scale defines five stages of injury and disability as five stages of disease progression, ranging from no symptoms to bedridden or wheelchair-bound without assistance. Furthermore, in relation to staging, this scale does not accurately capture the severity and complexity of swallowing deficits because they manifest early in the disease process, before diagnosis. Pathology before nigrostriatal dopamine depletion is included in Early Braak Stages (1–2); however, this model does not take into consideration peripheral involvement earlier in life, such as α-syn aggregation in muscles and organs. Moreover, Braak staging is more frequently documented in research studies than it is in clinical practice. While dysphagia usually gets worse as the disease progresses, this is not always linear and isn't always linked to a specific stage of the illness because PD has a heterogeneous presentation by nature and there aren't many clinical tools in neurology that include reliable assessments of swallowing function at different stages of the disease.
- ***Diagnosis of Dysphagia in PD:*** Despite the fact that dysphagia may be among the initial symptoms of PD, it is not frequently addressed in routine neurology consultations.

But only 20–40% of patients realize they have swallowing difficulties; this is partly due to impaired laryngeal sensation, which increases the risk of silent aspiration in this population. One important aspect of PD is deficits in proprioception in most sensorimotor domains. Thus, to detect swallowing abnormalities associated with PD in its early stages, a thorough approach to diagnosis is essential (Suttrup & Dysphagia, 2016).

- ***Clinical Screening and Evaluation:*** Standardized self-report questionnaires can be used as a preliminary screening tool for swallowing impairment and are useful in the diagnosis of swallowing dysfunction in PD. The most widely used questionnaire to evaluate the effect of dysphagia on the quality of life in Parkinson's disease patients is the dysphagia-specific Swallowing Quality of Life Questionnaire (SWAL-QOL). In clinical trials and research, the SWAL-QOL has proven to be a helpful instrument. Furthermore, the Sydney Swallow Questionnaire is a popular clinical and research tool. It is a 17-item visual-analog scale self-report questionnaire that assesses various aspects of a person's swallowing performance.

For the diagnosis of dysphagia in PD, clinical assessments of swallowing utilizing trials with solid and liquid boluses are also crucial. Methods like the "standard water swallow test" can be used to screen for aspiration or penetration; however, in order to diagnose dysphagia in this population as a whole, instrumented assessments are needed to determine the type and extent of impairment.

- ***Instrumented Evaluations:*** Unlike clinical screens and evaluations, instrumented assessments produce functional measurements of swallowing physiology impairments and enable visualization of oropharyngeal structures. Using instrumented tools, over 50% of PD patients without symptoms have swallowing dysfunction. The Fiberoptic Endoscopic Evaluation of Swallowing (FEES) and the Videofluoroscopic Swallow Study (VFSS) are the two methods most frequently used to assess oropharyngeal dysphagia.

With the use of video X-ray technology, the VFSS makes it possible to examine the swallow and see the oral, pharyngeal, and esophageal phases of the swallow, as well as the passage of the bolus through the upper esophageal sphincter. Furthermore, during VFSS, the entire esophagus can be seen to evaluate esophageal dysfunction, including achalasia. Small amounts of radiation are involved in this procedure, which is typically carried out in radiology (although mobile units can be used at the bedside). Anatomical and physiological swallowing impairments can be identified using lateral and anterior/posterior views. Oropharyngeal swallow deficits are common in PD patients, and they can exacerbate bolus clearance and airway compromise/aspiration problems.

Pharyngeal and laryngeal structures can be seen with FEES thanks to the use of a flexible endoscope that is passed through the hypopharynx and placed into the nasal passage. It is possible to evaluate the anatomy and physiology of the velopharynx, posterior pharyngeal wall, epiglottis, vocal folds, pyriform sinuses, and base of the tongue in addition to swallow safety (penetration/aspiration/

clearance after cough) and efficiency (pharyngeal residue). Additionally, respiration and secretions can be assessed, and sensory testing can be carried out. It can be argued that FEES is more sensitive than VFSS, particularly for penetration and aspiration.

High-Resolution Manometry (HRM) is a valuable tool for evaluating pressure and timing events in the pharynx and esophagus. A catheter containing pressure sensors is inserted through the nasal cavity into the esophagus to measure pressure and timing variations during swallowing. HRM is particularly beneficial for detecting subtle swallowing issues in the early stages of PD. When used with the Sydney Swallow Questionnaire, HRM has been shown to be an effective method for identifying even minor changes in swallowing function in individuals with early-stage PD, surpassing the accuracy of VFSS results. Additionally, intraluminal impedance can track the speed and direction of bolus movements and, when combined with pressure measurements, is a powerful tool for assessing motility and luminal content flow. The combination of manometry and impedance is commonly used to assess esophageal motility disorders and pharyngeal swallow function. Impedance, when paired with HRM pressure and timing measurements, is a reliable method for evaluating pharyngeal residue.

Deficits in airway protection frequently lead to worsening health outcomes that affect quality of life. For PD-associated dysphagia, a complete pulmonary and airway examination along with a cough function assessment is advised.

A variety of instruments, such as a comprehensive airway and cough examination, are frequently used for a detailed analysis of disruptions in the oral, pharyngeal, and esophageal phases of swallowing in PD. Oral residue, premature spillage, piecemeal deglutition, and repetitive tongue pumping are common oral phase findings in PD-associated dysphagia. Pharyngeal stage findings include reduced swallow rate during spontaneous swallowing, penetration, aspiration, residue in the pyriform sinuses and vallecula, and somatosensory deficits. Patients with Parkinson's disease frequently exhibit esophageal hypomobility, spasms, and contractions during the esophageal phase.

8.2.5. Treatment

Your swallowing disorder's type or underlying cause will determine how dysphagia is treated.

- **Oropharyngeal Dysphagia:** A speech or swallowing therapist may be recommended for treatment of oropharyngeal dysphagia. Possible therapeutic outcomes include:

i. Exercises for learning. You may be able to better coordinate your swallowing muscles or re-stimulate the nerves that initiate the swallowing reflex by doing specific exercises. acquiring skills in swallowing.

ii. In order to facilitate swallowing, you may also learn how to position your head and body and how to put food in your mouth. If diseases like Parkinson's or Alzheimer's are causing your dysphagia, exercises and new swallowing techniques may be helpful.

- **Esophageal Dysphagia:** Approaches to treating esophageal dysphagia could involve the following:

i. Esophageal dilation. Dilation is the process of inserting an endoscope into the esophagus and stretching it by blowing up a balloon that is attached. Achalasia, esophageal stricture, motility abnormalities, and Schatzki ring—an irregular ring of tissue at the junction of the esophagus and stomach—are treated with this therapy. To treat strictures and rings, long, flexible tubes with different diameters can also be placed into the esophagus through the mouth.

ii. Surgery. You may require surgery to clear your esophageal path if you have an esophageal tumor, achalasia, or pharyngoesophageal diverticulum.

iii. Medicines. Prescription medications that lower stomach acid can be used to treat GERD-related swallowing difficulties. It may take a while for you to get used to taking these medications.

It may be suggested to use corticosteroids for eosinophilic esophagitis. Smooth muscle relaxants may be helpful for esophageal spasm.

iv. Diet. Depending on what is causing your dysphagia, you might be prescribed a special diet to help with your symptoms. One possible treatment for eosinophilic esophagitis is diet.

- **Severe Dysphagia:** A feeding tube can be advised if your inability to swallow safely keeps you from eating and drinking enough, even after treatment. Nutrients can be given via a feeding tube without the need to swallow.
- **Surgery:** In order to treat swallowing issues brought on by obstructions or narrowing of the throat, surgery may be required. Bony outgrowths, paralysis of the vocal cord, pharyngoesophageal diverticula, GERD, and achalasia are examples of blockages. Esophageal cancer can also be treated surgically. Following surgery, speech and swallowing therapy are typically beneficial.

The cause of dysphagia determines the kind of surgical treatment that is needed. A few instances are:

i. **Laparoscopic Heller myotomy:** This entails severing the esophageal sphincter, a muscle located at the base of the esophagus. The esophageal sphincter malfunctions in achalasia patients, preventing food from being released into the stomach. Heller myotomy aids in the solution of this issue.

ii. **Peroralendoscopicmyotomy (POEM):** To treat achalasia, the POEM procedure entails making an incision in the esophageal lining. The lower esophageal sphincter's muscle is then cut by the surgeon or gastroenterologist, just like in a Heller myotomy.

iii. **Stentplacement:** A narrowed or obstructed esophagus may be propped open with a stent, which is a metal or plastic tube. For example, stents used in esophageal cancer patients are permanent, whereas other stents are eventually removed.

iv. **OnabotulinumtoxinA (Botox):** The esophageal sphincter, a muscle at the end of the esophagus, can be injected with this. It relaxes as a result, facilitating better swallowing in achalasia. Repeat injections may be necessary with this technique, which is less invasive than surgery. Further research is required.

8.2.6. Lifestyle Changes

Altering your food is another way to help manage dysphagia. If you find it difficult to swallow liquids, you can try using a food thickener. You may consider pureeing solid foods if they are causing issues. To determine what is most convenient for you, you can also experiment with larger and smaller portions of solid foods. Other approaches exist for the management of symptoms. A little over 70% of persons with Parkinson's disease drool. Sucking on hard candy—preferably sugar-free—is a simple way to stop drooling. This aids in encouraging swallowing, which momentarily lessens drooling. Although dysphagia can affect your life, there are ways to manage it. If you're worried about how you swallow or would like more information about your options, think about contacting your doctor.

8.3. Role of a Speech and Language Therapist in a Rehabilitation Team

The fields of speech and language pathologists, sometimes referred to as speech and language therapists, include voice, speech, language, hearing, feeding, swallowing, and the social and cognitive facets of communication. To help people reach their full potential, they offer evaluation, diagnosis, treatment, and support to those who struggle with swallowing, eating, and human communication at any stage of life. Within this framework, human communication includes all cognitive processes involved in understanding and expressing spoken and written language, in addition to nonverbal and/or alternative forms of communication. Swallowing and communication are general terms that cover a wide range of functional aspects.

- Speech production and fluency, language, cognition, voice, resonance, and hearing are all components of communication.
- All facets of swallowing are included in swallowing, including associated feeding behaviors.

The International Association of Communications Sciences and Disorders, a non-profit global organization of experts and scientists in communication, voice, speech-language pathology, audiology, and swallowing, oversees speech and language therapy on a global scale.

As an autonomous profession, speech-language pathologists can work alone or in an interdisciplinary setting, collaborating with audiologists, doctors, nurses, educators, dieticians, occupational therapists, physiotherapists, psychologists, child care providers, social workers, and communication health assistants, among others.

-They can also accept referrals from a variety of sources, including the patient themselves (self-referral) or from other individuals involved with the patient (Br Dent, 2022).

8.3.1. Where Speech and Language Therapists Work?

Speech-language pathologists collaborate with kids, adults, families, and caregivers to conduct evaluations and create individualized treatment plans that address each patient's swallowing and communication requirements. They operate in a broad range of settings and circumstances, such as outpatient clinics, children's centers, mainstream and special schools, assessment rooms, daycare centers, nursing homes, homes of clients, courtrooms, prisons, and facilities for young offenders.

- **Articulation Disorders:** An articulation disorder is the incapacity to pronounce some words correctly. A young person with this speech disorder may add, change, drop, or distort word sounds. Saying "thith" instead of "this" is an illustration of word distortion.

- **Fluency Disorders:** A fluency disorder impairs speech's rhythm, cadence, and flow. Fluency disorders include cluttering and stuttering. A stutterer finds it difficult to produce sounds, and they may repeat words entirely or in parts, or they may block or interrupt their speech. A clutterer frequently speaks quickly and blends words together.
- **Resonance Disorders:** When normal airflow in the nasal or oral cavities is blocked or obstructed, the vibrations that determine voice quality are altered, leading to a resonance disorder. It may also occur from an improper closure of the velopharyngeal valve. Neurological conditions, enlarged tonsils, and cleft palate are frequently linked to resonance abnormalities.
- **Receptive Disorders:** A receptive language disorder sufferer finds it difficult to comprehend and process other people's words. This may make you appear bored when someone is talking, make it difficult for you to follow instructions, or have a small vocabulary. Receptive language disorder can be brought on by other language disorders, autism, hearing loss, and head trauma.
- **Expressive Disorders:** Difficulty expressing or conveying information is a sign of expressive language disorder. You might find it difficult to construct correct sentences if you have an expressive disorder, for example, by using the wrong verb tense. It is linked to developmental disabilities like hearing loss and Down syndrome. In addition, a medical condition or head trauma may be the cause.
- **Cognitive-Communication Disorders:** Cognitive-communication disorder is the term used to describe communication difficulties resulting from damage to the area of the brain responsible for thought processes. It may cause difficulties with speaking or listening, memory, and problem solving. Biological issues, including aberrant brain development, specific neurological disorders, brain trauma, or stroke, may be the cause.
- **Aphasia:** A person's capacity to communicate and comprehend others is impacted by this acquired communication disorder. It frequently impairs a person's capacity to read and write as well. Although aphasia can also be caused by other brain disorders, strokes are the most common cause of it.
- **Dysarthria:** Speech that is slow or slurred as a result of a lack of strength or control in the speech muscles characterizes this condition. The most common causes are diseases of the nervous system, such as multiple sclerosis (MS), amyotrophic lateral sclerosis (ALS), and stroke, which result in facial paralysis or weakness of the tongue and throat.

8.3.2. Knowledge and Skills for Clinical Practice

1. **Assessment:** Speech-language pathologists are skilled in the differential diagnosis of swallowing and communication disorders. Disorders related to speech, language, swallowing, and communication can arise during development, as a complication of an illness, or independently, without any obvious underlying medical cause. They are not able to differentially diagnose medical conditions, but they can diagnose swallowing and communication disorders. The ICF framework is used in the assessment process, which evaluates participation, activity, structure, and function of the body in relation to personal and environmental factors. Culturally and linguistically appropriate behavioral observation, standardized and/or criterion-referenced tools, the use of instrumentation, a review of records, case histories, and previous test results, as well as interviews with the individual and/or family to inform decisions, are all possible components of the assessment process. It is possible to complete the assessment process in conjunction with other experts. Speech-language pathologists;

- use culturally and linguistically appropriate assessment protocols; conduct behavioral observation to gauge an individual's abilities in a naturalistic setting or context;
- diagnose communication and swallowing disorders; use endoscopy, video fluoroscopy, and other instrumentation to assess aspects of voice, resonance, velopharyngeal function, and swallowing;
- document assessment and trial results for choosing AAC interventions and technology, including speech-generating devices;
- administer standardized and/or criterion-referenced tools to compare individuals with their peers;
- review medical records to determine pertinent health, medical, and pharmacological information;
- interview individuals and/or family members to obtain case histories to identify specific concerns.

2. **Treatment:** Speech-language pathologists enhance people's capacity for swallowing and communication, which enhances their quality of life. They achieve this by developing and implementing treatment plans that address the symptoms and concerns of communication disorders, swallowing disorders, and related functional issues. Improving a person's functional outcomes is the ultimate aim of therapy.

provide services that are appropriate for the individual's culture and language;

- integrate the best available research evidence with practitioner expertise, individual preferences, and values to establish treatment goals;
- use treatment data to inform decisions and assess the efficacy

of services; incorporate academic materials and goals into treatment;

- administer treatment at the proper frequency and intensity using best practices;
- participate in activities related to treatment that fall within the purview of the professional's expertise; and
- work in conjunction with other professionals to deliver services.

3. **Intervention**

- Language Intervention
  - To encourage language development, speech and language therapists will engage a child in play and conversation while pointing out pictures, books, objects, or current events. To improve language skills, the therapist might employ repetition exercises and provide examples of proper vocabulary and grammar.
- Articulation Intervention
  - In articulation, or sound production, exercises, the speech-language pathologist demonstrates to the child—typically during play activities—the proper sounds and syllables in words and sentences. Age-appropriate play that takes into account each child's unique needs is being played out. The child will be demonstrated by the SLP how to produce specific sounds, like the "r" sound, and possibly even how to move their tongue to produce those sounds.
- Oral-motor/Feeding and Swallowing Interventions
  - To strengthen the mouth muscles used for eating, drinking, and swallowing, speech and language therapists employ a range of oral exercises, such as facial massage and different tongue, lip, and jaw exercises. During eating and swallowing, speech and language therapists may also introduce a variety of food textures and temperatures to help a child become more aware of their mouth.

4. **Modalities, Technology, and Instrumentation:** Advanced tools and technologies are used by speech-language pathologists to assess, treat, and care for patients with disorders of feeding, swallowing, and communication. To improve the caliber of the services they offer, speech-language pathologists apply their expertise in the use of cutting-edge equipment and technologies to research and develop new technologies. The use is just one example of the services that speech-language pathologists provide in this field:

- A variety of AAC technologies are available to assist individuals with communication impairments.
- These technologies include endoscopy, video fluoroscopy, fiber-optic evaluation of swallowing (voice, velopharyngeal function, swallowing), and other instruments to assess voice, resonance, and swallowing.

- Telehealth/tele practice services allow individuals to access specialists remotely.
- Ultrasound and biofeedback systems can help with speech sound production, voice, and swallowing disorders.
- Other modalities, such as American Sign Language, may also be used as needed (Simms, 2020).

A Closer Look

Rehabilitation

Exercise regimens are advised for PD patients. There is some evidence that rehabilitation can help with speech or mobility issues, but the quality and quantity of the studies are questionable. Frequent exercise can help maintain and enhance mobility, flexibility, strength, gait speed, and quality of life, whether or not physical therapy is involved. Compared to a self-supervised exercise program at home, there are greater improvements in motor symptoms, mental and emotional functioning, everyday living activities, and quality of life when an exercise program is carried out under the supervision of a physiotherapist. Clinical exercises could be a useful intervention for improving the general wellbeing of Parkinson's patients. Depression and improved motor function are possible outcomes. Generalized relaxation techniques, like gentle rocking, have been found to reduce excessive muscle tension and improve flexibility and range of motion for individuals experiencing stiffness. Other useful methods for fostering relaxation include diaphragmatic breathing, rhythmic initiation, slow rotations of the trunk and limbs, and meditation techniques. When it comes to gait and managing the symptoms of the disease, such as hypokinesia, shuffling, and reduced arm swing, physiotherapists employ a range of techniques to enhance functional mobility and safety. During rehabilitation programs, improving gait speed, the base of support, stride length, and trunk and arm-swing movement are areas of interest. Techniques include the use of verbal cueing (manual, visual, and auditory), exercises (marching and PNF patterns), assistive equipment (pole walking and treadmill walking), and environment modification (surfaces, inputs, open vs. closed). For individuals with primary muscular weakness and weakness related to inactivity with mild to moderate PD, strengthening exercises have been shown to improve both strength and motor function. However, reports have indicated an interaction between strength and the length of time patients took their medications. As a result, when able, persons with PD should exercise 45 to 1 hour after taking their medications. Exercises involving deep diaphragmatic breathing can help with respiratory dysfunctions in advanced Parkinson's disease as well as chest-wall mobility and vital capacity that are compromised by a forward-flexed posture. Constipation may get better with exercise. It is unclear whether physical fatigue in PD can be lessened by exercise. People with PD have demonstrated improved manual dexterity following strength training exercises using manual putty. Enhancements in manual dexterity and strength can positively affect individuals with Parkinson's disease by promoting greater independence in daily tasks that involve holding objects. One of the most popular treatments for speech problems linked to Parkinson's disease is the Lee Silverman voice treatment (LSVT). SVT in particular, or speech therapy, may help with speech. Occupational therapy (OT) assists individuals with the disease in engaging in a significant portion of their daily activities in an effort to improve their quality of life and overall health. Though there is some evidence that OT may improve motor skills and quality of life during the course of therapy, there have been few and poorly quality studies on the subject.

Summary

- If you have PD, you probably notice that people ask you to repeat what you just said more than they used to. In addition, speaking clearly and intelligibly becomes a little more difficult when you have PD.
- The most common speech problems experienced by people with PD involve reduced volume (hypophonia), reduced pitch range (monotone), and difficulty with the articulation of sounds or syllables (dysarthria). In essence, you can't speak as loudly as others, you find it more difficult to convey emotion when you do speak, and you find it difficult to form the words you are trying to pronounce.
- Besides the frustrating speech and voicing problems of PD, there may also be language problems. These language problems very likely make the speech problems more difficult to deal with, so it is important to identify these language difficulties when they appear.
- Effective communication is fundamental to human connection and quality of life. Spoken and written communication is our primary means of conveying thoughts, emotions, and intentions.
- Changes in the brain in people with Parkinson's mean that your movements become smaller and less forceful than before. This can lead to problems with your speech and communication. Issues may relate to making sure your voice is loud enough, making your pronunciation clear enough and getting the right tone to your voice.
- If speech disturbances are suspected, the patient should consult with a Speech-Language Pathologist (SLP) experienced in treating people with PD, for a diagnosis. The clinician will take the patient's medical history and complaints, and identify the specific type of speech and voice disturbance. The patient's occupation, daily activities, and social background will also be discussed as they relate to how the patient uses their voice in their daily life.
- Many people with Parkinson's disease have a hard time swallowing because they lose control of their mouth and throat muscles. As a result, chewing and managing solid foods can be difficult.
- Early intervention for dysphagia is important. Beginning treatment early can reduce your risk of complications and death.
- Dysphagia can cause malnutrition or dehydration. It can also cause aspiration, the medical term for "food going down the wrong pipe." Aspiration can lead to aspiration pneumonia, which is the leading cause of death for people with PD. This is a type of lung infection that occurs when food, saliva, liquids, or vomit is breathed into the lungs or airways leading into the lungs, instead of being swallowed.
- The heterogeneous clinical presentation of PD complicates the diagnostic procedure. Diagnosis is primarily based on the presence of hallmark motor signs (*i.e.,* resting tremor, bradykinesia, muscle rigidity, postural instability), response to dopamine replacement, and brain imaging.

References

1. Alcalay, R. N., Mirelman, A., Saunders-Pullman, R., Tang, M. X., Mejia-Santana, H., Raymond, D., & Bar-Shira, A. (2013). Parkinson disease phenotype in Ashkenazi Jews with and without LRRK2 G2019S mutations. *Movement Disorders, 28*(14), 1966–1971. https://doi.org/10.1002/mds.25647.
2. Antony, P. M. A., Diederich, N. J., Krüger, R., & Balling, R. (2013). The hallmarks of Parkinson's disease. *FEBS Journal, 280*(23), 5981–5993. https://doi.org/10.1111/febs.12335.
3. Argolo, N., Sampaio, M., Pinho, P., Melo, A., & Nóbrega, A. C. (2015). Swallowing disorders in Parkinson's disease: Impact of lingual pumping. *International Journal of Language & Communication Disorders, 50*(5), 659–664. https://doi.org/10.1111/1460-6984.12158.
4. Armstrong, M. J., & Okun, M. S. (2020). Diagnosis and treatment of Parkinson disease: A review. *JAMA, 323*(6), 548–560. https://doi.org/10.1001/jama.2019.22360.
5. Ball, N., Teo, W. P., Chandra, S., & Chapman, J. (2019). Parkinson's disease and the environment. *Frontiers in Neurology, 10*, 218. https://doi.org/10.3389/fneur.2019.00218.
6. Beattie, D. T., & Smith, J. A. M. (2008). Serotonin pharmacology in the gastrointestinal tract: A review. *Naunyn-Schmiedeberg's Archives of Pharmacology, 377*(2–4), 181–203. https://doi.org/10.1007/s00210-008-0276-9.
7. Bieger, D., & Neuhuber, W. (2006). Neural circuits and mediators regulating swallowing in the brainstem. *GI Motility Online*, 1–19. https://doi.org/10.1038/GIMO74.
8. Blauwendraat, C., Nalls, M. A., & Singleton, A. B. (2020). The genetic architecture of Parkinson's disease. *The Lancet Neurology, 19*(2), 170–178. https://doi.org/10.1016/S1474-4422(19)30287-X.
9. Borghammer, P., Horsager, J., Andersen, K., Van Den Berge, N., Raunio, A., Murayama, S., & Myllykangas, L. (2021). Neuropathological evidence of body-first vs brain-first Lewy body disease. *Neurobiology of Disease, 161*, 105557. https://doi.org/10.1016/j.nbd.2021.105557.
10. Braak, H., De Vos, R. A. I., Bohl, J., & Del Tredici, K. (2006). Gastric α-Synuclein immunoreactive inclusions in Meissner's and Auerbach's Plexuses in cases staged for Parkinson's disease-related brain pathology. *Neuroscience Letters, 396*(1), 67–72. https://doi.org/10.1016/j.neulet.2005.11.012.
11. Braak, H., del Tredici, K., Rüb, U., de Vos, R. A. I., Jansen Steur, E. N. H., & Braak, E. (2003). Staging of brain pathology related to sporadic Parkinson's disease. *Neurobiology of Aging, 24*(2), 197–211. https://doi.org/10.1016/S0197-4580(02)00065-9.
12. Braak, H., Ghebremedhin, E., Rüb, U., Bratzke, H., & del Tredici, K. (2004). Stages in the development of Parkinson's disease-related pathology. *Cell and Tissue Research, 318*(1), 121–134. https://doi.org/10.1007/s00441-004-0956-9.
13. Del Tredici, K., & Braak, H. (2013). Dysfunction of the locus coeruleus-norepinephrine system and related circuitry in Parkinson's disease-related dementia. *Journal of Neurology, Neurosurgery, and Psychiatry, 84*(7), 774–783. https://doi.org/10.1136/jnnp-2011-301817.
14. Farri, A., Accornero, A., & Burdese, C. (2007). Social importance of dysphagia: Its impact on diagnosis and therapy. *Acta Otorhinolaryngologica Italica, 27*(2), 83–86.

15. Fernandez, H. H., & Lapane, K. L. (2002). Predictors of mortality among nursing home residents with a diagnosis of Parkinson's disease. *Medical Science Monitor, 8*(6), 241–246.

16. Findley, L. J. (2007). The economic impact of Parkinson's disease. *Parkinsonism & Related Disorders, 13*(Suppl 8), S8–S12. https://doi.org/10.1016/j.parkreldis.2007.06.003.

17. Gillies, G. E., Pienaar, I. S., Vohra, S., & Qamhawi, Z. (2014). Sex differences in Parkinson's disease. *Frontiers in Neuroendocrinology, 35*, 370–384. https://doi.org/10.1016/j.yfrne.2014.02.002.

18. Haaxma, C. A., Bloem, B. R., Borm, G. F., Oyen, W. J. G., Leenders, K. L., Eshuis, S., & Horstink, M. W. I. M. (2007). Gender differences in Parkinson's disease. *Journal of Neurology, Neurosurgery, and Psychiatry, 78*(8), 819–824. https://doi.org/10.1136/jnnp.2006.103788.

19. Healy, D. G., Falchi, M., O'Sullivan, S. S., Bonifati, V., Durr, A., Bressman, S., & Zabetian, C. P. (2008). Phenotype, genotype, and worldwide genetic penetrance of LRRK2-associated Parkinson's disease: A case-control study. *The Lancet Neurology, 7*(7), 583–590. https://doi.org/10.1016/S1474-4422(08)70117-0.

20. Heijmans, M., Habets, J. G. V., Herff, C., et al. (2019). Monitoring Parkinson's disease symptoms during daily life: A feasibility study. *npj Parkinson's Disease, 5*, 21. https://doi.org/10.1038/s41531-019-0100-1.

21. Iwaki, H., Blauwendraat, C., Leonard, H. L., Makarious, M. B., Kim, J. J., Liu, G., & van Nimwegen, M. (2021). Differences in the presentation and progression of Parkinson's disease by sex. *Movement Disorders, 36*(1), 106–117. https://doi.org/10.1002/mds.28312.

22. Jones, C. A., & Ciucci, M. R. (2016). Multimodal swallowing evaluation with high-resolution manometry reveals subtle swallowing changes in early and mid-stage Parkinson disease. *Journal of Parkinson's Disease, 6*(1), 197–208. https://doi.org/10.3233/JPD-150687.

23. Kalf, J. G., de Swart, B. J. M., Bloem, B. R., & Munneke, M. (2012). Prevalence of oropharyngeal dysphagia in Parkinson's disease: A meta-analysis. *Parkinsonism & Related Disorders, 18*(4), 311–315. https://doi.org/10.1016/j.parkreldis.2011.11.006.

24. Kempster, P. A., O'Sullivan, S. S., Holton, J. L., Revesz, T., & Lees, A. J. (2010). Relationships between age and late progression of Parkinson's disease: A clinicopathological study. *Brain, 133*(6), 1755–1762. https://doi.org/10.1093/brain/awq059.

25. Kim, Y. H., Oh, B. M., Jung, I. Y., Lee, J. C., Lee, G. J., & Han, T. R. (2015). Spatiotemporal characteristics of swallowing in Parkinson's disease. *The Laryngoscope, 125*(2), 389–395. https://doi.org/10.1002/lary.24869.

26. Mahler, L. A., Ramig, L. O., & Fox, C. (2013). Evidence-based treatment of voice and speech disorders in Parkinson disease. *Current Opinion in Otolaryngology & Head and Neck Surgery, 23*(3), 209–215.

27. Marras, C., & Chaudhuri, K. R. (2016). Nonmotor features of Parkinson's disease subtypes. *Movement Disorders, 31*(8), 1095–1102. https://doi.org/10.1002/mds.26510.

28. Marras, C., Chaudhuri, K. R., Titova, N., & Mestre, T. A. (2020). Therapy of Parkinson's disease subtypes. *Neurotherapeutics, 17*(4), 1366–1377. https://doi.org/10.1007/s13311-020-00894-7.

29. Martinez-Martin, P., Pecurariu, C. F., Odin, P., van Hilten, J. J., Antonini, A., Rojo-Abuin, J. M., & Brooks, D. J. (2012). Gender-related differences in the burden of non-motor symptoms

in Parkinson's disease. *Journal of Neurology, 259*(8), 1639–1647. https://doi.org/10.1007/s00415-011-6392-3.

30. Miller, I. N., & Cronin-Golomb, A. (2010). Gender differences in Parkinson's disease: Clinical characteristics and cognition. *Movement Disorders, 25*(16), 2695. https://doi.org/10.1002/mds.23388.
31. Mu, L., Chen, J., Sobotka, S., Nyirenda, T., Benson, B., Gupta, F., & Beach, T. G. (2015). Alpha-synuclein pathology in sensory nerve terminals of the upper aerodigestive tract of Parkinson's disease patients. *Dysphagia, 30*(4), 404–417. https://doi.org/10.1007/s00455-015-9612-7.
32. Mu, L., Sobotka, S., Chen, J., Su, H., Sanders, I., Adler, C. H., & Beach, T. G. (2013). Alpha-synuclein pathology and axonal degeneration of the peripheral motor nerves innervating pharyngeal muscles in Parkinson disease. *Journal of Neuropathology and Experimental Neurology, 72*(2), 119–129. https://doi.org/10.1097/NEN.0b013e3182801cde.
33. Nienstedt, J. C., Bihler, M., Niessen, A., Plaetke, R., Pötter-Nerger, M., Gerloff, C., & Pflug, C. (2019). Predictive clinical factors for penetration and aspiration in Parkinson's disease. *Neurogastroenterology & Motility, 31*(6), e13524. https://doi.org/10.1111/nmo.13524.
34. Pagano, G., Ferrara, N., Brooks, D. J., & Pavese, N. (2016). Age at onset and Parkinson disease phenotype. *Neurology, 86*(15), 1400–1407. https://doi.org/10.1212/WNL.0000000000002461.
35. Pflug, C., Bihler, M., Emich, K., Niessen, A., Nienstedt, J. C., Flügel, T., & Gerloff, C. (2018). Critical dysphagia is common in Parkinson disease and occurs even in early stages: A prospective cohort study. *Dysphagia, 33*(1), 41–50. https://doi.org/10.1007/s00455-017-9831-1.
36. Plowman-Prine, E. K., Sapienza, C. M., Okun, M. S., Pollock, S. L., Jacobson, C., Wu, S. S., & Rosenbek, J. C. (2009). The relationship between quality of life and swallowing in Parkinson's disease. *Movement Disorders, 24*(9), 1352–1358. https://doi.org/10.1002/mds.22617.
37. Postuma, R. B., Berg, D., Stern, M., Poewe, W., Olanow, C. W., Oertel, W., & Lang, A. E. (2015). MDS clinical diagnostic criteria for Parkinson's disease. *Movement Disorders, 30*(12), 1591–1601. https://doi.org/10.1002/mds.26424.
38. Potulska, A., Friedman, A., Królicki, L., & Spychała, A. (2003). Swallowing disorders in Parkinson's disease. *Parkinsonism & Related Disorders, 9*(6), 349–353.
39. Ramig, L. O., Fox, C., & Sapir, S. (2008). Speech treatment for Parkinson's disease. *Expert Review of Neurotherapeutics, 8*(2), 297–309.
40. Rothrie, S., Fitzgerald, E., Brady, G. C., & Roe, J. W. G. (2022). The role of the speech and language therapist in the rehabilitation of speech, swallowing, voice and trismus in people diagnosed with head and neck cancer. *British Dental Journal, 233*(9), 801–805.
41. Samii, A., Nutt, J. G., & Ransom, B. R. (2004). Parkinson's disease. *The Lancet, 363*(9423), 1783–1793. https://doi.org/10.1016/S0140-6736(04)16305-8.
42. Schapira, A. H. V., Chaudhuri, K. R., & Jenner, P. (2017). Non-motor features of Parkinson disease. *Nature Reviews Neuroscience, 18*(7), 435–450. https://doi.org/10.1038/nrn.2017.62.
43. Shannon, K. M., Keshavarzian, A., Mutlu, E., Dodiya, H. B., Daian, D., Jaglin, J. A., & Kordower, J. H. (2012). Alpha-synuclein in colonic submucosa in early untreated Parkinson's disease. *Movement Disorders, 27*(6), 709–715. https://doi.org/10.1002/mds.23838.
44. Simms, M. D. (2020). Language development and communication disorders. In R. M. Kliegman, J. W. St. Geme, N. J. Blum, S. S. Shah, R. C. Tasker, & K. M. Wilson (Eds.), *Nelson Textbook of*

Pediatrics (21st ed., chap. 52). Philadelphia, PA: Elsevier.

45. Sioka, C., Fotopoulos, A., & Kyritsis, A. P. (2010). Recent advances in PET imaging for evaluation of Parkinson's disease. *European Journal of Nuclear Medicine and Molecular Imaging, 37*(8), 1594–1603. https://doi.org/10.1007/s00259-009-1357-9.
46. Smith, K. M., & Caplan, D. N. (2018). Communication impairment in Parkinson's disease: Impact of motor and cognitive symptoms on speech and language. *Brain and Language, 185*, 38–46. https://doi.org/10.1016/j.bandl.2018.08.002.
47. Sung, H. Y., Kim, J. S., Lee, K. S., Kim, Y. I., Song, I. U., Chung, S. W., & Lee, I. S. (2010). The prevalence and patterns of pharyngoesophageal dysmotility in patients with early-stage Parkinson's disease. *Movement Disorders, 25*(14), 2361–2368. https://doi.org/10.1002/mds.23290.
48. Suttrup, I., & Warnecke, T. (2016). Dysphagia in Parkinson's disease. *Dysphagia, 31*(1), 24–32. https://doi.org/10.1007/s00455-015-9671-9.
49. Swan, M., Doan, N., Ortega, R. A., Barrett, M., Nichols, W., Ozelius, L., & Sarva, H. (2016). Neuropsychiatric characteristics of GBA-associated Parkinson disease. *Journal of the Neurological Sciences, 370*, 63–69. https://doi.org/10.1016/j.jns.2016.08.059.
50. Umemoto, G., Tsuboi, Y., Kitashima, A., Furuya, H., & Kikuta, T. (2011). Impaired food transportation in Parkinson's disease related to lingual bradykinesia. *Dysphagia, 26*(3), 250–255. https://doi.org/10.1007/s00455-010-9296-y.
51. Zajac, D. J. (2018). Evaluation and management of speech disorders for the patient with cleft palate. In R. J. Fonseca (Ed.), *Oral and Maxillofacial Surgery* (3rd ed., chap. 32). St. Louis, MO: Elsevier.

Chapter 9

MALNUTRITION AND RELATED DISORDERS

Contents

Introduction

Among people with Parkinson's disease (PD), malnutrition is a serious issue because of the disease and the symptoms it causes. Parkinson's disease (PD) frequently affects motor abilities, such as swallowing and chewing, which makes eating difficult and causes people to eat less. Furthermore, the illness may cause changes in metabolism and an increase in energy expenditure, which could make patients' nutritional status even more problematic. As a result, weight loss and malnutrition are common in people with Parkinson's disease (PD), which can worsen the disease's course and have an adverse effect on general health. Furthermore, malnutrition in Parkinson's disease (PD) is caused by both decreased food intake and nutritional deficiencies. Medication used to treat Parkinson's disease symptoms, like levodopa, can affect how well certain nutrients are absorbed. Levodopa can cause problems with how well proteins and some vitamins are absorbed. Deficiencies in vital nutrients, such as vitamin B12 and vitamin D, which are critical for general health and neurological function, may result from this medication-related malabsorption.

Moreover, there is a link between PD patients who are malnourished and a higher chance of developing related disorders. For example, osteoporosis and bone fractures are more common in people with Parkinson's disease (PD), in part because of inadequate diet and vitamin D deficiency. Inadequate protein intake can also lead to muscle weakness and frailty, which increases the risk of falls and injuries. A multimodal approach is necessary to address malnutrition in Parkinson's disease patients. Despite swallowing difficulties and decreased appetite, healthcare providers frequently recommend dietary adjustments to ensure an adequate intake of nutrients. It is also possible to prescribe nutritional supplements to address particular deficiencies. Furthermore, as the disease advances, caregivers and medical professionals are essential in monitoring the nutritional status of patients with Parkinson's disease and modifying interventions.

Malnutrition and associated nutritional disorders have a substantial impact on Parkinson's disease patients, affecting both the course of the disease and general health outcomes. In order to address these issues and maintain patients' quality of life and optimal nutritional status, a thorough understanding of how the disease affects nutrition is necessary.

Orientation and Directional Terms:

Terms	Definition	Illustration
Undernutrition	Undernutrition is a deficiency of calories or of one or more essential nutrients.	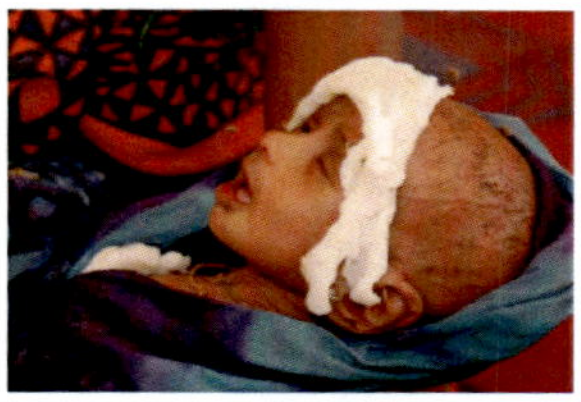
Overnutrition	Overnutrition is a form of malnutrition in which the intake of nutrients is oversupplied.	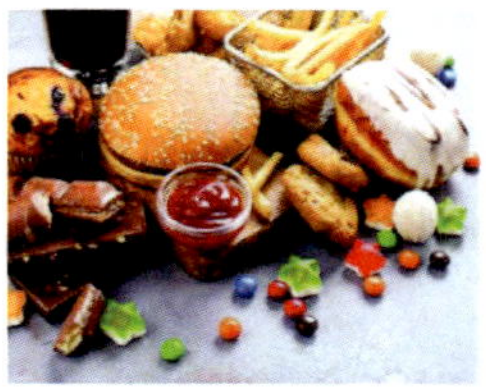
Micronutrient	Micronutrients are vitamins and minerals needed by the body in very small amounts. However, their impact on a body's health are critical, and deficiency in any of them can cause severe and even life-threatening conditions.	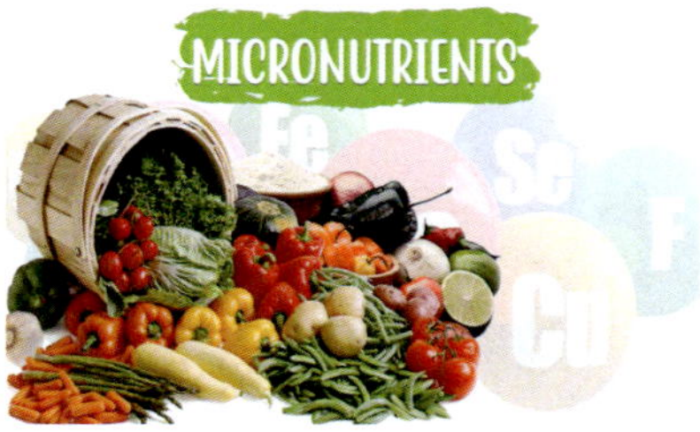
Hypothyroidism	Hypothyroidism is a common condition where the thyroid doesn't create and release enough thyroid hormone into your bloodstream.	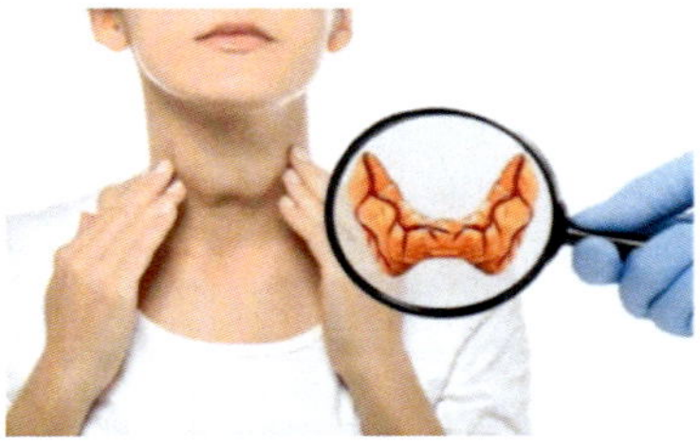
Dementia	Dementia is not a specific disease but is rather a general term for the impaired ability to remember, think, or make decisions that interferes with doing everyday activities.	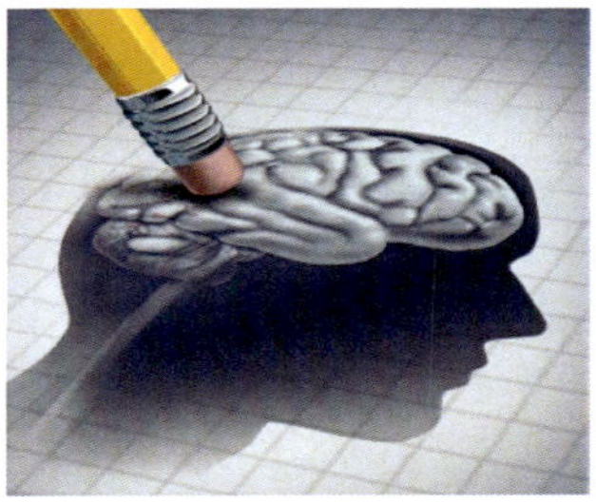

9.1. Overview of Malnutrition

The complex problem of malnutrition among people with Parkinson's disease (PD) is impacted by both socioeconomic factors and disease-related factors. Numerous motor and non-motor symptoms of Parkinson's disease (PD) can have an immediate effect on one's nutritional status. For example, patients with dysphagia (difficulties with chewing and swallowing) may find it difficult to eat enough food. Further complicating their dietary intake, tremors and rigidity may impair their ability to cook or eat on their own. Furthermore, non-motor symptoms like anxiety and depression frequently coexist with Parkinson's disease (PD) and can lower appetite or interest in food, which can result in unintentional weight loss and nutritional deficiencies. The side effects of medications used to treat Parkinson's disease (PD) can include nausea, taste loss, and changes in appetite. These side effects can also lead to nutritional issues. Social factors can increase the risk of malnutrition in people with Parkinson's disease (PD). These factors include restricted access to nutrient-dense food, financial constraints, or reduced social interactions due to mobility issues. Additionally, because Parkinson's disease (PD) is progressive, nutritional requirements may vary over time, necessitating continuous monitoring and dietary intervention adjustments. In order to address malnutrition in Parkinson's disease patients, a multidisciplinary team comprising neurologists, dietitians, and caregivers must create individualized nutrition plans that take into account each patient's unique needs and challenges. Healthcare professionals can enhance the quality of life and general health outcomes for people with Parkinson's disease by addressing these factors in their entirety.

An organism experiences malnutrition when it receives too few or too many nutrients, which can lead to health issues. In particular, it is an excess, deficit, or imbalance of energy, protein, and other nutrients that negatively impacts the structure and tissues of the body. Not getting enough nourishment is known as malnutrition. Undernutrition and overnutrition are included in the category of diseases known as malnutrition. Lack of nutrients can cause undernutrition, which can manifest as underweight, wasting, and stunted growth. Overnutrition brought on by an abundance of nutrients can lead to obesity. Overnutrition in the form of obesity is starting to manifest in the same communities as undernutrition in certain developing nations.

A complex worldwide health problem, malnutrition is defined by excesses, imbalances, or deficiencies in one or more critical nutrients. It can have detrimental effects on one's development, general well-being, and health in people of all ages. Malnutrition covers a wider range of illnesses, including both undernutrition and overnutrition, despite being frequently linked to starvation and undernutrition.

Perhaps the most well-known type of malnutrition is undernutrition. It happens when people don't eat enough calories or vital nutrients to meet their body's requirements. Chronic undernutrition can cause wasting, stunted growth, and deficiencies in certain micronutrients, which can harm the immune system, impair cognitive and physical development, and raise the risk of illness and infection. Undernutrition can have long-term effects on a child's capacity to learn, develop, and thrive. Conditions like kwashiorkor and marasmus, which are characterized by severe wasting, edema, and muscle loss, can result from undernutrition in extreme circumstances.

Overnutrition is becoming increasingly worrisome in various regions around the world, especially in affluent countries and cities. It occurs when people consume too many calories, usually from sugary, fatty, and processed foods, without getting the necessary nutrients. This can result in obesity and health problems like type 2 diabetes, heart disease, and certain cancers. Interestingly, both overnutrition and undernutrition can occur simultaneously in a population, creating a double burden of malnutrition where some people suffer from hunger and lack of nutrients while others face obesity and diet-related illnesses.

Another important component of malnutrition is deficiencies in micronutrients. People may not get enough vitamins and minerals, even in cases where they eat enough calories, for optimal bodily function. Iron deficiency, which can cause anemia and impair oxygen transport; vitamin A deficiency, which can impair vision and weaken the immune system; and iodine deficiency, which can cause thyroid issues and cognitive impairments, are common micronutrient deficiencies. The cycle of poverty and malnutrition is exacerbated by micronutrient deficiencies, which disproportionately affect vulnerable populations such as infants, young children, and pregnant women.

Additionally, there are wider social, economic, and environmental effects of malnutrition. It can impede social and economic advancement by sustaining cycles of poverty and inequality. People who are malnourished are more likely to suffer from poor health, be less productive, and have lower earning potential, which keeps them stuck in a cycle of deprivation and poverty. Furthermore, because unsustainable agricultural practices and food systems put a strain on ecosystems and natural resources, malnutrition contributes to environmental degradation and resource depletion. Malnutrition must be addressed with an all-encompassing, integrated strategy that takes into account its underlying causes and determinants. This entails expanding access to wholesome food, supporting nursing and appropriate complementary feeding methods, boosting food security and agricultural productivity, and fortifying social safety nets and health systems. Additionally crucial are behavior modification programs and nutrition education, which enable people and groups to choose healthful foods and follow healthy eating habits.

Malnutrition is a complicated, multidimensional global health issue with far-reaching effects. It undermines human potential, development, and health, affecting people individually, in families, and in communities all over the world. We can work toward creating a world where everyone has access to the nutrients they need to live healthy, active, and fulfilling lives by placing a high priority on nutrition and funding comprehensive interventions.

9.1.1. Types of Malnutrition

Malnutrition can refer to either excessive or insufficient nourishment. It may also indicate an imbalance in micronutrients, such as vitamins and minerals, or macronutrients, such as proteins, carbs, and fats.

- **Undernutrition:** When most people think of malnutrition, they think of undernutrition. A lack of nutrients is called undernutrition. If your body has problems absorbing enough nutrients from your food or if your diet is inadequate, you may be undernourished. Undernutrition can result in both visible and invisible loss of muscle and fat. It is possible to be malnourished and overweight.

i. ***Macronutrient Undernutrition:*** This undernutrition of proteins, carbs, and fats is also referred to as protein-energy undernutrition. The primary dietary components known as macronutrients are those that your body uses to create energy in order to function. Your body quickly starts to disintegrate without them, or even just one of them. It breaks down tissues and stops doing things it doesn't need to in order to save its limited energy.

ii. ***Micronutrient Undernutrition:*** Minerals and vitamins comprise micronutrients. Although your body requires them in smaller quantities, it still needs them for a variety of processes. Many suffer from mild deficiencies in specific vitamins and minerals as a result of eating a diet that is not very varied. A mild vitamin deficiency may not seem to be affecting you, but when micronutrient undernutrition worsens, it can start to cause major problems that take time to heal.

- **Overnutrition:** In order to acknowledge the potentially harmful health effects of consuming too many nutrients, the World Health Organization has recently included overnutrition in its definition of malnutrition. This includes the consequences of being overweight or obese, as these conditions are closely linked to a number of noncommunicable diseases (NCDs). It also covers the potential toxicity brought on by taking too much of a particular micronutrient.

i. ***Macronutrient Overnutrition:*** Your body stores extra protein, carbohydrate, and/or fat calories as fat cells in your adipose tissue when it doesn't need them. However, the fat cells themselves must proliferate when the body runs out of tissue in which to store fat. Larger fat cells are linked to a number of ensuing metabolic diseases as well as persistent inflammation. These may result in NCDs like stroke, coronary artery disease, and diabetes mellitus.

ii. ***Micronutrient Overnutrition:*** Supplementing with too many vitamins and minerals is possible. To understand how this occurs and how much of a particular vitamin or mineral is too much, more research is required. Micronutrient overnutrition generally happens infrequently and is not the result of diet alone. However, taking excessive amounts of some supplements can have harmful consequences. Consult your healthcare provider first, if possible.

Malnutrition, in its broadest sense, affects everyone. Malnutrition is frequently caused by a lack of knowledge about nutrition, a lack of access to a wide variety of foods, sedentary modern lifestyles, and financial hardships. Some forms of malnutrition are more common in certain populations.

Populations more at risk of undernutrition include:

- **Poor and Low Income**: Whether in a developed country like the U.S. or in developing countries with fewer resources overall, poorer communities have less access to adequate nutrition.
- **Children**: Children have greater nutritional needs than adults in order to grow and develop. Disadvantaged children are especially at risk of undernutrition and its consequences.
- **Chronically Ill**: Many chronic illnesses can directly affect appetite and/or calorie absorption. Some increase your caloric needs.

Spending time in the hospital is also a risk factor for undernutrition.

- **Elderly**: As adults advance in age, their nutrition can deteriorate for several reasons, including reduced mobility, institutionalization, reduced appetite and reduced absorption of nutrients.

Populations more at risk of overnutrition include:

- **Poor and Low Income**: In developed countries, poorer communities often have easier access to fast foods, which are high in calories but low in nutritional value, than they have to nutritious whole foods. This can lead to macronutrient overnutrition with micronutrient undernutrition.
- **Sedentary**: Desk jobs, family obligations, health and social factors that keep people sitting all day instead of out and moving about can lead to significant weight gain.

9.1.2. What Happens to the Body During Malnutrition?

Undernutrition in macronutrients (also known as protein-energy undernutrition) causes your body to run out of energy. It starts disintegrating its own tissues and stopping its operations as a way to make up for it. Its body fat reserves come first, followed by the muscles, skin, hair, and nails. Undernutrition in protein and energy frequently results in obvious emaciation. Children's development and growth may be stunted.

The immune system is among the first to start malfunctioning. People who are malnourished are therefore more vulnerable to disease and infection and heal more slowly. Heals are slower for wounds. Moreover, there is a slowdown in cardiac activity, which results in low blood pressure, body temperature, and heart rate. Folks may experience weakness, faintness, and apathy toward life. They might become less hungry, and certain parts of their digestive system might atrophy.

It is common for those who are malnourished in macronutrients to also be malnourished in micronutrients. Low calorie intake generally has an impact on vitamin and mineral levels as well. Certain vitamin deficiencies cause some of the consequences of severe undernutrition conditions, like kwashiorkor and marasmus. For instance, low levels of vitamin A can lead to visual issues, while low levels of vitamin D can result in soft bones. While some individuals may eat a lot of calories, they may not get enough vitamins and minerals. The consequences of malnutrition could be less noticeable in these situations. Individuals may be overweight as a result of macronutrient overconsumption, but a deficiency in minerals or vitamins can cause anemia symptoms such as weakness, fatigue, and fainting. Overnourished individuals may exhibit signs of the metabolic syndrome, including hypertension and insulin resistance.

9.1.3. Symptoms

The main symptom of malnutrition (undernutrition) is unintentional weight loss, although this is not always obvious.

- ***What are the Signs and Symptoms of Malnutrition?***

The signs and symptoms of malnutrition can vary, depending on the type. The most common symptom of malnutrition, undernutrition is unintentional weight loss, but people may also have one or several of these symptoms:

- Loss of fat and muscle mass
- Hollow cheeks and sunken eyes

- A swollen stomach
- Delayed wound healing
- Dry hair and skin
- Fatigue
- Difficulty concentrating
- Depression and anxiety

Other symptoms and indicators exist, but they differ according to the kind of malnutrition and the stage of life that is impacted. Other symptoms include weak bones, impaired brain development, impaired immunity, frequent infections, changes in intestinal mucosa, changes in hair and skin, and stunted physical growth.

Undernutrition leads to serious physical growth restriction and health problems and because of this, it can increase your risk of infection and death.

Undernutrition may look like:

- Low body weight, prominent bones, depleted fat and muscle.
- Thin arms and legs with edema (swelling with fluid) in your belly and face.
- Stunted growth and intellectual development in children.
- Weakness, faintness and fatigue.
- Irritability, apathy or inattention.
- Dry, inelastic skin, rashes and lesions.
- Brittle hair, hair loss and hair pigment loss.
- Frequent and severe infections.
- Low body temperature, unable to get warm.
- Low heart rate and blood pressure.

Overnutrition might look like the following:

- Obesity.
- High blood pressure.
- Insulin resistance.
- Heart disease.

9.2 Nutritional Health and the role of the Registered Dietician

Parkinson's disease (PD), a progressive neurodegenerative disease with both motor and non-motor symptoms, is largely controlled by nutritional health. A Registered Dietitian's (RD) ability to translate nutritional science into workable dietary plans that can reduce symptoms and enhance general health outcomes makes them essential to the management of Parkinson's disease (PD).

Parkinson's disease (PD) frequently affects motor abilities like balance and movement, but it also has an impact on non-motor abilities like mood, digestion, and thought processes. These symptoms may affect the amount of food consumed and the absorption of nutrients, making it difficult to maintain a healthy diet.

RDs are experts at determining each person's unique nutritional requirements based on their PD's particular symptoms and course. They can create customized meal plans that meet these requirements while taking into account things like drug interactions and gastrointestinal problems that are frequently linked to Parkinson's disease (PD).

For example, dysphagia (difficulty swallowing) or constipation are common in people with Parkinson's disease (PD), and they can have an impact on food intake and nutrient absorption.

Foods with altered textures or dietary supplements can be suggested by an RD to guarantee sufficient nutrient intake without aggravating these symptoms. Furthermore, some drugs used to treat Parkinson's disease symptoms may alter appetite or interact with nutrients, necessitating dietary changes that a registered dietitian (RD) can skillfully manage. A balanced diet high in vitamins, minerals, and antioxidants is often recommended by registered dietitians (RDs) as a way to support brain health and reduce oxidative stress, which is linked to the advancement of Parkinson's disease (PD).

In order to maximize the benefits of medication and general health, they might also offer advice on the significance of staying hydrated and keeping a healthy weight.

Beyond providing basic nutrition counseling, RDs are essential members of the healthcare team who work in tandem with neurologists, therapists, and other healthcare providers to improve the quality of life for people with Parkinson's disease (PD). RDs enable patients to make educated dietary decisions that can improve symptom management and overall health outcomes in Parkinson's disease through their specialized knowledge and personalized approach.

- There are many obstacles and frank barriers to nutritional health among people with PD. These can be due to the nature of the disease, to disabilities resulting from the disease, or to the medications needed to treat it.
- Nutrient depletion can weaken the immune system, lead to depression, unplanned weight loss, cognitive impairment, protein-energy malnutrition, bone fractures, dehydration, pressure ulcers, and other serious conditions, often requiring hospitalization.
- These can seriously impact on the health and quality of life of the individual.
- Hence, a registered dietician's medical nutrition therapy is a crucial part of a multidisciplinary treatment plan. It can lower hospitalization rates and health-related costs, improve quality of life, and help prevent malnutrition. As soon as possible after a PD diagnosis, a registered dietician should be involved.

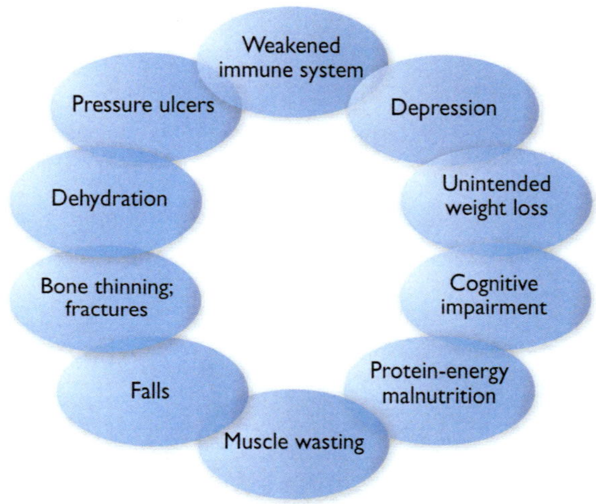

Figure 9.1. ***Malnutrition***. Potential effects of poor nutrition which can affect PD patients

Source: https://www.google.co.in/books/edition/Parkinson_s_Disease/K-EXhIJ6-sYC?hl=en&gbpv=0

9.2.1 Nutritional Disorders Related to Autonomic Effects of PD

PD may have an impact on the autonomic nervous system, which could slow the GI tract's motility. This may have an effect on one or more GI tract sections, creating numerous obstacles to nutrient replacement. The common nonmotor issues associated with autonomic dysfunction in Parkinson disease include constipation, dysphagia, sialorrhea, rhinorrhea, urinary difficulties, and sexual dysfunction.

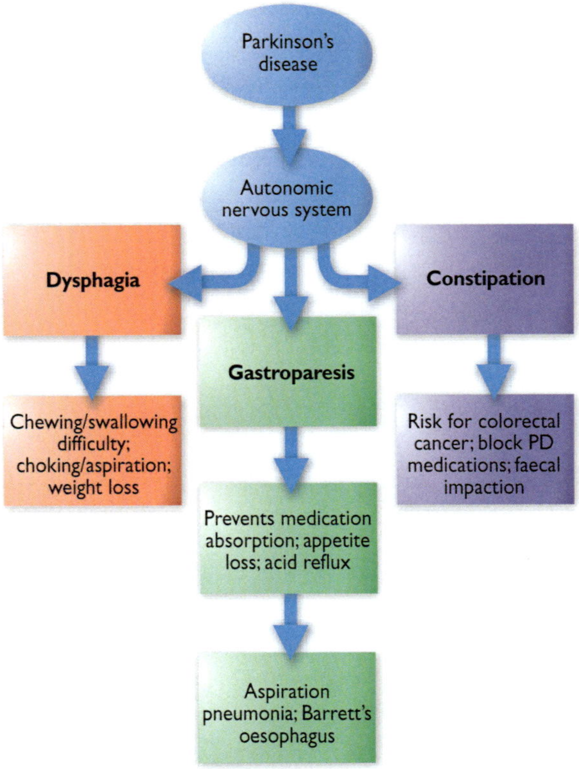

Figure 9.2. ***Autonomic effects.*** Involvement of the autonomic nervous system in reducing nutrient intake in PD patients

Source: https://www.google.co.in/books/edition/Parkinson_s_Disease/K-EXhIJ6-sYC?hl=en&gbpv=0

Dysphagia

- Chewing and swallowing difficulties.
- Choking, and/or aspiration of foods, liquids, refluxed stomach contents, and saliva.
- Unfavourably impacts on energy and nutrient intake:
- Unplanned weight loss.
- Malnutrition.
- Aspiration pneumonia.

Administration. if necessary, a referral to a speech-language pathologist for a swallowing assessment and altered food consistency. For a nutrition assessment and suitable diet planning, the person should be referred to a registered dietician if the speech and language therapist finds that pureed or thickened liquids are necessary.

Gastroparesis

- Delays the passage of food into the small intestine.
- May prevent or slow the absorption of medication.
- Causes early satiety, loss of appetite, inability to finish meals.
- Can cause gastro-oesophageal reflux disease:
  - May lead to injury of oesophagus and lower oesophageal sphincter.
  - Can cause Barrett's oesophagus, a precancerous condition.
  - If dysphagia is present, there is increased risk for aspiration of refluxed stomach contents, and aspiration pneumonia.
  - Medications used to treat gastro-oesophageal reflux disease by raising gastric pH can interfere with the metabolism of some nutrients, including vitamin B12 and iron.
- *Management.* It is best to have a lot of tiny meals and snacks that are high in nutrients and moderate in fat and fiber. Levodopa should be taken approximately 30 minutes prior to each small morning, midday, and evening meal. Protein needs should be evaluated and distributed equally among these meals. Between

these meals, low-protein snacks should be consumed in order to meet total caloric requirements. When stomach emptying is slowed, using "liquid Sinemet," Parcopa (USA), or Madopar Dispersible (Europe) may be beneficial.

- If gastro-oesophageal reflux disease is present, use of small meals and avoidance of 'trigger foods,' i.e. caffeine, citrus, tomatoes, alcohol, should be helpful. The day's final meal should be consumed at least 4 hr before bedtime, so that the stomach is empty before lying down.

Constipation

- May predate diagnosis of PD by as much as several years; may even be an early symptom of PD.
- Elevates risk for colorectal cancer.
- Can block effectiveness of PD medications.
- Chronic laxative use, including senna and cascara sagrada, may damage the colon.
- Dysregularion of autonomic nervous system may cause pelvic floor dysfunction, with inability to evacuate the stool.
- Chronic or prolonged constipation may cause faecal impaction.
- *Management.* Talk to the patient about the symptoms of faecal impaction and the availability of colorectal cancer screening. As ability allows, physical activity is preferred. Insoluble fiber from food sources—at least 25 g per day—when combined with six to eight 250 ml glasses of liquids can speed up colon transit time and increase the volume of stool produced. It may be beneficial to take probiotics and prebiotics together with meals of foods high in fiber, like kiwifruit and prunes. The dietician should evaluate the amount of fiber and liquids consumed and offer tailored guidance as necessary.
    - In the event that dietary interventions are ineffective in causing bowel movement, pelvic floor dysfunction should be taken into account, and medical intervention may be required. To prevent the need for long-term laxative use, the best way to manage constipation should instead focus on dietary and lifestyle modifications.

9.2.2 Nutritional Disorders Related to Mental Aspects of PD

Parkinson's disease may also affect mental and emotional health and energy level; this can have an impact on nutrient repletion.

- *Management.* Assess status of B1 (thiamine), B2 (riboflavin), B3 (niacin), B6 (pyridoxine), B12, and folate, all of which are implicated in cognitive impairment, memory loss, confusion, and dementias. Assess dietary intake, and provide advice where needed. Consider use of fortified foods or vitamin/mineral supplements. The carer will be of primary importance in helping to guard against malnutrition, and careful instruction and education of the carer are required.

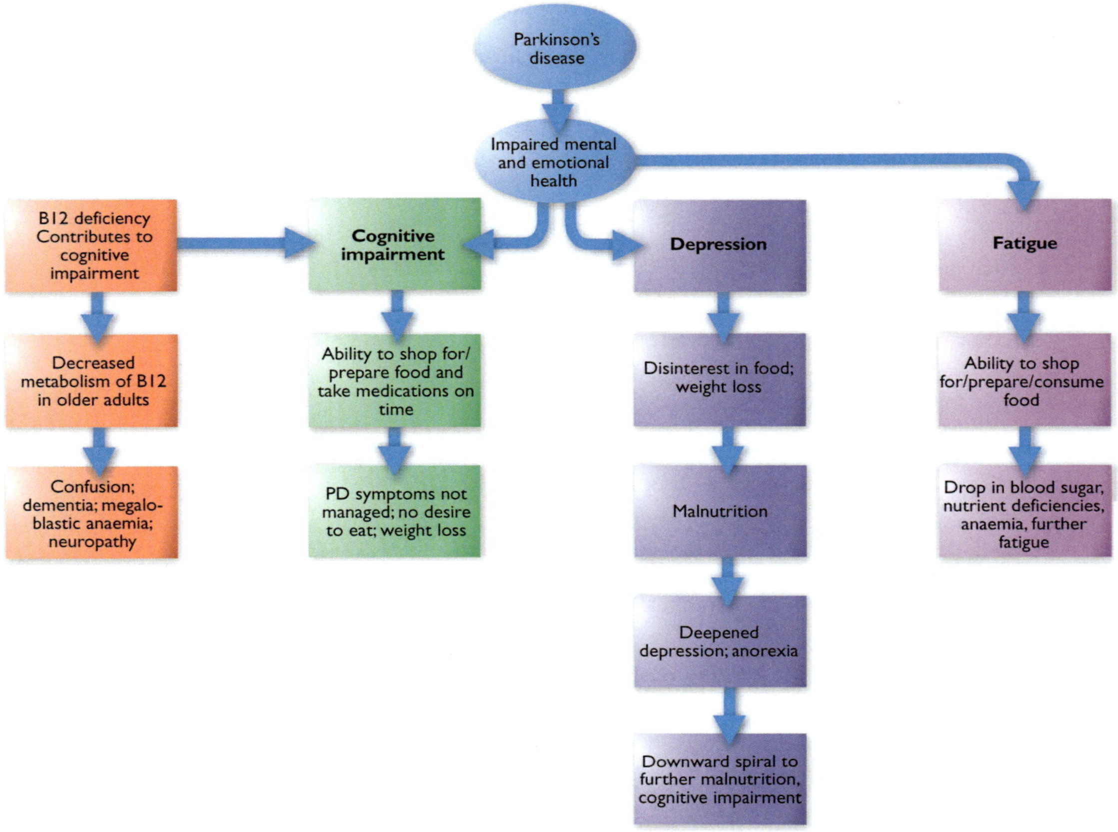

Figure 9.3. ***Mental and emotional health.*** Involvement of mental and emotional health and its impact on nutritional status in PD.

Source: https://www.google.co.in/books/edition/Parkinson_s_Disease/K-EXhIJ6-sYC?hl=en&gbpv=0

Depression

- Affects about 40% of patients.
- May be endogenous or exogenous.
- May range from sadness to major depression.
- May predate diagnosis of PD by several years.
- Depression can impact on nutritional health:
- Significantly affects functional ability.
- May adversely affect the appetite and desire to eat.
- Results in narrowed range of food choices, diminished food intake, unplanned weight loss.
- Ensuing nutritional deficiencies can exacerbate existing depression, anorexia, and unwillingness to eat.
- Creates a downward spiral to malnutrition.
- Anxiety or panic attacks may accompany, or be independent of, depression.

- Management. It will be important to determine both the form and degree of depression, and whether it will be best treated by therapeutic counselling, dietary measures, or medication. Addition of antidepressants, particularly in older adults, and more particularly those already using two or more medications, may produce adverse side-effects.
- Consider referral to a registered dietician for assessment of dietary intake, particularly if unplanned weight change has occurred. If diet is inadequate, fortified foods or a multivitamin/mineral supplement may be helpful. Additionally, provision of omega-3 fatty acids, via fish oil capsules, may be helpful.
- Also consider referral to a qualified therapist who can provide counselling and prescribe an antidepressant if needed.
- If anxiety or panic attacks are reported, determine whether these occur regularly, particularly if before meals, or at the same time of day. If so, hypoglycemia should be ruled out as a causative factor.

Fatigue

- Complaints of exhaustion and sleepiness are common among patients. This may alter the ability to shop for, prepare, and eat food.
- Can be an effect of PD.
- May be a side-effect of medications, with additive effects from multiple medications.
- May be dietary causes:
- Decreased food intake can result in drop in blood glucose, with attendant fatigue.
- Prolonged reduction in caloric intake may result in deficiencies of B vitamins and iron, and fatigue.
- The various anaemias can result in fatigue, shortness of breath, dizziness, confusion.
- *Management*. Rule out dietary causes. Reports of recent weight loss along with fatigue are an indication of nutrition-related etiology.
- Determine if energy intake is adequate (particularly if unplanned weight loss has occurred).
- Rule out deficiencies of folate, B6, B12, iron.
- Rule out hypoglycemia.
- Test for anaemia (iron-deficiency, macrocytic megaloblastic).
- If insomnia is present, discuss avoidance of caffeine and alcohol after late afternoon; regular practice of meditation, or yoga; a light snack before bedtime, such as a cracker with a teaspoonful of peanut butter, or half a banana. A calcium–magnesium supplement at bedtime may help with relaxation: 100–200 mg calcium, 50 mg magnesium.

9.2.3 Other Effects of PD on Nutritional Health

PD affects physical abilities and sensory functions, which can indirectly impact on nutritional health.

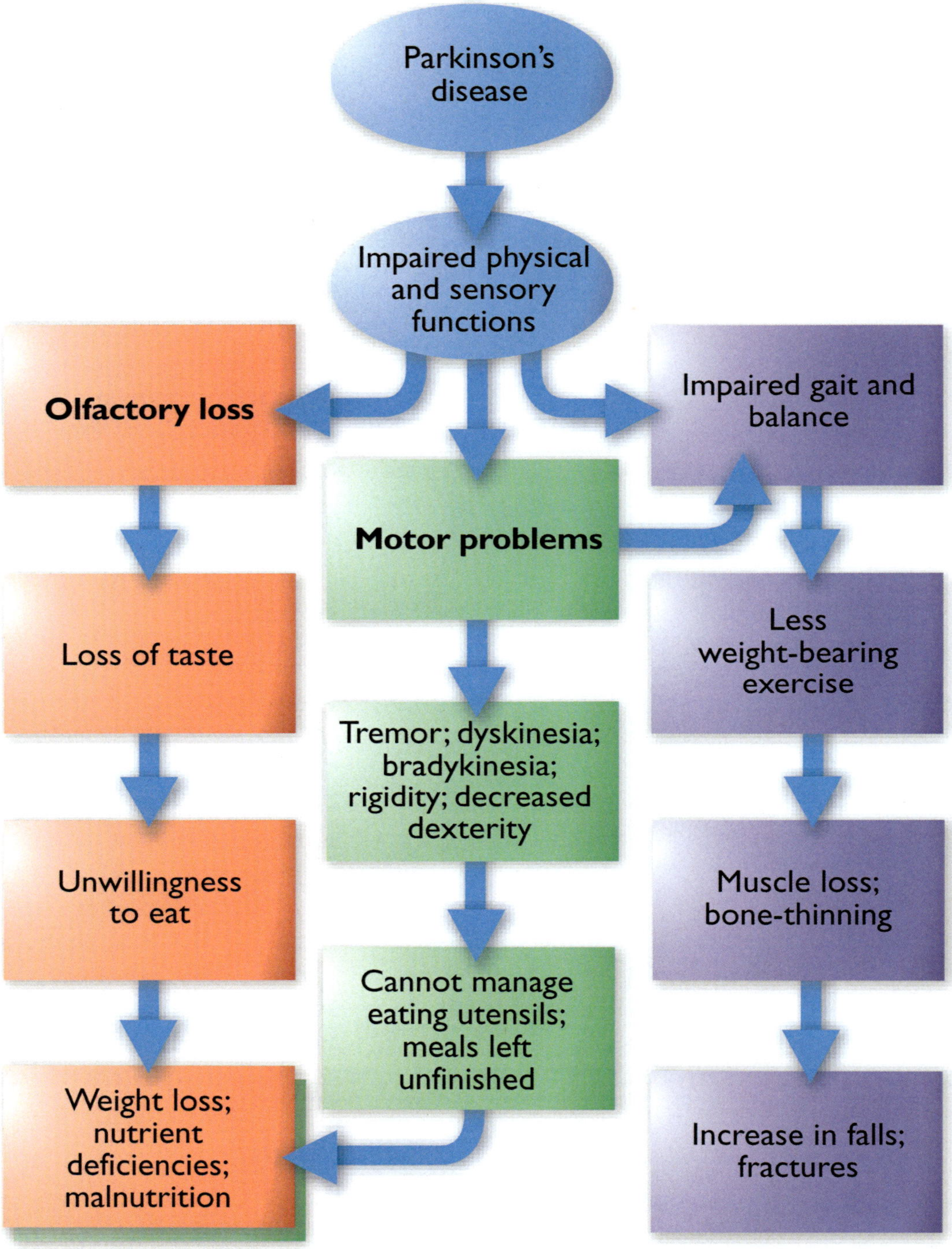

Figure 9.4. Physical and sensory functions. The physical symptoms of PD and their impact on nutritional status.

Source: https://www.google.co.in/books/edition/Parkinson_s_Disease/K-EXhIJ6-sYC?hl=en&gbpv=0

Physical impairment

- Symptoms include tremor, dyskinesia, rigidity, bradykinesia, decreased manual dexterity.
- These affect the ability to manipulate eating utensils.
- The patient may require hours to finish a meal.
- The patient cannot ingest sufficient food to maintain weight or nutrient repletion.
- *Management*. Determine whether patient is taking medications on time; if forgetful, may be undermedicated. Thus, PD symptoms will not be well controlled, and swallowing may be more difficult.
- Consider a referral to an OT, who may provide special eating utensils.
- Consider a referral to a registered dietician, for help choosing foods that can be eaten out of the hand, or that require less chewi

Impaired gait and balance

- Impaired gait and balance lead to a decrease in weight-bearing exercise.
- This results in muscle wasting and bone thinning.
- There is an increased likelihood of falls and increased likelihood of subsequent fractures.
- If diet is lacking in protein and nutrients, the probability of muscle wasting and bone thinning is further increased.
- Management. Encourage as much physical activity as ability permits. Consider referral to a physical therapist for help with appropriate exercises.
- Consider a referral to a registered dietician to determine adequacy of calcium, magnesium, vitamins D and K, for bone health; assessment of protein needs for muscle maintenance.
- If bone density baseline has not been established, order fall risk assessment and fracture risk assessment, including dual energy X-ray absorptiometry (DEXAscan), to determine baseline bone density.
- Advise patient and family regarding use of hip protectors, to help prevent fractures in case of falls.

Loss of olfaction

- This is common among PD patients.
- It is usually accompanied by loss of the sense of taste.
- In combination with other factors such as depression or medication-induced appetite loss, it can produce unwillingness to eat.
- This can seriously affect energy and nutrient intake.
- Management. Consider referral to a registered dietician who can help patient and family select preferred foods. Numerous small meals or nourishing snacks may be better than three large meals daily

9.2.4 Effects of PD Medication

The nutritional concerns related to effects of PD medications.

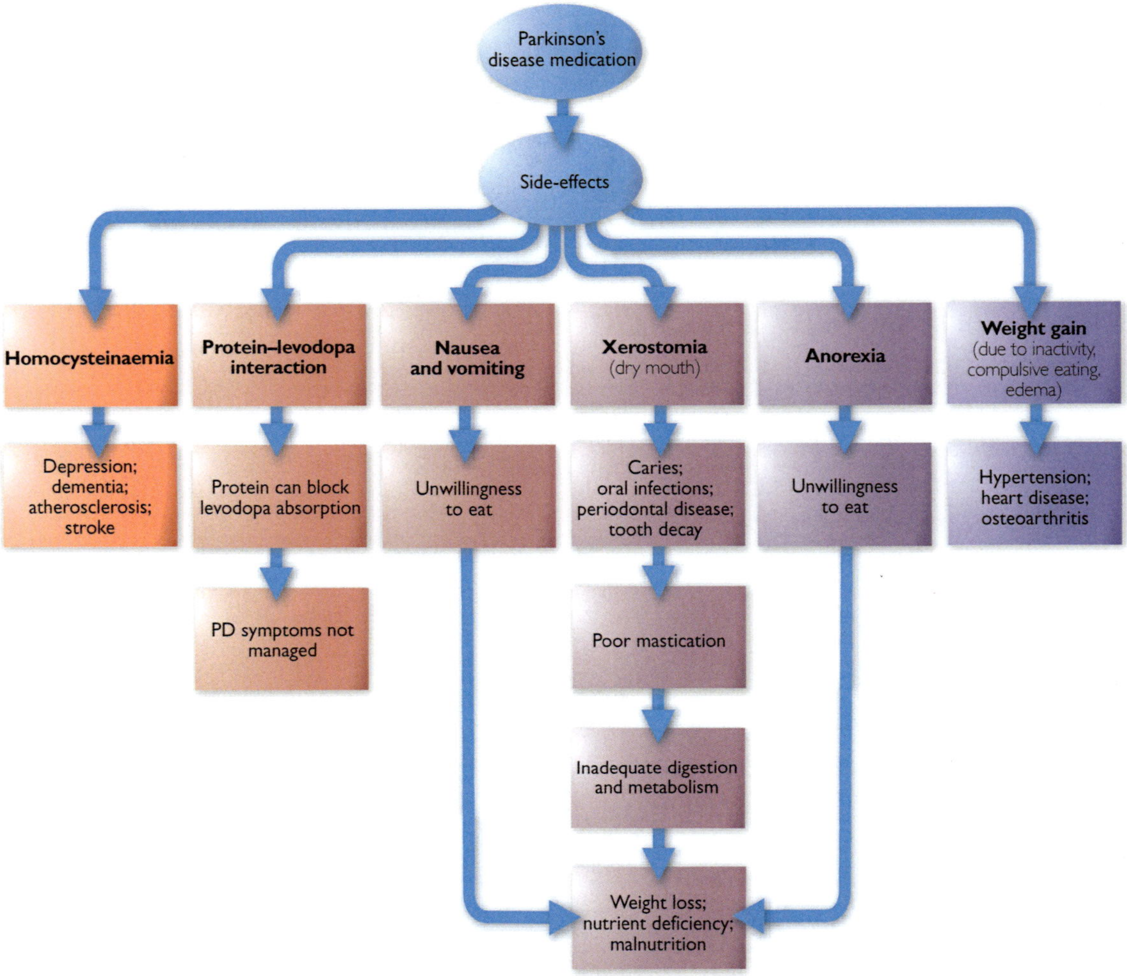

Figure 9.5. Medication side-effects. Various aspects of medication can have an impact on the nutritional status of PD patients.

Source: https://www.google.co.in/books/edition/Parkinson_s_Disease/K-EXhIJ6-sYC?hl=en&gbpv=0

Nausea/vomiting

- May need to take medications with meals until nausea has diminished, usually a few weeks. At that time, levodopa should be taken 30–60 minutes prior to meals.
- Many people find use of ginger tea, or chewing crystallized ginger, helps to manage nausea.
- Some cases may require medication, such as carbidopa (Lodosyn, available in the USA) or domperidone (available in Europe), to combat nausea/vomiting. Avoid use of prochlorperazine or metoclopramide; these may exacerbate PD symptoms and are contraindicated for those with PD.

Protein–levodopa interaction

- Both from the gut, and at the blood–brain barrier, levodopa competes for absorption with the large neutral amino acids, which are breakdown products of ingested proteins.
- Patients using quick-release formulations, such as Sinemet or Madopar (or their generic forms) should take these about 30 minutes prior to meals.
- The CR formulation may be taken with meals; however, more time is required before it takes effect. Thus, if motor fluctuations or gastroparesis are of concern, or if the individual is particularly protein-sensitive, it is best to take the CR form well ahead of meals also.
- If motor fluctuations are not controlled by taking levodopa prior to meals, further adjustment may be necessary.
- Initially, it was recommended that patients who experienced fluctuations abstain from protein during the day, when it was crucial for them to be mobile. Then, at the evening meal, all of the protein from the day was consumed. The allowed range for protein was 0.5–0.8 g/kg of body weight. But this unnatural eating regimen can lead to a lack of appetite, which can lead to unintended weight loss and malnourishment. Furthermore, the patient's PD symptoms won't go away at night, making it difficult for them to go to the bathroom or turn in bed. This causes them to avoid protein at dinner. Protein-energy malnutrition is the outcome.
- Of further concern, it is now known that older adults and people suffering from disorders such as PD have increased protein requirements.
- *Management*. A safe, simple, and effective method of management is for a dietician to assess the patient's calorie and protein needs, allotting 1.0–1.2 g protein/kg body weight.
  - Conditions such as unplanned weight loss, osteopenia/osteoporosis, sarcopenia, pressure ulcers, and fever, may increase protein needs.
  - The day's protein should be divided evenly among the morning, midday, and evening meals. Levodopa can then be taken 30 minutes before each meal, and between meals if necessary, without protein interaction.

Unplanned weight gain

- This can be due to:
  - Inactivity, brought on by decreased physical ability.
  - Edema.
  - PD medications, in particular the agonists, may result in weight gain. In some individuals, this is due to edema (fluid retention), which may dissipate over time. Persistence of marked edema and weight gain may lead to hypertension and other weight-related disorders.
  - Compulsive eating. PD medications, often the agonists, may lead to OCDs, and in some this results in overeating.

- *Management*. Encourage as much physical activity as ability permits.
- Regarding edema, a natural diuretic eating plan referred to as the DASH diet (dietary approach to stop hypertension) was developed to combat both edema and hypertension and studies have suggested benefit. The DASH diet can be adapted by the registered dietician for individual use. Resources are available on the Internet and can be downloaded at no charge
- If weight gain is due to compulsive overeating, the individual may benefit from counselling by a therapist, as well as referral to a dietician. Sometimes DA therapy will need to be discontinued.
- Whether the weight gain is due to edema or overeating, the patient should be carefully monitored. Some individuals respond favorably to a change in medication.

Unplanned weight loss

The etiology of unplanned weight loss can include:

- Medication side-effects, particularly in the older adult: nausea, anorexia, taste changes, depression.
- Dysphagia: difficulty chewing, swallowing.
- Gastroparesis, early satiety.
- Cognitive impairment.
- Decreased manual dexterity.
- *Management*. See previous sections for managing the above causes. Consider referral to a registered dietician for help with appropriate assessment and medical nutrition therapy.

Xerostomia

- Xerostomia (dry mouth) is of concern because it may lead to candidiasis, periodontal disease, caries, and other oral diseases; oral diseases may interfere with mastication.

It may result from:

- Side-effect of medications.
- Mouth breathing.
- Rarely, Sjögren's syndrome.
- *Management*. Xerostomia may be difficult to address. Patients often have difficulty with brushing and flossing. Also, may have limited success with dentures. Tremor, dystonia, and/or dyskinesia may interfere with dental care.
- Inquire about dry mouth and oral health, educate regarding need for fluids, and recommend consultation with a dentist in order to prevent tooth loss and oral disease.

Homocysteinaemia

- Elevated plasma homocysteine may occur with long-term use of levodopa.
- Homocysteinaemia is associated with depression, dementia, atherosclerosis, stroke.
- Serum homocysteine requires the combined action of vitamins B6, B12, and folate for clearance from the bloodstream. Elevation can occur with deficiency of one or more of these.

- Most PD patients are older adults; many elderly people produce less intrinsic factor, needed for absorption of B12 in the ileum, which may result in pernicious anaemia.
- Many elderly suffer from atrophic gastritis: the stomach secretes less of the acid needed to cleave B12 from food proteins, resulting in megaloblastic anaemia.
- Changed eating habits may, over time, result in B-vitamin deficiencies, the signs of which closely resemble, and may exacerbate, symptoms of PD: paresthesia, impaired gait, personality or behaviour changes, sore or burning mouth or tongue, burning feet, dementia, and depression.
- An excess of folate may mask B12, thus B12 status must be measured independently, testing for methylmalonic acid
- Because of the prevalence of cognitive impairment and dementia in PD, serum homocysteine should be assessed, along with B6, B12, and folate status, and tests for megaloblastic and pernicious anaemias.
- In order to assess whether the diet is sufficient, a registered dietician should periodically ask for a three-day food and medication diary. If not, the doctor should be notified and laboratory testing should be ordered. To return levels to normal, an intramuscular injection or B-complex supplement may be required.

9.3 Prevalence and Risk Factors for Malnutrition in Patients with Parkinson's disease

One chronic degenerative neurodegenerative disease is Parkinson's disease (PD). In China, the prevalence of Parkinson's disease (PD) is less than 2% among those over 65, making up over 40% of all PD patients worldwide. Every year, the prevalence rises. PD places elderly people's physical and mental health in grave danger and has significant negative social and economic effects. According to certain research, certain lifestyle interventions, like behavior therapy, better sleep, happier moods, and physical activity, may enhance the quality of life for people with Parkinson's disease. Nevertheless, the impact of nutritional status on the quality of life of Parkinson's disease patients has not been extensively studied. According to a study, total fat mass and the degree of motor impairment in PD patients are negatively correlated. Another study revealed that PD patients' malnutrition can lead to gustatory and olfactory dysfunction. Nutritional risk assessment is becoming more and more crucial in Parkinson's disease. Therefore, in order to more accurately forecast the prognosis and course of PD, we assessed the cross-sectional association between nutritional status and PD.

9.3.1 Prevalence of Malnutrition in Parkinson's Disease

Patients with Parkinson's disease (PD) may be more vulnerable to malnourishment due to the disease's symptoms and the adverse effects of the medications used to treat it. A reduction in nutritional status is linked to a number of unfavorable health and life quality outcomes. The degree to which malnutrition currently affects this population is unknown, though. This review set out to methodically evaluate the findings and methodology of studies that reported on the prevalence of malnutrition in patients with Parkinson's disease. Included were studies that used body mass index, weight change, anthropometric measurements, nutritional screening and assessment scores, and other methods to try and categorize participants with Parkinson's disease (PD) into nutritional risk and/or malnutrition categories. Between 0 and 24 percent of Parkinson's disease (PD) patients had malnutrition, and between 3 and 60 percent of PD patients were considered to be at risk for it.

After Alzheimer's disease, Parkinson's disease (PD) is the second most common neurodegenerative disorder. It typically affects adults over 50, with a sharp rise in incidence after age 60. It has been estimated that the disease affects 1 percent of people over 65 worldwide, with a crude age-adjusted global incidence of 9–13 cases per 100,000 people annually.

People with Parkinson's disease (PD) have been found to be more susceptible to malnutrition than people of the same age because of the nature of the disease. A malnutrition-related imbalance in energy, protein, and other nutrients can lead to abnormal body composition, size, or shape, as well as abnormal clinical results and function.

For the purposes of this review, malnutrition is defined as a deficit in protein and energy rather than an excess, or protein-energy malnutrition. A lower quality of life and worse health outcomes, such as increased mortality, weakened immunity, delayed wound healing, more frequent and prolonged hospital stays, a higher risk of osteoporosis, and a higher chance of falling, are linked to malnutrition. Although it is widely acknowledged that people with Parkinson's disease (PD) have poorer nutritional status, it is unclear how much of this population is undernourished or at risk of malnutrition.

9.3.2 Increased risk of Malnutrition in Parkinson's disease

Individuals with Parkinson's disease (PD) have been found to have significantly lower body weight and body mass indices (BMIs) as well as higher rates of unintentional weight loss when compared to age-matched controls. The length, stage, and severity of a disease all cause a significant decrease in body weight/BMI. Due to inadvertent weight loss and a sedentary lifestyle that can begin as early as two to four years before diagnosis, people with Parkinson's disease (PD) are also more likely to experience an accelerated course of age-related sarcopenia, which is defined as a loss of muscle mass, composition, and quality.

Effect of symptoms on nutritional status

Individuals with Parkinson's disease (PD) have been found to have significantly lower body weight and body mass indices (BMIs) as well as higher rates of unintentional weight loss when compared to age-matched controls. The length, stage, and severity of a disease all cause a significant decrease in body weight/BMI. Due to inadvertent weight loss and a sedentary lifestyle that can begin as early as two to four years before diagnosis, people with Parkinson's disease (PD) are also more likely to experience an accelerated course of age-related sarcopenia, which is defined as a loss of muscle mass, composition, and quality.

In PD, neuropsychiatric symptoms like apathy, confusion, depression, anxiety, and dementia are more common than in age-matched populations. It has been discovered that these neuropsychiatric symptoms are linked to older adults' reduced food intake and consequent weight loss. Constipation, dysphagia, olfactory decline, early satiety, decreased gastric transit time, nausea, sweating, sleep disturbances, and sialorrhea are some other prevalent non-motor symptoms of Parkinson's disease (PD). Additionally, compared to age-matched controls, PD patients experience the majority of these symptoms more frequently.

Effect of Pharmaceutical Therapy on Nutritional Status

Apart from the inborn symptoms of Parkinson's disease (PD), pharmacological treatment for symptoms also affects nutritional status. Levodopa is typically used in dopamine replacement therapy, which is a common treatment used to relieve Parkinson's disease symptoms. Nausea, vomiting, and weight loss are side effects. Lower BMIs have been linked to higher levodopa intakes. Furthermore, levodopa use may cause motor fluctuations, or "off" periods, when weariness, apathy, and anxiety may intensify. Involuntary movements, or dyskienesias, are another side effect of dopamine replacement therapy that can raise energy needs and expenditure.

Appropriate screening and assessment of malnutrition in this population is particularly crucial for early interventions and improved outcomes, given the elevated presence of malnutrition risk factors in Parkinson's disease (PD). Giving precise estimates of the rate of malnutrition in this population will help allocate resources in the right order. As a result, the purpose of this review is to methodically evaluate the design and findings of research on the prevalence of malnutrition in Parkinson's disease (PD).

9.3.3 Parkinson's disease: the Nutrition Perspective

Estimated to affect 1% of adults over 60, Parkinson's disease (PD) is the second most common neurodegenerative condition. In his 1817 work "An Essay on the Shaking Palsy," James Parkinson detailed the condition's non-motor as well as motor aspects. Akinesia, stiffness, tremor, and postural instability are the symptoms of Parkinsonism; the latter is more likely to manifest as the disease worsens. Neuropsychiatric, sleep, and autonomic dysfunction symptoms are examples of non-motor symptoms that frequently precede the onset of motor signs. When it comes to managing the disease, nutrition is a factor that is frequently disregarded but holds significant importance. The aetiology of dysfunction is always complex, with various features emerging over the course of the illness and varying in their impact on quality of life (Fig. 9.6).

The most common cause of Parkinsonism is idiopathic Parkinson's disease (PD), which is diagnosed clinically when at least two of the four clinical signs listed by the UK Queens sq\. Brain Bank criteria are present. Imaging is helpful, especially when characteristics like dysautonomia, rapid progression, lack of tremor, early falls, or non-reaction to levodopa suggest a different diagnosis. The primary goal of therapy is to make up for the dopamine that is lost initially due to presynaptic degeneration of dopaminergic cells in the substantia nigra and striatum. Especially in the early stages of the disease, dopaminergic medications provide a satisfying response. Because of the disease's heterogeneity, selecting a treatment plan requires careful consideration of individual circumstances.

Stages 1 through 5 involve unilateral involvement and little to no functional impairment; at stage 5, the person is confined to a wheelchair or bed. These stages might not correspond with pathophysiological stages, but the goal of this scale is to be useful in real-world situations and consistent across scores from various clinicians. The most popular clinical rating scale for Parkinson's disease (PD) is the Movement Disorder Society-Unified Parkinson's Disease Rating Scale, which assesses motor signs, the effect of motor and non-motor symptoms on daily living, and motor complications. In order to characterize the clinical course of Parkinson's disease (PD), Macmahon and Thomas proposed a scale that starts with the "diagnostic" phase and progresses through a relatively stable "maintenance" phase, "complex" phase, which is marked by motor fluctuations, the onset of cognitive impairment, and the appearance of axial symptoms, such as falls, dysphagia, and freezing of gait, before ending in a palliative phase. It is now understood that a number of symptoms, known as premotor symptoms, such as depression, anosmia, constipation, and rapid-eye movement sleep behavior disorder, may manifest years before motor symptoms do, during a period known as the "prodromal" phase.

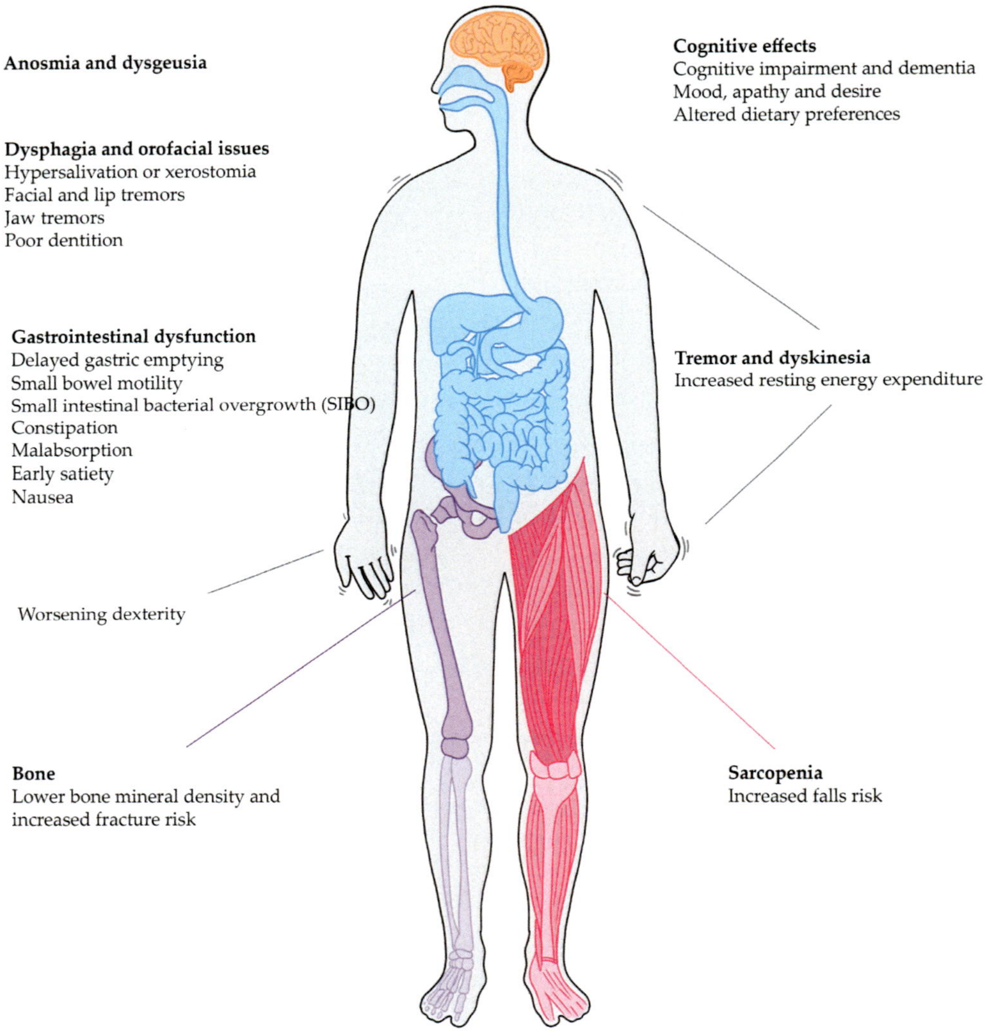

Figure 9.6. Nutrition-related issues faced by patients with Parkinson›s disease.

Source: https://static.cambridge.org/binary/version/id/urn:cambridge.org:id:binary:20220627180529995-0783:S0029665121003645:S0029665121003645_fig1.png?pub-status=live

Pathophysiology and Aetiology of Parkinson's Disease

The pathological hallmark of Parkinson's disease (PD) is the loss of dopaminergic neurons in the substantia nigra, which is believed to be caused by aggregated forms of the protein α-synuclein, or Lewy bodies, building up within the neurons. A sequential progression of neuronal damage throughout the nervous system, categorised into six neuropathological stages, was described by Braak and colleagues by studying post-mortem brains from individuals with and without prior symptoms of parkinsonism. Stage 1 consisted of lesions in the dorsal motor nucleus of the glossopharyngeal and vagal nerves, which later progressed to reach the brainstem, and finally involved the cerebral cortex in stage 6. Crucially, it was observed that the development of PD's hallmark lesions preceded the clinical manifestation of both motor and non-motor dysfunction. The myenteric and submucosal plexuses, which are collections of neurons that make up the enteric nervous system that regulates the function of the gastrointestinal (GI) tract, were found to contain Lewy bodies by Braak and colleagues in a later neuropathological study. This has given rise to the "dual-hit hypothesis," which postulates that a neurotropic pathogen that causes Parkinson's disease may enter the central nervous system through both the nose and the stomach. A small percentage of PD patients have the Mendelian form of the illness, in which the illness is brought on by the inheritance of a single causative gene (e.g. PARK2, SNCA, LRRK2, and PINK1) in a pattern that is either autosomal dominant or recessive.

These familial parkinsonian cases are uncommon, though, and most cases of Parkinson's disease (PD) are thought to be the result of a confluence of environmental and genetic factors. Searching for variations throughout the genome, genome-wide association studies try to find out if any found SNPs have a different frequency in PD cases compared to controls. Numerous loci have been suggested as potential causes of Parkinson's disease (PD); these low penetrance variants, each with a negligible effect on risk, may add up to increase an individual's risk. Comparably, a large number of observational studies have looked at the influence of environmental factors on the risk of Parkinson's disease (PD). These factors include dietary factors like caffeine and alcohol intake; exposure to environmental toxins like pesticides; biomarkers like BMI; drugs; co-occurring illnesses; and lifestyle factors like smoking. However, because of the possibility of reverse causation and residual confounding, apparent associations might not actually reflect a causal relationship. Additionally, there might be interactions between environmental and genetic risk factors, modifying the effect of any environmental factor by the genetic risk that exists in the background.

A Closer Look

Malnutrition

Parkinson's disease (PD) patients are at high risk for malnutrition because of a number of factors that impact dietary intake and metabolism. The illness itself may cause symptoms like dysphagia, poor chewing, and decreased appetite, all of which increase the risk of consuming insufficient amounts of nutrients. Furthermore, nausea is one of the side effects of some PD medications, which further reduces appetite. In addition, if proper nutritional intake is not maintained, the motor symptoms of Parkinson's disease (PD), such as tremors and rigidity, can increase energy expenditure and cause inadvertent weight loss. Malnutrition risk may increase as a result of difficulties people may have preparing meals, grocery shopping, and eating on their own as the illness worsens.

Healthcare professionals, dietitians, and caregivers must work together in a multidisciplinary manner to effectively manage malnutrition in people with Parkinson's disease. Nutritional supplements, altered diets to address swallowing issues, and help with meal planning are some strategies to ensure enough calorie and nutrient intake despite Parkinson's disease's challenges.

Summary

- Parkinson's disease (PD) frequently affects motor abilities, such as swallowing and chewing, which makes eating difficult and causes people to eat less. Furthermore, the illness may cause changes in metabolism and an increase in energy expenditure, which could make patients' nutritional status even more problematic.
- The complex problem of malnutrition among people with Parkinson's disease (PD) is impacted by both socioeconomic factors and disease-related factors. Numerous motor and non-motor symptoms of Parkinson's disease (PD) can have an immediate effect on one's nutritional status.
- Undernutrition in macronutrients causes your body to run out of energy. It starts disintegrating its own tissues and stopping its operations as a way to make up for it.
- Parkinson's disease (PD), a progressive neurodegenerative disease with both motor and non-motor symptoms, is largely controlled by nutritional health.
- Patients with Parkinson's disease (PD) may be more vulnerable to malnourishment due to the disease's symptoms and the adverse effects of the medications used to treat it.
- Apart from the inborn symptoms of Parkinson's disease (PD), pharmacological treatment for symptoms also affects nutritional status. Levodopa is typically used in dopamine replacement therapy, which is a common treatment used to relieve Parkinson's disease symptoms.

References

1. Adams, M. S., Khan, N. Z., Begum, S. A., Wirz, S. L., Hesketh, T., & Pring, T. R. (2012). Feeding difficulties in children with cerebral palsy: Low-cost caregiver training in Dhaka, Bangladesh. *Child: Care, Health and Development, 38*(6), 878–888. https://doi.org/10.1111/j.1365-2214.2011.01309.x.
2. Ali, M. S., Kassahun, C. W., & Wubneh, C. A. (2020). Overnutrition and associated factors: A comparative cross-sectional study between government and private primary school students in Gondar Town, Northwest Ethiopia. *Journal of Nutrition and Metabolism, 12*, 1–12. https://doi.org/10.1155/2020/3152481.
3. Avery, A. (2021). Food insecurity and malnutrition. *Kompass Nutrition and Dietetics, 1*(2), 41–43.
4. Brazier, Y. (2020). Malnutrition: What you need to know UK. Brighton, UK: Healthline Media UK Ltd.
5. Burgess, A. (2008). Undernutrition in adults and children: Causes, consequences and what we can do? *Southern Sudan Medical Journal.*
6. Farhadi, S., & Ovchinnikov, R. S. (2018). The relationship between nutrition and infectious diseases: A review. *Biomedical and Biotechnology Research Journal (BBRJ), 2*(3), 168–172. Retrieved from: https://bbrj.org.
7. Gottlieb, C. A., Maenner, M. J., Cappa, C., & Durkin, M. S. (2009). Child disability screening, nutrition, and early learning in 18 countries with low and middle incomes: Data from the

third round of UNICEF's Multiple Indicator Cluster Survey (2005–06). *The Lancet, 374*(9704), 1831–1839. https://doi.org/10.1016/S0140-6736(09)61873-4.

8. Groce, N., Challenger, E., Berman-Bieler, R., Farkas, A., Yilmaz, N., Schultink, W., & Kerac, M. (2014). Malnutrition and disability: Unexplored opportunities for collaboration. *Pediatrics and International Child Health, 34*(4), 308–314. https://doi.org/10.1179/2046905514Y.0000000160.
9. Jonsson, U. (1993). *Nutrition and the United Nations Convention on the Rights of the Child*. Italy: UNICEF.
10. Kerac, M., Bunn, J., Chagaluka, G., Bahwere, P., Tomkins, A., et al. (2014). Follow-up of post-discharge growth and mortality after treatment for severe acute malnutrition (FuSAM Study): A prospective cohort study. *PLoS One, 9*(4), e96030. https://doi.org/10.1371/journal.pone.0096030.
11. Kerac, M., Postels, D. G., Mallewa, M., Alusine Jalloh, A., Voskuijl, W. P., Groce, N., & Heikens, G. T. (2014). The interaction of malnutrition and neurologic disability in Africa. *Seminars in Pediatric Neurology, 21*(1), 42–49. https://doi.org/10.1016/j.spen.2014.01.003.
12. Mandal, A. (2019). Causes of Malnutrition. Retrieved from: https://www.news-medical.net/health/Causes-of-malnutrition.aspx (accessed on 12 July 2024).
13. Mathur, P., & Pillai, R. (2019). Overnutrition: Current scenario & combat strategies. *The Indian Journal of Medical Research, 149*(695), 11. https://doi.org/10.4103/ijmr.IJMR_2388_18.
14. Murray, C. J., Vos, T., Lozano, R., Naghavi, M., Flaxman, A. D., Michaud, C., & Lopez, A. D. (2012). Disability-adjusted life years (DALYs) for 291 diseases and injuries in 21 regions, 1990–2010: A systematic analysis for the global burden of disease study 2010. *The Lancet, 380*(9859), 2197–2230. https://doi.org/10.1016/S0140-6736(12)61689-4.
15. Olusanya, B. O. (2010). Is undernutrition a risk factor for sensorineural hearing loss in early infancy? *British Journal of Nutrition, 103*(9), 1296–1301. https://doi.org/10.1017/S0007114510000193.
16. Pridmore, P., & Hill, R. C. (2009). Addressing the underlying and basic causes of child undernutrition in developing countries: What works and why? In *Minister of Foreign Affairs of Denmark* (Ed.), Denmark: Ministry of Foreign Affairs of Denmark.
17. Sablah, M. (2019). Causes and impacts of undernutrition over the life course. In *Nutrition*. New York: UNICEF.
18. Sandesh, A. (2017). Malnutrition, its causes and types of malnutrition. World Press Theme. Retrieved from: https://www.publichealthnotes.com/author/sandesh/ (accessed on 12 July 2024).
19. Saunders, J., & Smith, T. (2010). Malnutrition: Causes and consequences. *Clinical Medicine, 10*(6), 4.
20. The Use of Epidemiological Tools in Conflict-Affected Populations: Open-Access Educational Resources for Policy-Makers. (2009). London: London school of hygiene and tropical medicine. Retrieved from: http://conflict.lshtm.ac.uk/page_138.htm (accessed on 12 July 2024).
21. Tuzun, E. H., Guven, D. K., Eker, L., Elbasan, B., & Bulbul, S. F. (2013). Nutritional status of children with cerebral palsy in Turkey. *Disability and Rehabilitation, 35*(5), 413–417. https://doi.org/10.3109/09638288.2012.691141.

22. U.S. Department of Health & Human Services, National Institutes of Health, Office of Dietary Supplements. (2021). Iron. Retrieved from: https://ods.od.nih.gov/factsheets/Iron-HealthProfessional/ (accessed on 12 July 2024).

23. U.S. Department of Health & Human Services, National Institutes of Health, Office of Dietary Supplements. (2021). Vitamin B6. Retrieved from: https://ods.od.nih.gov/factsheets/VitaminB6-HealthProfessional/ (accessed on 12 July 2024).

24. Walker, S. P., Wachs, T. D., Gardner, J. M., Lozoff, B., Wasserman, G. A., Pollitt, E., et al. (2007). Child development: Risk factors for adverse outcomes in developing countries. *The Lancet, 369*(9556), 145–147. https://doi.org/10.1016/S0140-6736(07)60076-2.

25. Yalçın, N., Armut, M., Çakır, B. K., & Demirkan, K. (2019). Drug-induced nutritional disorders. *Clinical Science of Nutrition, 1*(3), 10.

26. Young, H. (2020). Nutrition in Africa's drylands: A conceptual framework for addressing acute malnutrition. Boston: Feinstein International Center, Tufts University.

27. Younis, K., Ahmad, S., & Badpa, A. (2015). Malnutrition: Causes and strategies. *Journal of Food Processing & Technology, 6*(4), 8. https://doi.org/10.4172/2157-7110.1000437.

Chapter 10

COMPLEMENTARY MEDICINE AND PD

Contents

Introduction

PD is a complex neurodegenerative disorder characterized by a range of motor and non-motor symptoms that significantly impact quality of life. While conventional treatments such as medication and surgery are essential for managing symptoms and slowing disease progression, they may not address all aspects of the condition or may cause side effects.

As a result, many individuals with PD turn to complementary medicine, which encompasses a diverse range of therapies and practices that complement conventional treatments by addressing physical, emotional, and spiritual well-being. Complementary medicine offers additional avenues for symptom management, rehabilitation, and support, often focusing on holistic approaches that consider the interconnectedness of body, mind, and spirit. In the context of PD, complementary medicine encompasses various modalities, including acupuncture, massage therapy, yoga, dietary supplements, and mind-body practices, each offering unique benefits and potential synergies with conventional treatments. This introduction provides an overview of complementary medicine in PD, highlighting its role in enhancing overall health and well-being for individuals living with this challenging condition (Zhou and Benharash, 2014).

Orientation and Directional Terms:

Term	Definition	Illustration
Massage therapy	Massage therapy is used to help manage a health condition or enhance wellness. It involves manipulating the soft tissues of the body.	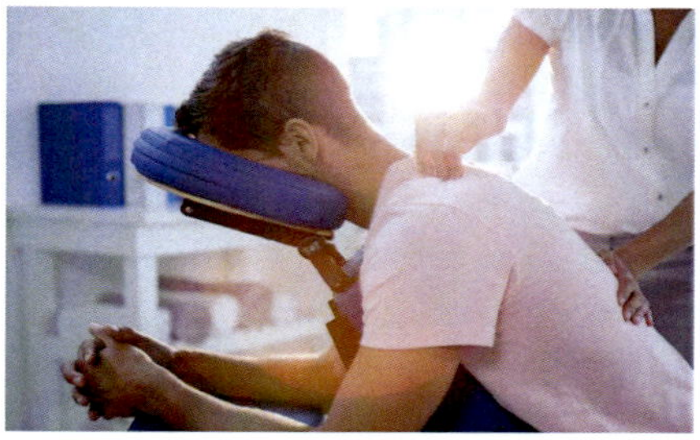
Yoga	Yoga brings the body and mind together and is built on three main elements – movement, breathing and meditation. Yoga has many physical and mental health benefits including improved posture, flexibility, strength, balance and body awareness.	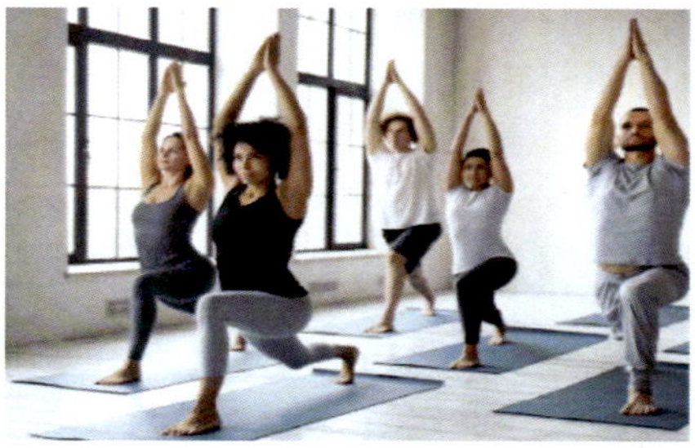
Meditation	Meditation is a practice that involves focusing or clearing your mind using a combination of mental and physical techniques.	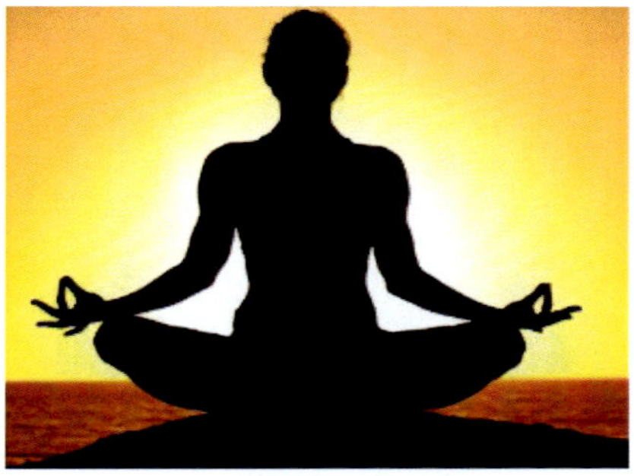
Tai chi	It is an internal Chinese martial art practiced for self-defense and health. Known for its slow, intentional movements, tai chi has practitioners worldwide and is particularly popular as a form of gentle exercise and moving meditation, with benefits to mental and physical health	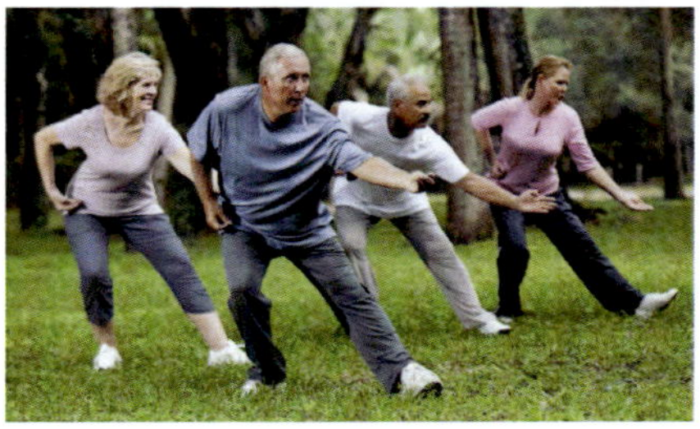
Dietary Supplements	Dietary supplements are intended to add to or supplement the diet and are different from conventional food. Generally, to the extent a product is intended to treat, diagnose, cure, or prevent diseases, it is a drug, even if it is labeled as a dietary supplement.	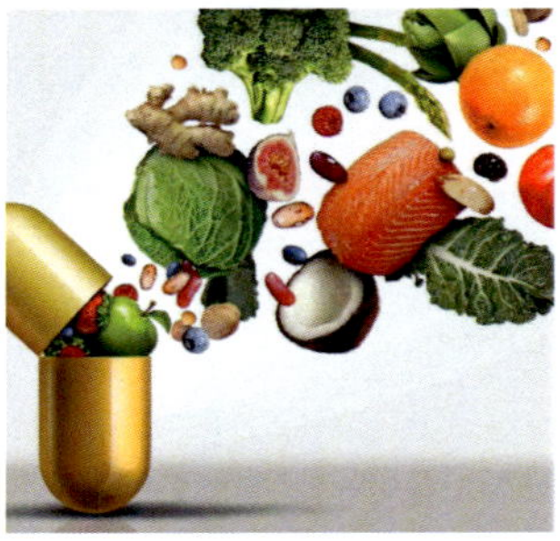

10.1. Acupuncture

Acupuncture is a traditional Chinese medicine that involves inserting tiny needles into the skin at specific locations known as acupoints to regulate the body's qi (energy flow). It is predicated on the idea that numerous meridians, each representing a distinct organ system, are interconnected by these points and run the length of the body. Certain diseases that result from disruption along the meridians can therefore be treated or cured by stimulating acupoints with heat, pressure, or needles. Despite being a popular treatment method in Eastern medicine for millennia, acupuncture is still debatable because of conflicting evidence regarding its effectiveness. However, it is now widely used in Western medicine as a complementary therapy for a wide range of illnesses, including numerous neurologic disorders. Early open-label trials of acupuncture for PD patients showed that the treatment was safe and might be effective for both motor and non-motor symptoms (Leiet al, 2023).This led to the need for more research using randomized, controlled trials (Table 10.1).

Table 10.1. *Reported Clinical Trials of Acupuncture for Patients with Parkinson's Disease*

Collected data (Legends: NA = not applicable; EA = electroacupuncture; PD = Parkinson's disease; fMRI = functional magnetic resonance imaging).

Study Details	Participants	Study Design	Control Group	Interventions (GE)	Outcomes Measures	Results/ Conclusions	Side Effect
A Clinical Study of Integrating acupuncture and western medicine in treating patients with Parkinson's disease *The American Journal of Chinese Medicine*	**Inclusion Criteria:** Diagnosed with PD for over 6 months (criteria of the core assessment program for intracerebral transplantation (CAPIT). **Exclusion Criteria:** Severe diseases of the heart, brain, liver, kidneys, endocrine, or hematopoietic system, psychosis, or dementia and who did not agree to participate in the study. **Dropout:** NA **Randomization:** Non-random sample	Effects of acupuncture treatment in PD patients N = 40	Drug Therapy Levodopa N = 20	Acupuncture Treatment + Drug Therapy **19 points:** DU20 (unilateral), GB20, LI11, LI10, LI4, GB31, ST32, GB34, GB38 (bilateral) Frequency: 2×/week - short-term (18 weeks—36 sessions) n = 20 - long-term (36 weeks—72 sessions) n = 13 Depth of insertion: 5–30 mm Needle stimulation: manual ("De-Qi": soreness, numbness, distention and pain) Time: 15 min Needle type: 0.27 mm × 25/40 mm	**3 Assessment Moments:** before, in the middle and at the end of the study. - Unified Parkinson's Disease Rating Scale (UPDRS) - Beck Anxiety Inventory (BAI) - Beck Depression Inventory-Version 2 (BDI-II) - WHO quality of life (WHOQOL)	Acupuncture treatment: -reduces symptoms and signs of mind, behavior, mood, depression - complications of therapy - reduce UPDRS scores - improve the quality of life	NO

Study Details	Participants	Study Design	Control Group	Interventions (GE)	Outcomes Measures	Results/ Conclusions	Side Effect
A pilot clinical trial to objectively assess the efficacy of electroacupuncture on Gait in Patients with Parkinson's Disease Using Body Worn Sensors *PLoS ONE*	**Inclusion Criteria:** (1) Community-dwelling aged 55 years or older with a diagnosis of PD; (2) patients who can walk 20 m without walking assistance; and (3) patients who are stable without anti-PD medication(s) change for at least 1 month. **Exclusion Criteria:** Patients who (1) have received previous acupuncture; (2) DBS; (3) with any clinically significant medical condition, psychiatric condition, drug or alcohol abuse, or laboratory abnormality that would, in the judgment of the investigators, interfere with the ability to participate in the study; and (4) with non-PD related gait disorders **Dropout:** zero dropout rate **Randomization:** drawing pieces of paper from a bag	Efficacy of EA for gait disorders using body-worn sensor technology in patients with PD N = 15	Sham Acupuncture Insertion less than 4 mm, under the skin at non-acupuncture points, without needle manipulation N = 5	EA Treatment **11 points:** in Foot Motor Sensory Area, Balance Area, GV20, GV14, LI4, ST36, GB34, BL40, SP6, KI3, LR3 Frequency: 3×/week Depth of insertion: 0.25 × 40–50 mm—Transversely in GV20, Balance Area, Foot Motor Sensory Area and Perpendicularly in the rest Needle stimulation: from 4 to 100 Hz. The pulse was an asymmetric biphasic square wave with a pulse width of 100 microseconds (μS). "De-qi" was achieved with needle manipulation. Three pocket portable electric stimulators (ITO ES-130, Japan) were used for EA stimulation. Time: 30-min sessions Needle type: Sterile disposable, surgical stainless steel acupuncture needles (Seirin, L type, Japan) N = 10	**2 Assessment Moments:** At baseline and after completion of treatments. - Unified Parkinson's Disease Rating Scale (UPDRS) - SF-12 health survey - Short Falls Efficacy Scale-International (FES-I) - Visual analogue scale (VAS) - Steady-state gait speed (stride length, cadence, double support, and midswing angular velocity)	All gait parameters were improved in the experimental group in response to EA treatment.	YES
Acupuncture as Adjuvant Therapy for Sleep Disorders in Parkinson's Disease *Journal of Acupuncture and Meridian Studies*	**Inclusion criteria:** (1) patients with idiopathic PD according to the UK Parkinson's Disease Society Brain Bank criteria (2) Stage I e III PD, according to the Hoehn e Yahr scale (3) age 35 e 80 years; (4) minimum score of 18 on the Mini-Mental State Examination for a low academic level or a minimum score of 26 for high academic level and (5) a stable dose of anti-Parkinsonian medication for 2 months. **Exclusion criteria:** another neurological condition or who had received physiotherapy **Dropout:** NA **Randomization:** The patients were enumerated and allocated to experimental or control groups according to a simple raffle.	Effects of acupuncture on sleep disturbances N = 11	No Intervention **N = 11**	Acupuncture Treatment **8 points:** LR3, SP6, LI4, TE5, HT7, PC6, LI11, GB20. Frequency: 1×/week for 8 weeks Time: 30 min N = 11	**2 Assessment Moments:** Prior to the start of the study and after. - MMSE - HY scale - PDSS (Parkinson's Disease Sleep Scale)	A therapeutic benefit of acupuncture in sleep disorders in patients with PD.	NO

Study Details	Participants	Study Design	Control Group	Interventions (GE)	Outcomes Measures	Results/ Conclusions	Side Effect
Madopar combined with acupuncture improves motor and non-motor symptoms in Parkinson's disease patients: A multicentre randomized controlled trial. *European Journal of Integrative Medicine*	**Inclusion:** (1) met the diagnostic criteria; (2) aged between 40–75 years; (3) patients with the revised Hoehn–Yahr stage 1–4; (4) Madopar dosage could be maintained for ≥3 months with a stable medical condition or first-consult patients who had not been treated for Parkinson's disease in the past; (5) inpatients or outpatients who were able to follow up; (6) conscious with normal communication; and (7) signed informed consent form. **Exclusion:** Patients with (1) Hoehn–Yahr stage 4–5; (2) Parkinson's syndrome (3) merged with other serious diseases, such as diseases of the heart, liver, kidney, endocrine and hematopoietic system; (4) mental illness or dementia; (6) allergic patients; or (7) non-first-consult patients.	Effect of integrated therapy on improving motor and nonmotor symptoms in PD patients. N = 76	Drug Therapy Madopar only	Acupuncture Treatment + Drug Therapy (Madopar) Jin's three-needle therapy: GV17, GB19^A^, Sishenzhen and temporal three-needle midpoint of the posterior hairline, the depression above the *protuberantia occipitalis externa*. Frequency: 4 days per week; 12 weeks—2×/week (four-week follow-up) Time: 30 min per day	**3 Assessment Moments:** In Week 0. within (Week 4), and after (Week 8) - Unified Parkinson's Disease Rating Scale (UPDRS) - Modified Webster Scale - Parkinson's Disease Sleep Scale (PDSS) - Self-rating Depression Scale (SDS)	Integrated therapy showed a greater advantage, with earlier non-motor symptom improvement. Acupuncture had a certain long-term effect.	NO
Acupuncture for motor symptom improvement in Parkinson's disease and the potential identification of responders to acupuncture treatment *Integrative Medicine Research*	**Inclusion:** a stable dosage of anti-PD medication for at least two months without adverse effects and diagnosed by a neurologist according to the UK Parkinson's Disease Society Brain Bank criteria **Exclusion:** Parkinson-plus syndrome or secondary Parkinson's syndrome	Effectiveness of EA and explore its mechanisms in PD patients when used as adjunctive therapy to conventional drugs. N = 50	Drug Therapy	EA + drug **4 points:** GB20 + LI4 and central GV16 + GV14 Frequency: 8 weeks—20 session sessions that occur every 3 days Needle stimulation: 9 V, 1 A, 9 W, and 100 Hz Time: 30 min	**Assessment Moments:** 12 h after the latest intake of medication. - Unified Parkinson's Disease Rating Scale (UPDRS) III and IV - Hoehn–Yahr (H-Y) stage -Nonmotor Symptoms Quest (NMSQ) -Parkinson's Disease Quality of Life Questionnaire (PDQ) 39 items - Hamilton Depression Scale (HAMD) - Pittsburgh Sleep Quality Index (PSQI) - Hamilton Anxiety Scale (HAMA) - Neuroinflammatory factors: nitric oxide, tumour necrosis factor, interleukin-1, and prostaglandin – Neurotransmitters: dopamine, acetylcholine, norepinephrine, and 5-hydroxytryptamine.	Acupuncture improves motor symptoms and quality of sleep	NO

Study Details	Participants	Study Design	Control Group	Interventions (GE)	Outcomes Measures	Results/ Conclusions	Side Effect
Acupuncture in the treatment of fatigue in Parkinson's disease: A pilot, randomized, controlled, study. *Brain and Behavior*	**Inclusion:** (1) diagnosis of PD based on criteria developed by Gelb, Oliver, and Gilman (1999) which is adopted by the National Institute of Neurological Disorders and Stroke, US National Institute of Health, (2) age 21–85 years old, (3) presence of moderately severe fatigue as defined by a score of ≥10 on the General Fatigue Domain of the Multidimensional Fatigue Inventory (Smets, Grasen, Bonke, and De Haes, 1995), and (4) no acupuncture treatment in the past 6 months. **Exclusion:** (1) significant cognitive, language or psychiatric illnesses which prevent the subject from understanding instructions and participating in the study, (2) needle phobia, (3) comorbidity with a bleeding disorder, (4) known anaemia with hemoglobin level < 10 g/dl, (5) known congestive cardiac failure and/or end-stage renal disease, (6) female subjects of childbearing age, and (7) presence of symptomatic postural hypotension.	Efficacy of acupuncture in patients with PD-related fatigue N = 40	Sham Acupuncture Needles developed by Jongbae Park (Park Sham Device, PSD)—When pressed onto the skin, it telescopes into the handle and the blunt tip stay on the skin instead of penetrating it. The plastic tube with adhesive foot-plate is placed on the skin to hold it in place	Real Acupuncture **11 acupoints:** right PC 6, left PC 6, right LI 4, left LI4, right ST 36, left ST 36, right SP 6, left SP 6, right KI 3, left KI 3, and CV 6. Frequency: 10 sessions—5 weeks—2×/week Time: 20 min	**3 Assessment Moments:** at baseline, 5 and 9 weeks. - General Fatigue Score of the Multidimensional Fatigue Inventory (MFI-GF) - MFI-Total Score - Unified Parkinson's Disease Rating Scale Motor score (UPDRS Motor) - Parkinson's Disease Questionnaire-39 (PDQ 39) - Geriatrics Depression Scale (GDS) - Epworth Sleepiness Scale ESS)	Both real and sham acupuncture are equally effective in improving PD-related fatigue, and this is likely due to nonspecific or placebo effects this improvement was maintained up to 4 weeks after completion of treatment.	YES—3

Study Details	Participants	Study Design	Control Group	Interventions (GE)	Outcomes Measures	Results/ Conclusions	Side Effect
Acupuncture Modulates the Cerebello-Thalamo-Cortical Circuit and Cognitive Brain Regions in Patients of Parkinson's Disease with Tremor *Frontiers Aging Neuroscience*	**Inclusion:** diagnosed based on the UK PD Society Brain Bank clinical diagnostic criteria, and tremor at rest in at least one upper or lower extremity on either side was assessed by item 20 of the Unified Parkinson's Disease Rating Scale **Exclusion:**secondary Parkinsonism, atypical Parkinsonian disease, advanced PD stage (H-Y ≥ 4), age less than 45 or greater than 80 years, history of other neurological disorders or head trauma, left-handedness, cognitive impairment (Mini-Mental State Examination (MMSE) score < 24), depression tendency (Beck Depression Inventory (BDI) score > 4), and any contraindications for fMRI.	Effect of acupuncture on PD patients with tremor and its potential neural mechanism by fMRI N = 41	Sham Acupuncture (0.2 cm deep and 0.5cun next to the points) + Waiting Group (True acupuncture was performed after final evaluation)	True acupuncture group DU20, GB20, and the Chorea-Tremor Controlled Zone Needle stimulation: The reinforcing-reducing method conducted by twirling was performed every 10 min Time: 30 min needle retention time	**2 Assessment Moments:** Before and after the treatment course. - fMRI scans of the patients' brains - UPDRS II and III subscales	Acupuncture reduces tremor	NO
Acupuncture on GB34 activates the precentral gyrus and prefrontal cortex in Parkinson's disease *BMC Complementary and Alternative Medicine*	**Inclusion:** Diagnosed with clinically definite idiopathic PD by a neurologist from the Kyung Hee Medical Hospital. **Exclusion:** Atypical Parkinsonian disorder, other neurological or major medical conditions (head injury, stroke) or current psychiatric problems.	Evaluate the influence of GB 34 in brain areas And compare brain activity between PD patients and healthy participants N = 24	Healthy Participants N = 12	PD Patients **1 Point:** Right GB 34 (frequently used acupoint for motor function treatment in the oriental medical field needle) Depth of insertion: 1.0 cm Needle type: 0.25 × 40 mm N = 12	**Assessment Moments** - fMRI experiment - Edinburg Handedness Inventory - Hoen and Yahr stage - Korean Mini-Mental State Examination - Beck Depression Inventory	GB 34 seems to be a suitable acupoint	NO

Study Details	Participants	Study Design	Control Group	Interventions (GE)	Outcomes Measures	Results/ Conclusions	Side Effect
Does Integrative Medicine Enhance Balance in Aging Adults?—Proof of Concept for Benefit of Electro-acupuncture Therapy in Parkinson's Disease *Gerontology* [**29**]	**Inclusion:** Aging adults aged 55 years or older with idiopathic PD diagnosed by movement disorder specialists based on the UK Brain Bank criteria. **Exclusion:** Any type of neurological disorder other than PD or if they have prior experience with EA therapy.	Assess EA improvement in postural balance in PD patients N = 56	Sham Acupuncture (With the insertion of needles just under the skin at non-acupuncture points) stimulation with minimal intensity compared to real EA (just turning on the light of the stimulator) Healthy Participants	**EA treatment 20 points:** GV20, GV14 on the midline and bilateral Foot Motor Sensory Area, Balance Area, bilateral ST36, LI4, GB34, LR3, KI3, SP6, BL40. Frequency: 1×/week—3 weeks Needle stimulation: Electrical stimulation frequency: 4 Hz or 100 Hz with intensity just below the level that induces visible muscle contraction. Time: 30 min N = 15	**2 Assessment Moments:** At baseline and after the final therapy. In the "off medication stage" (>12 h after their last PD medication dose). - Balance assessment (Medial-lateral centre of gravity sway to anterior-posterior sway and ankle-to-hip sway during eyes-open, eyes-closed, and eyes-open dual-tasks trials) - Unified Parkinson's Disease Rating Scale (UPDRS) - Visual analogue scale (VAS) - SF-12 health survey - Short Falls Efficacy Scale-International (SHORT FES-I) - Mini-Mental State Examination (MMSE) - Hoehn and Yahr staging	Improvement in rigidity and balance following EA	NO
Effect and Potential Mechanism of Electroa-cupuncture Add-On Treatment in Patients with Parkinson's Disease *Evidence-Based Complementary and Alternative Medicine*	**Inclusion:** a stable dose of anti-Parkinsonian medication for at least 2 months and did not report adverse events. Patients were diagnosed with PD according to UK Parkinson's Disease Society Brain Bank criteria. **Exclusion:** secondary Parkinson's syndromes, Parkinson-plus syndromes, infectious disease in central and peripheral systems, dysarthria, severe psychiatric diseases affecting expression, malignant tumour, disability, and other serious somatic diseases.	Effectiveness and mechanisms of EA add-on treatment in PD patients N = 50	Drug Therapy	Drug + EA **6 points:** bilateral GB20 and LI4 and central Du14 and Du16 Frequency: 20 sessions every 3 days and lasted 2 months Depth of insertion: 2.0–2.5 cm Needle stimulation: inserted obliquely electrical pulses of 9 V, 1 A, 9 W, and 100 Hz Time: 30 min Needle type: 0.25 mm × 40 mm	**2 Assessment Moments** Before and after. GC was reevaluated on the first day after 2 months of drug treatment. Evaluated 12 h after Parkinsonian drugs. - Unified Parkinson's Disease Rating Scale (UPDRS) III - Hamilton Depression Rating Scale (HAMD-) - Pittsburgh Sleep Quality Index - Anxiety Scale- (HAMA-) - Nonmotor Symptoms Quest (NMSQ) - Montreal Cognitive Assessment - Mini-Mental State Examination	EA dramatically reduces motor symptoms of PD patients and nonmotor symptoms, especially sleep quality and depression	NO

Study Details	Participants	Study Design	Control Group	Interventions (GE)	Outcomes Measures	Results/ Conclusions	Side Effect
Effectiveness of acupuncture and bee venom acupuncture in idiopathic Parkinson's disease *Parkinsonism and Related Disorders*	**Inclusion:** adults with idiopathic Parkinson's disease who had been on a stable dose of anti-Parkinsonian medication for at least 1 month. The study neurologist diagnosed each patient with IPD based on symptoms, medications, and brain imaging. **Exclusion:** patients with severe previous or current psychiatric or organic brain disorders other than PD (including secondary Parkinsonism), atypical Parkinsonism, somatic diseases, alcohol abuse, or narcotic abuse.	Effectiveness of both acupuncture and bee venom acupuncture as adjuvant therapies for idiopathic Parkinson's disease N = 35	No Intervention N = 9	1. Acupuncture Treatment 2. Bee Venom Acupuncture Treatment **10 points:** GB 20, LI11, GB34, ST36, LR3 bilateral Frequency: 16 total sessions—twice a week for 8 weeks Depth of insertion: $1.0 \times 10^{1.5}$ cm Needle stimulation: rotated at 2 Hz for 10 s to achieve Deqi Time: 20 min. Needle type: 0.25mm × 0.30 mm N = 13 each	**2 Assessment Moments** Before and after the treatment. - Unified Parkinson's Disease Rating Scale - Parkinson's Disease Quality of Life Questionnaire - Beck Depression Inventory - Berg Balance Scale - Time and number of steps required to walk 30 m	Both acupuncture and bee venom acupuncture showed promising results as adjuvant therapies for Parkinson's disease	NO
Effects of Acupuncture and Qigong Meditation on Nonmotor Symptoms of Parkinson's Disease *Journal of Acupuncture Research*	**Inclusion:** idiopathic PD (based on UK Parkinson's Disease Society Brain Bank criteria), who were taking an anti- Parkinson's medication **Exclusion:** NA	Whether Qigong and acupuncture affect nonmotor symptoms of PD N = 21	Qigong Meditation Only	Acupuncture and Qigong Meditation **6 points:** bilateral GB20, LI4 and central Du14 and Du16 + Healing breathing, Kwanjeong Meditation, and Qigong healing—repeated 12 times Frequency: 12 treatments—5 min until De qi was achieved Depth of insertion: 2.0–2.5 cm obliquely Time: 50 min Needle type: 0.25 × 40 mm	**2 Assessment Moments** Before and after 12 treatments at baseline and 1 month after 12 treatments. - Unified Parkinson's Disease Rating Scales (UPDRS 1) - Test of Smell Identification (TSI)	The combination of Qigong and acupuncture and Qigong alone was shown to improve the nonmotor symptoms and olfactory function of PD.	NA

Study Details	Participants	Study Design	Control Group	Interventions (GE)	Outcomes Measures	Results/ Conclusions	Side Effect
Efficacy of Combined Treatment with Acupuncture and Bee Venom Acupuncture as an Adjunctive Treatment for Parkinson's Disease *The Journal of Alternative and Complementary Medicine*	**Inclusion:** Stable dose of anti-Parkinsonian medication for at least 1 month; Hoehn and Yahr scale I–IV; More than 1 point in two or more items in the UPDRS part III; Mini-Mental State Examination-Korean version score greater than 24 points (out of 30); Consent to the study after full description. **Exclusion:** Severe psychiatric or organic brain disorders other than PD, previous or current; Secondary Parkinsonism due to medication, cerebrovascular disease, tumour, infection, etc; Atypical Parkinsonism or Parkinson-plus syndrome; Somatic disease; Alcohol or narcotic abuse; Expecting a baby; Determined to be inappropriate for participation by the investigator. **Dropout:** Skipped more than 8 of the total 24 treatment sessions in the study or control group; Not able to continue the study because of serious adverse events or aggravation of the condition; Withdrawal of the consent; Impossible to complete the scheduled study as planned by the judgment of the principal investigator. **Randomization:** Double-blind	Efficacy of acupuncture and bee venom acupuncture for idiopathic Parkinson's disease. Duration of the effects by follow-up assessments at the end of the treatment N = 63	Drug Therapy Anti-Parkinsonian drugs without additional intervention Sham Acupuncture received a normal saline injection (shallow minimal acupuncture stimulation was performed at the same points using the same acupuncture needles for 15 min without de qi)	Acupuncture Treatment **10 points:** GB20, LI11, GB34, ST36, and LR3 bilateral Frequency: twice a week for 12 weeks Depth of insertion: 1.0–1.5 cm Needle stimulation: rotated at 2 Hz for 10 s to achieve de qi Time: 15 min Needle type: 0.25 × 30 mm	**4 Assessment Moments** At baseline and at 12, 16, and 20 weeks. Performed in the medication "on" - Unified Parkinson's Disease Rating Scale (UPDRS) part II and part III score - Postural instability—posturography using the Balance Master System - Gait disturbance (PIGD) score - Gait speed and number - Parkinson's Disease Quality of Life Questionnaire - Beck Depression Inventory	Combined treatment of acupuncture and BVA might be a safe and useful adjunctive treatment	NO

Study Details	Participants	Study Design	Control Group	Interventions (GE)	Outcomes Measures	Results/ Conclusions	Side Effect
Comparative study of the efficacy of the usual therapy for Parkinson's disease plus auricular acupuncture and the usual therapy without acupuncture *Revista Internacional de Acupuntura*	**Inclusion:** Diagnosis of idiopathic PE confirmed by a neurologist. Symptomatic PE with a duration of between 1 and 15 years before entering the study. Age between 30 and 75 years at the time of diagnosis. **Exclusion:** Major motor disabilities (only a la EP). Psychiatric illnesses such as: Clinically diagnosed depression (severe depression will be considered to have 30 points or more on the Beck scale), generalised anxiety, social phobia, etc.—Cortical dementia with synamnesia, aphasia, or any other typical Alzheimer's symptom.—Parkinsonism (Parkinsonian syndromes), isolated phenomena, cerebellar syndrome.	Efficacy of the routine treatment in Parkinson's disease (PD) plus permanent auricular acupuncture versus routine treatment without acupuncture N = 32	Sham Acupuncture	100–120 needles Depth of insertion: 2 mm Needle type: titanium needles	**2 Assessment Moments** Before and 12 weeks after. - Unified Parkinson's Disease Rating Scale	The efficacy of the *Forever Needles*, compared to those of the group without permanent insertion for the treatment of PD, could not be established in this study.	NA
Evaluation of Rehabilitation and MRI Results of the Combined Therapy of *Bushenzhichan* Formula and Needle Embedding for Parkinson's Disease *Indian Journal of Pharmaceutical Sciences*	**Inclusion:** Diagnostic criteria of the Motor Disorder and (PD) Group of the Chinese Medical Association Neurology Chapter **Exclusion:** NA	Evaluate Parkinson's disease patients using combined therapy of *Bushenzhichan* formula and needle embedding and analysing the Magnetic resonance imaging test results N = 180	Drug Therapy Madopar Only (100/1500 mg, 3–4 times a day) N = 90	Madopar as well as combined therapy of *Bushenzhichan* formula and needle embedding. The constituents of *Bushenzhichan* formula are as follow up 9 g deer antler glue, 9 g *Zhigancao*, 20 g raw tortoise plastron, 20 g *fructus cannabis*, 20 g *codonopsis*, 20 g raw turtle shell, 12 g gelatin, 12 g *gastrodiaelata*, 12 g pulp of cornus, 30 g *Fructus Lycii*, 30 g *Radix Paeoniae alba*, 30 g dries *Radix Rehmanniae*, 30 g *cistanche*, 30 g *uncaria*, 15 g *Radix Ophiopogonis*, 10 g *polygonatum*. It is considered a single Chinese herb free from decoction, which could be dissolved in 400 mL of boiled water, once a day, and used as a tea after lunch and dinner while warm **Points:** *Baihui (GV 20), Sishencong (EX-HN 1), Fengchi (GV 20), Taichong (LR 3), Yanglingquan (GB 34), Sanyinjiao (BP6), Hegu (LI4), Ganshu (BL18), Shenshu (BL23)* and the chorea-trembling controlled area. N = 90	**Assessment Moments** - MRI test results - UPDRS	The combined therapy of *Bushenzhichan* formula and needle embedding could significantly improve the therapeutic efficacy and promote recovery in Parkinson's disease patients	NA

Study Details	Participants	Study Design	Control Group	Interventions (GE)	Outcomes Measures	Results/ Conclusions	Side Effect
Gait Disturbance Improvement and Cerebral Cortex Rearrangement by Acupuncture in Parkinson's Disease: A Pilot Assessor-Blinded, Randomized, Controlled, Parallel-Group Trial *Neurorehabilitation and Neural Repair*	**Inclusion: WI Exclusion: WI Randomization:** Not blinding	Effects of acupuncture on gait disturbance N = 26	Drug Therapy	Acupuncture Treatment + Drug Therapy 8 treatments—2×/week for 4 weeks **Points:** WI	**Assessment Moments** Assessments in the "on" state intervention phase (4 weeks) and a follow-up phase (4 weeks). - Gait parameters—GAITRite system and hemodynamic responses in the cerebral cortices using functional near-infrared spectroscopy - Unified Parkinson's Disease Rating Scale (UPDRS) scores - Neurotransmitter levels	Acupuncture tended to improve hypometric gait and rearranged activation of the cerebral cortex	NA
Randomized, Controlled Trial of Acupuncture for Fatigue in Parkinson's Disease *Movements Disorders*	**Inclusion:** UK Brain Bank criteria for probable PD10; age 40 to 99 years; fluent in English; stable medication uses for 30 days; and self-reported moderate or severe fatigue using the International Parkinson's and Movement Disorder Society UPDRS fatigue item. **Exclusion:** dementia or a score below 24 on the Montreal Cognitive Assessment (MoCA) presence of another medical condition expected to produce fatigue; active depression or Hospital Anxiety and Depression Scale (HADS) depression subscale score greater than 10; the presence of an untreated sleep disorder; or exposure to acupuncture within the past 6 months.	Determine whether a 6-week course of acupuncture could improve PD-related fatigue N = 94	Sham Acupuncture (non-acupuncture points, located 0.5 in lateral to the real)	Acupuncture Treatment **11 points:** GV20, GV24, CV6, unilateral, LI 10, HT 7, ST36, SP 6 bilateral Frequency: 2/ week during 6 weeks = 12 Treatments Depth of insertion: 0.5 to 1 cm Needle stimulation: The needle was twisted three times to the right Time: 30 min	**Assessment Moments:** - Modified Fatigue Impact Scale at 6 weeks - Sleep, mood, quality of life, and maintenance of benefits at 12 weeks - Parkinson's Disease Sleep Scale (PDSS) - Epworth Sleepiness Scale (ESS) - Apathy Evaluation Scale (AES). - Quality of life (QOL) - Parkinson's Disease Questionnaire (PDQ-39)	Acupuncture may improve PD-related fatigue, but real acupuncture offers no greater benefit than sham treatments.	YES—constipation

Source: Pereira CR, Machado J, Rodrigues J, de Oliveira NM, Criado MB, Greten HJ. Effectiveness of Acupuncture in Parkinson's Disease Symptoms—A Systematic Review. Healthcare. 2022; 10(11):2334. https://doi.org/10.3390/healthcare10112334.

10.1.1. Acupuncture for Motor Symptoms of Parkinson's Disease

Since the Unified Parkinson's Disease Rating Scale, motor subscale (mUPDRS) is one of the four cardinal motor features used to diagnose PD, measures of motor dysfunction have been used in many acupuncture trials to assess efficacy. One of the first double-blind, sham-controlled, randomized studies on electroacupuncture (EA) in PD patients was conducted in 2005 by Cristian and colleagues.

They found non-significant trends toward improvement on a number of motor and non-motor measures. Ten acupuncture sessions were used in a different randomized, controlled trial carried out in China, and the average levodopa dose was significantly lower than that of the controls. In their comparison of standard acupuncture, bee venom acupuncture (BVA), and a third non-intervention control group, Cho and colleagues discovered that both treatments significantly raised the participants' initial mUPDRS scores.

The same group compared BVA with conventional medical treatment and sham acupuncture (twice weekly saline injections combined with acupuncture in sham acupoints) in a follow-up trial. When compared to controls on the mUPDRS, both the acupuncture and sham groups demonstrated a significant improvement after 12 weeks.

The BVA group showed improvement from baseline in the mUPDRS, the number of steps to walk 20 meters, the Beck Depression Inventory (BDI), the Parkinson's Disease Quality of Life Questionnaire (PDQL), and the postural instability and gait disturbance (PIGD) score; however, this difference was not statistically significant when compared to the sham acupuncture group. Li and colleagues randomized 41 PD patients into waiting, sham, and acupuncture groups. They discovered that the active treatment group significantly improved on the mUPDRS, particularly the tremor scores. According to conventional Chinese theory, the acupuncture targeted acupoints DU20, GB20, and the chorea-tremor controlled zones, all of which are said to reduce tremor (Cho et al., 2018).

10.1.2. Acupuncture for Gait and Balance in Parkinson's Disease

Apart from addressing general motor disability associated with PD, certain trials have concentrated more on the particular problems of gait dysfunction and balance impairment. In 27 PD patients, an open-label acupuncture trial showed an instant improvement of 10% in gait speed, 8% in step length, 11% in floor reaction force, and an additional 2% in steps per minute on cadence testing. Toosizadeh and colleagues conducted a small, sham-controlled trial and discovered that weekly EA treatments over a 3-week period led to improved rigidity scores in the mUPDRS (specifically, balance measurements) and significant improvements in balance when compared to patients receiving the treatment at non-acupuncture points. After three weekly electroacupuncture sessions, the same group used wearable sensors on 15 patients to show improvement in gait, as measured by gait speed (9–19% improvement on various measures), stride length (9% improvement), and mid-swing velocity (6% improvement). Although these are encouraging results, longer-term, blinded trials are needed to confirm them.

10.1.3. Acupuncture for Non-Motor Symptoms of Parkinson's Disease

Many of these trials have included non-motor scales as secondary outcomes in addition to motor function monitoring. Open-label trials consistently show improvements in depression, sleep, and quality of life. In certain controlled trials, the experimental group experienced improvements in activities of daily living (ADLs), depression on the BDI, and quality of life as measured by the 39-item Parkinson's Disease Questionnaire (PDQ-39).

Since fatigue is a common complaint among patients with PD, two randomized, controlled trials have assessed the effects of acupuncture specifically on fatigue. Kluger and colleagues compared the effects of real versus sham acupuncture in 94 PD patients who reported mild to moderate fatigue. Although both groups had significantly improved from baseline, there was no difference in the scores on the Modified Fatigue Impact Scale (MFIS) at six and twelve weeks. A more recent study involving 40 patients also found no differences in measures of fatigue between the groups, although both the acupuncture and sham groups experienced improvements in fatigue by week five, which continued until week nine.

After eight weekly sessions, Aroxa et al. observed a significant improvement in the overall Parkinson's Disease Sleep Scale (PDSS), particularly in the domains of general sleep quality, nocturnal psychosis, and nocturnal motor symptoms when compared to medication-only controls. This research involved 22 patients with Parkinson's disease.

Finally, a recent study examined the effectiveness of acupuncture specifically in treating PD. This treatment has been the subject of extensive research. 16 patients who self-selected into an acupuncture or non-intervention control group based on their personal preference were those who scored above zero on the King's Parkinson's Disease Pain Scale (KPPS) and had not received acupuncture within the previous three months. When compared to controls, patients who received acupuncture showed a significant improvement in their KPPS and overall UPDRS score, but not in their depressive symptoms (Yu et al, 2019).

10.1.4. Imaging and Acupuncture in Parkinson's Disease

Researchers have evaluated the effects of acupuncture on PD patients using a variety of imaging modalities, such as resting-state fMRI, functional magnetic resonance imaging (fMRI), and single-photon emission computerized tomography (SPECT) imaging. Data on five PD patients receiving levodopa and five PD patients receiving levodopa plus acupuncture were published by Huang and colleagues in 2009. The data revealed increased glucose metabolism in the bilateral frontal and occipital lobes, as well as in the temporal lobes, thalamus, and cerebellum on the side with less impairment. Ten PD patients who received five weeks of EA showed an increase in cerebral blood flow in the more affected hemispheres of the brain, including the frontal lobe, occipital lobe, basal ganglia, and cerebellum, when compared to ten patients receiving levodopa alone. Using 99mTc-TRODAT-1 SPECT imaging, this failed to demonstrate any alteration in basal ganglia dopamine transporter activity, indicating that acupuncture is ineffective in addressing the pathophysiologic mechanisms underpinning Parkinson's disease.

Ten PD patients were studied by Chae and colleagues following acupuncture, covert placebo, and overt placebo; fMRI was performed following each procedure, which the patients received at different times. After receiving acupuncture as opposed to a covert placebo, there was an increase in activity in the putamen and primary motor cortex, indicating that the treatment may modify the basal ganglia–thalamocortical circuit and alleviate motor symptoms. Specifically targeting the GB34 acupoint, which is believed to cure diseases of the lower extremities (including pain and weakness), muscles, and gallbladder, Yeo and colleagues conducted a small, randomized, sham-controlled trial comparing twelve PD patients to healthy controls. Furthermore, neuroprotection in MPTP mouse models has been shown in this area. Their findings demonstrate that patients with PD and healthy controls differ in terms of baseline activation and response to acupuncture, with PD patients exhibiting higher levels of activation in the precentral gyrus, prefrontal cortex, and putamen. After that, they conducted an open-label assessment of the benefits of acupuncture at right GB34 and LR3, two acupoints that can help with walking difficulties as well as lower extremity weakness, numbness, and pain. They also added other acupoints based on the symptoms of each patient. Numerous brain regions showed changes in fMRI, but thalamic response showed a statistically significant increase that correlated with the change in mUPDRS. PD patients enrolled in a 2018 trial were randomly assigned to receive standard medical therapy, sham acupuncture, or actual acupuncture. The cerebello-thalamo-cortical circuit was modulated in the fMRI, in addition to demonstrating a 3.6 and 4.4 point improvement on the UPDRS II and III subscales, respectively. This functional alteration was consistent with the notable improvement in the mUPDRS tremor score. The research conducted by Yu and colleagues. that assessed pain in PD patients revealed enhanced connectivity via four connections: between the left middle temporal and precentral gyri, right postcentral and precentral gyri, right supramarginal and precentral gyri, and right medial temporal gyrus and insular cortex—all regions implicated in emotion and sensory discrimination.

10.2. Tai Chi

For centuries, people have used taiji quan, also known as tai chi, a traditional Chinese martial art, to improve their physical and mental health. The phrase alludes to the idea of yin and yang, which combines breathing, meditation, and intricate, controlled movements to create dynamic balance. Numerous medical conditions, including Parkinson's disease, have been the subject of extensive research on Tai Chi. A review of Tai Chi for general health and fitness found strong evidence that it improves endurance and balance. Tai Chi open-label trials indicate that patients with PD may benefit in terms of movement awareness and obstacle negotiation. The effects of Tai Chi on motor and non-motor symptoms have been further examined in a number of randomized, controlled trials.

Table 10.2 shows son natural products studies conducted on animal or cell models of PD.

Table 10.2. *Natural Products for Parkinson's Disease*

Origin of Extraction	Mechanism	Cell or Animal Model	Inducer	Mode of Action and Target Signal
Duzhong Fang	Inflammation	C57bl/6 mice	MPTP	↓ locomotor dysfunction, inflammation, Iba1, microglia reactivity state ↑ striatal dopamine content, dopaminergic neurons, TH

Origin of Extraction	Mechanism	Cell or Animal Model	Inducer	Mode of Action and Target Signal
KOK	Inflammation	C57BL/6 mice	MPTP ML385	↓ neurological dysfunction and motor impairments, the loss of dopaminergic neurons and fibers, Iba1, the upregulation of inflammatory mediators (IL-6, TNF-α, COX-2, and iNOS), neurotoxicity (microglial activation and inflammatory response ↓), BBB disruption markers (PECAM-1 and GFAP), neurotoxicity and inflammation (phosphorylated forms of ERK, JNK, and p38 & IκB and NF-κB ↓), ROS, MAPKs and NF-κB signaling pathways ↑ Nrf2 signaling (decreases the expression levels of Keap1 (a repressor protein that binds to Nrf2), and increases the expression levels of Nrf2 transcription factor, Nrf2 targeting genes HO-1 and NQO-1)
DBYW	Mitochondrial dysfunction	Rat PC-12 cells	pDJ-1 trans fection MPP^+	↓ DJ-1, mitochondrial dysfunction ↑ mitochondrial mass, total ATP content, the Akt phosphorylation
BvPLA2	Inflammation	Human A53T α-Syn Transgenic mice	A53T Transgenes	↓ motor dysfunction, α-Syn, the activation and numbers of microglia, and the ratio of M1/M2
Hesperetin	Inflammation	Wistar rats	6-OHDA	↓ astrogliosis (GFAP ↓), apoptosis (nigral DNA fragmentation ↓), the loss of SNC dopaminergic neurons ↑ striatal catalase activity and GSH content, Bcl2
Paeonol	Inflammation	C57BL/6 mice	MPTP	↓ motor dysfunction, oxidative stress (the activity levels of SOD, CAT, and GSH ↑), neuroinflammation(the number of Iba1-positive and IL-1β-positive cells ↓), ↑ TH-positive neurons, BDNF, dopaminergic neurons protection

Origin of Extraction	Mechanism	Cell or Animal Model	Inducer	Mode of Action and Target Signal
Gastrodin	Mitochondrial dysfunction	Drosophila melanogaster	PINK1 gene mutant	↓ the loss of dopaminergic neurons, the onset of Parkinson-like phenotypes ↑ lifespan, climbing ability, resistance to oxidative stress, enzyme activities of superoxide dismutase (SOD) and catalase (CAT), the expression of anti-oxidative genes
Trehalose	Lysosomal Disorders	Human A53T α-Syn Transgenic mice	A53T Transgenes	↓ α-Synuclein-Induced Behavioral Impairment, α-Synuclein Accumulation ↑ DA Neuronal Survival, protection against the reduction of TH protein expression, autophagosome formation, LC3-II levels
BSJDF	Lysosomal Disorders	Pheochromocytoma12 (PC12)	MPP+ (MPTP)	improved cell survival in the PC12 cell PD model activated the autophagic process in PC12 cells. increased expression of Atg12 and LC3 proteins and upregulated Atg12 mRNA.
NRD	inflammation	Wistar rats	Rotenone	↑ level of superoxide dismutase, catalase, and glutathione ↓ level of malondialdehyde inhibited the release of proinflammatory cytokines and inflammatory mediators prevented ROT-induced glial cell activation and the loss of dopaminergic neurons and nerve fibers attenuated rotenone-induced dopaminergic neurodegeneration.

Origin of Extraction	Mechanism	Cell or Animal Model	Inducer	Mode of Action and Target Signal
Vanillic acid	Mitochondrial dysfunction	Sprague Dawley rats	Rotenone	↓ Weight gain, Catalepsy, Rearing TBARS level (at 25 mg/kg and 50 mg/kg) SAG(superoxide anion generation) ↑ behavior, CAT
Vanillin	Inflammation	Male Wistar rats	6-OHDA	↓ apomorphine-induced rotations, free radical release, expression of pro-inflammatory cytokines, lipid peroxidation ↑ striatal dopamine content, glutathione and superoxide dismutase enzyme protection of dopaminergic neurons

Source: So Y-J, Lee J-U, Yang G-S, Yang G, Kim S-W, Lee J-H, Kim J-U. The Potentiality of Natural Products and Herbal Medicine as Novel Medications for Parkinson's Disease: A Promising Therapeutic Approach. International Journal of Molecular Sciences. 2024; 25(2):1071. https://doi.org/10.3390/ijms25021071.

10.2.1. Tai Chi for Motor Symptoms and Postural Instability of Parkinson's Disease

The investigation into Tai Chi's potential benefits for PD motor symptoms during the previous 20 years has yielded conflicting findings. For comparison, non-exercise controls have been used in numerous studies. After 20 one-hour Tai Chi sessions, Hackney and Earhart found improvement in the mUPDRS compared to those receiving usual care; Choi and colleagues found improvement after 36 sessions compared to baseline within the Tai Chi group, but not in comparison to controls. When compared to the baseline, two groups' mUPDRS scores did not significantly improve; however, one study did observe improvements in balance on the Berg Balance Scale (BBS). Similar to this, Vergara-Diaz and colleagues compared participants in a biweekly Tai Chi intervention with non-exercise controls. Although they did not find a significant difference between the pre- and post-intervention on the mUPDRS, the Tai Chi group showed non-significant trends toward improvement in the Activity-Specific Balance Confidence scale (ABC), Timed Up and Go (TUG) test, dual-task gait stride-time variability, and PDQ-39 (Hackney and Earhart, 2008).

In an attempt to ascertain whether benefits are unique to Tai Chi rather than the overall effects of exercise, other studies have used exercise comparator groups. When patients were randomized to Tai Chi, a combined exercise control group, or a non-exercise control group, Cheon and colleagues observed that upper limb strength and agility significantly improved in both exercise groups when compared to the non-exercise controls. Although cardiovascular endurance was improved in both groups when compared to baseline, the combined exercise group outperformed the Tai Chi group by a significant margin.

Zhang et al. randomized twenty patients to a multimodal exercise group and twenty patients to a Tai Chi intervention. They observed no differences between the groups on the BBS, mUPDRS, gait velocity, stride length, and the TUG test, but both groups had improved significantly from baseline. Kurt and colleagues conducted a study wherein they contrasted land-based exercise with Ai Chi, an aquatic form of Tai Chi. The results indicated that both types of exercise improved the participants' dynamic balance, BBS, TUG test, mUPDRS, and PDQ-39 from baseline; however, the Ai Chi group's improvement was statistically greater.

The largest Tai Chi randomized, controlled trial to date was published in the New England Journal of Medicine. Li and team enlisted 195 Parkinson's disease patients, then randomly assigned them to Tai Chi, resistance training, or stretching. In the predetermined primary outcome measure of postural stability, the Tai Chi group outperformed the resistance training and stretching groups in terms of maximum excursion (a measure of one's ability to stretch beyond one's comfort zone) and directional control (a measure of movement accuracy). In addition, the Tai Chi group performed better than the stretching group in all secondary outcomes, such as the TUG test, the mUPDRS, and gait (walking velocity and stride length) and strength tests.

Crucially, at three months, the Tai Chi group continued to record fewer falls than either of the control groups. The eight-item Parkinson's Disease Questionnaire (PDQ-8) was used to measure quality of life improvements.

More importantly, these findings imply that Tai Chi is a helpful intervention to address postural instability and reduce fall risk in this population.

Specifically, Tai Chi is at least as effective as other forms of exercise at improving the motor symptoms of Parkinson's disease. Numerous other studies have examined the impact of Tai Chi on postural stability and balance, and they have shown improvements in a range of balance metrics, such as the BBS, the ABC scale, one-foot balancing, and the overall number of falls.

10.2.2. Tai Chi for Non-Motor Symptoms of Parkinson's Disease

In their 2009 study, Hackney and Earhart randomized a sizable group of 61 PD patients to a range of exercise interventions specifically designed to assess quality of life. In this study, participants in the Tai Chi, waltz/foxtrot, and control groups did not significantly improve from baseline on any of the PDQ-39 quality of life measures; only the tango group did. In a smaller study, Nocera and team randomized twenty-one individuals to either Tai Chi or a non-contact control group, in which participants were free to choose to exercise at home on their own volition without the guidance of a teacher. They discovered that the emotional well-being subscale and the PDQ-39 total score were considerably higher for those in the Tai Chi group.

Yang and colleagues investigated whether group-based Tai Chi might be more beneficial for non-motor symptoms than individual Tai Chi, but after 13 weeks, they found no discernible difference between the two types of interventions. While neither group demonstrated improvement in depressive symptoms on the

Hamilton Depression Rating Scale (HAM-D), both did show improvement from baseline in global non-motor symptoms (NMSs) and sleep.

10.3. Qi Gong

Qi Gong is a traditional Chinese practice that enhances the flow of qi through movement, posture, breathing, and meditation. It is similar to Tai Chi. Qi Gong is a practice that predates Tai Chi study and has been practiced for nearly 5000 years in China, despite being less popular in Western culture. The recentness of randomized clinical trials suggests that there is growing interest in this treatment, even though few studies have been done to assess its impact on PD (Table 10.3).

Table 10.3. *Physical Activity for Patients with Parkinson's Disease*

(i) Exercise mode and improvement for motor symptoms of Parkinson's disease			
Symptom	**Exercise Mode**	**Improvement**	**References: Grade** [2]
Freezing of gait	Running, swimming, cycling, hiking, aerobic dancing, jogging skipping rope, running, cycling, kick-boxing, playing tennis heel-to-toe walk tai chi	Walking speed ↑ [1] step and stride length ↑ motor performance ↑ cadence ↑ cardiovascular endurance ↑ gait speed ↑ balance ↑ weight shifting ability ↑ movement control ↑ trunk rotation ↑ multidirectional stepping ability ↑ maintenance of postures ↑ walking speed and steps ↑	[**21**]: A, [**22**]: C, [**23**]: C, [**24**]: B, [**25**]: D, [**26**]: A
Motor skill dysfunction	Kick-boxing playing tennis push-ups and pull-ups calf raises	Cardiovascular endurance ↑ muscle strength ↑ stretch and calf muscle strength ↑	[**21**]: A, [**27**]: A, [**28**]: A, [**29**]: B, [**30**]: B, [**31**]: A
Weak muscles	Lunges and bicep curls using dumbbells weight training high-intensity interval training functional training, eccentric training, interval training sprinting training mid back squeezes planks squats burpees pendulum lunges	Muscle strength ↑ muscle resistance ↑ muscle strength ↑ muscle strength ↑ firm muscle ↑ back muscle strength ↑ core muscle strength ↑ core and thigh muscle strength ↑ core and whole-body muscle strength ↑ core and thigh muscle strength ↑	[**32**]: D, [**33**]: C, [**34**]: A, [**35**]: B

(i) Exercise mode and improvement for motor symptoms of Parkinson's disease			
Symptom	**Exercise Mode**	**Improvement**	**References: Grade [2]**
Imbalance	Standing on one foot, BOSU ball [3] movements Brisk walking Tai Chi dance cycling	Balance ↑ walking speed and steps ↑ weight shifting ability ↑ movement control ↑ trunk rotation ability ↑ multidirectional stepping ↑ maintenance of postures ↑ dynamic balance ↑ backward walking ↑ turning and multitasking skills ↑ walking speed and steps ↑	[**20**]: A, [**22**]: C, [**23**]: C, [**36**]: D
Rigidity	The shimmy [4] bridge press easy standing body transition exercise yoga rotation whole body stretching snow angels hamstring stretch hip flexor stretch calf stretch shoulder shrugs chin tucks	Coordination and relaxation ↑ core strength and body strength ↑ body balance and coordination ↑ stretching ↑ body balance and coordination ↑ coordination ↑ stretching ↑ muscle relaxation ↑ stretching ↑ stretching ↑ stretching ↑ stretching ↑ neck stiffness improvement ↑	[**27**]: A, [**37**]: A, [**38**]: A

[1] " ↑ " represents increase; " ↓ " represents decrease. [2] The level of evidence of each reference is graded as A: overwhelming data from randomized controlled trials (RCTs); B: quasi-experimental design; C: results stem from uncontrolled, nonrandomized, and/or observational studies; D: review or evidence insufficient for categories A to C. [3] BOSU stands for Bionic Oscillatory Stabilization Unit, which is an inflated rubber hemisphere device using for balance training. [4] A dance move that requires shoulders quickly alternated back and forth with body holding still.

(ii) Exercise mode and improvement for non-motor features (except cognitive dysfunction) of Parkinson's disease			
Symptom	**Exercise Mode**	**Improvement**	**References: Grade [4]**
Constipation	Physical therapy incorporating abdominal massage [1]	Abdominal movement range ↑ [2]	[**42**]: D, [**43**]: B, [**44**]: C

(ii) Exercise mode and improvement for non-motor features (except cognitive dysfunction) of Parkinson's disease			
Symptom	**Exercise Mode**	**Improvement**	**References: Grade** [4]
Depression	Tai Chi, Yoga	Flexibility ↑ [3]	[**27**]: A, [**45**]: A, [**46**]: A, [**47**]: B
Drooling	Expiratory muscle strength training	Muscle strength ↑	[**32**]: A, [**48**]: A, [**49**]: D
Fatigue	Tango, High-intensity exercise training	Blood circulation ↑ Metabolism ↑	[**50**]: A, [**51**]: D, [**52**]: B
Orthostatic hypotension	Leg-holding exercises	Circulation ↑	[**33**]: C, [**42**]: D
pain	Tai Chi, Breathing exercises, Yoga	Flexibility ↑ Resistance ↑ Balance ↑	[**27**]: A, [**37**]: A, [**38**]: A, [**45**]: A, [**46**]: A, [**53**]: D, [**54**]: D
Psychosis (hallucinations or delusions)	Aerobic exercise, Yoga	Focus ↑ Cardiovascular ↑ Muscle strength ↑ Body coordination ↑	[**33**]: C, [**34**]: A, [**35**]: B
Sexual dysfunction	Qigong, Cycle ergometer exercise training	Focus ↑ Depression symptoms ↓	[**46**]: A, [**55**]: A, [**56**]: D
Anorexia, nausea, vomiting	General exercise	Neural apoptosis ↓ Neurodegeneration process ↓ PD development and symptoms ↓	[**57**]: D, [**58**]: D, [**59**]: D
Sleep problems	Nordic Walking Aerobic training Weight lifting exercise Yoga	Muscle strength ↑ Coordination ↑ Physical capacity ↑ Cardiorespiratory fitness ↑	[**28**]: A, [**31**]: A, [**42**]: D, [**60**]: C, [**61**]: B, [**62**]: A, [**63**]: A, [**64**]: A, [**65**]: A

(ii) Exercise mode and improvement for non-motor features (except cognitive dysfunction) of Parkinson's disease			
Symptom	**Exercise Mode**	**Improvement**	**References: Grade [4]**
Urinary problems	Exercise-based, biofeedback-assisted behavioral intervention Pelvic floor muscle exercise	Muscle strength ↑	[**29**]: B, [**30**]: B, [**66**]: A

Source: Cheng Y-C, Su C-H. Evidence Supports PA Prescription for Parkinson's Disease: Motor Symptoms and Non-Motor Features: A Scoping Review. International Journal of Environmental Research and Public Health. 2020; 17(8):2894. https://doi.org/10.3390/ijerph17082894.

[1] To use massage techniques for pwPD with constipation problems. [2] " ↑ " represents increase; " ↓ " represents decrease. [3] Studies have shown that yoga can be considered as a therapy in treating depressive and anxiety disorders. Following along from the suggested exercise mode that targets the alleviation of the symptoms pwPD have, physical improvements then appear. [4] The level of evidence of each reference is graded as A: overwhelming data from randomized controlled trials (RCTs); B: quasi-experimental design; C: results stem from uncontrolled, nonrandomized, and/or observational studies; D: review or evidence insufficient for categories A to C.

10.3.1. Qi Gong for Motor Symptoms of Parkinson's Disease

Six randomized controlled trials have assessed how Qi Gong interventions affect motor symptoms in Parkinson's disease. In three studies, Qi Gong was compared to non-exercise controls and resulted in significant improvements in a number of motor outcomes, including the percentage of patients with improved mUPDRS scores, changes in mUPDRS and total UPDRS from baseline to 8 weeks, a reduction in muscle hardness measured by myometry, and improvement on the TUG test. While there was an improvement on the 6-min walking test (6MWT) following aerobic exercise, neither group showed an improvement in motor function on the mUPDRS in a 7-week cross-over study comparing Qi Gong followed by aerobic exercise to aerobic exercise followed by Qi Gong.

Xiao and Zhuang found that 45 PD patients who completed 6 months of Qi Gong showed significant improvements in the mUPDRS, motor symptoms at night (a PDSS subscale), 6MWT, TUG test, gait speed, and BBS when compared to daily walking. When Baduanjin Qi Gong, a particular type of medical Qi Gong, was contrasted with traditional physical therapy, the results showed that although the intervention group's BBS, ABC, TUG test, and 6MWT scores significantly improved from baseline, they did not differ significantly from the controls.

It is surprising that, given the practice's heavy emphasis on balance, no studies have explicitly examined Qi Gong's effects on it as a primary endpoint.

An open-label study found that practicing Qi Gong for six weeks reduced double-support time, a gauge of postural stability.

In the extensive study of 98 Parkinson's disease patients previously detailed, participants experienced a reduction in falls and fractures following the intervention in comparison to their baseline assessment, and this was nearly significant when compared to the group receiving traditional physical therapy (Xiao et al, 2016).

10.3.2. Qi Gong for Non-Motor Symptoms of Parkinson's Disease

Multiple trials have also disclosed secondary non-motor outcomes, yielding inconsistent outcomes that could be attributed to differences in the comparator groups, treatment frequency, and trial design. Eight weeks of twice weekly Qi Gong sessions resulted in a decrease in constipation, pain, and daytime sleepiness compared to controls in Schmitz-Hubsch and colleagues' study.

Compared to controls who did not exercise, tai chi (qi dance) improved the PDQL. However, neither group showed any discernible improvement over a 7-week period, nor did a study comparing Qi Gong to aerobic exercise show any improvement in the PDQ-39.

Clinical trials have focused most of their attention on sleep. An open-label study of seven patients who practiced Qi Gong for six weeks revealed some improvement in sleep quality at the conclusion of the program.

Xiao and Zhuang presented a secondary outcome in their large-scale randomized trial that showed improvement in the PDSS after practicing Qi Gong as opposed to walking every day. Moon et al. focused on how Qi Gong affected sleep patterns and TNF-α levels, an inflammatory cytokine implicated in the sleep-wake cycle and thought to contribute to the degeneration of dopaminergic cells in Parkinson's disease.

Ten patients were randomly assigned to practice Qi Gong or sham Qi Gong (traditional movements without breathing exercises or meditation) in this pilot study. The patients reported a significant improvement in their PDSS and nighttime symptoms, which was correlated with a decrease in TNF-α.

10.4. Yoga and Meditation

Yoga is a traditional Indian spiritual and meditation practice that has gained popularity as a physical fitness routine in recent years. It entails a series of breathing exercises and meditation with an emphasis on the mind-body connection. These ideas suggest that yoga, like traditional exercise regimens, may help with motor symptoms of PD, but with an added emphasis on non-motor outcomes. Although meditation has not been independently studied, it is frequently included in randomized trials of yoga to assess the impact of these interventions on Parkinson's disease symptoms (Hall et al, 2011) (Figure 10.1.)

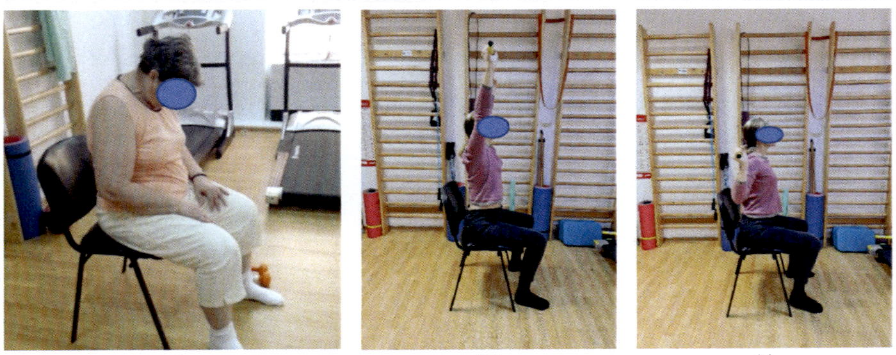

(a) (b) (c)

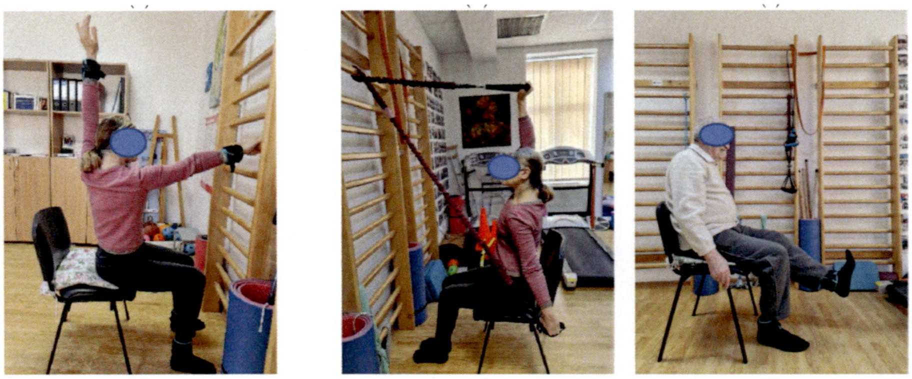

(d) (e) (f)

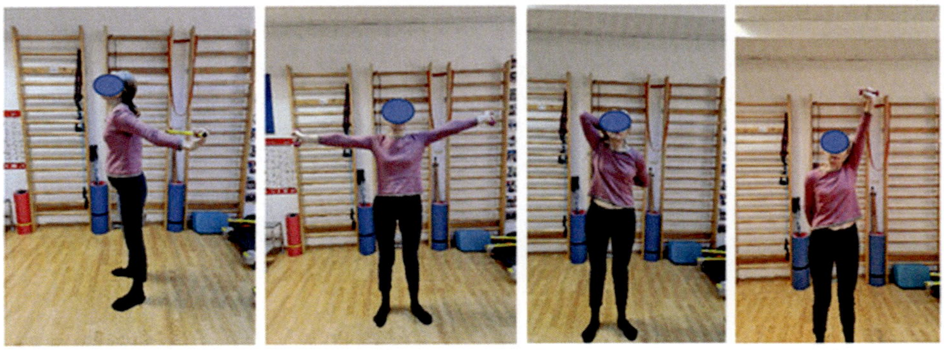

(a) (b) (c) (d)

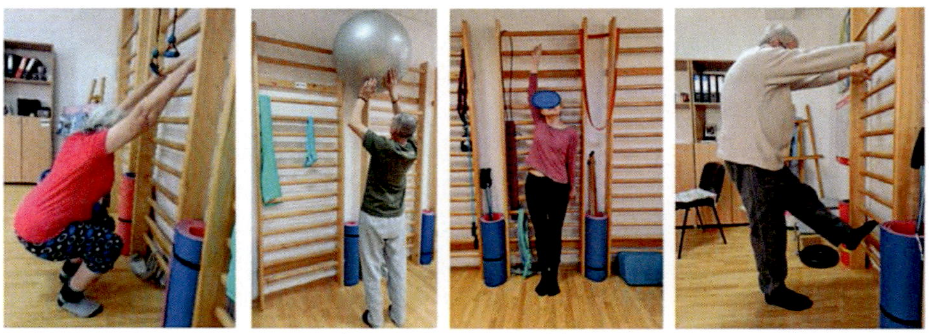

(a) (b) (c) (d)

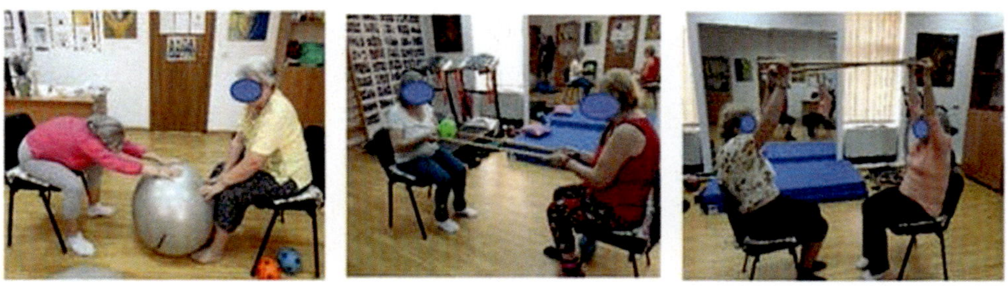

(e) (f) (g)

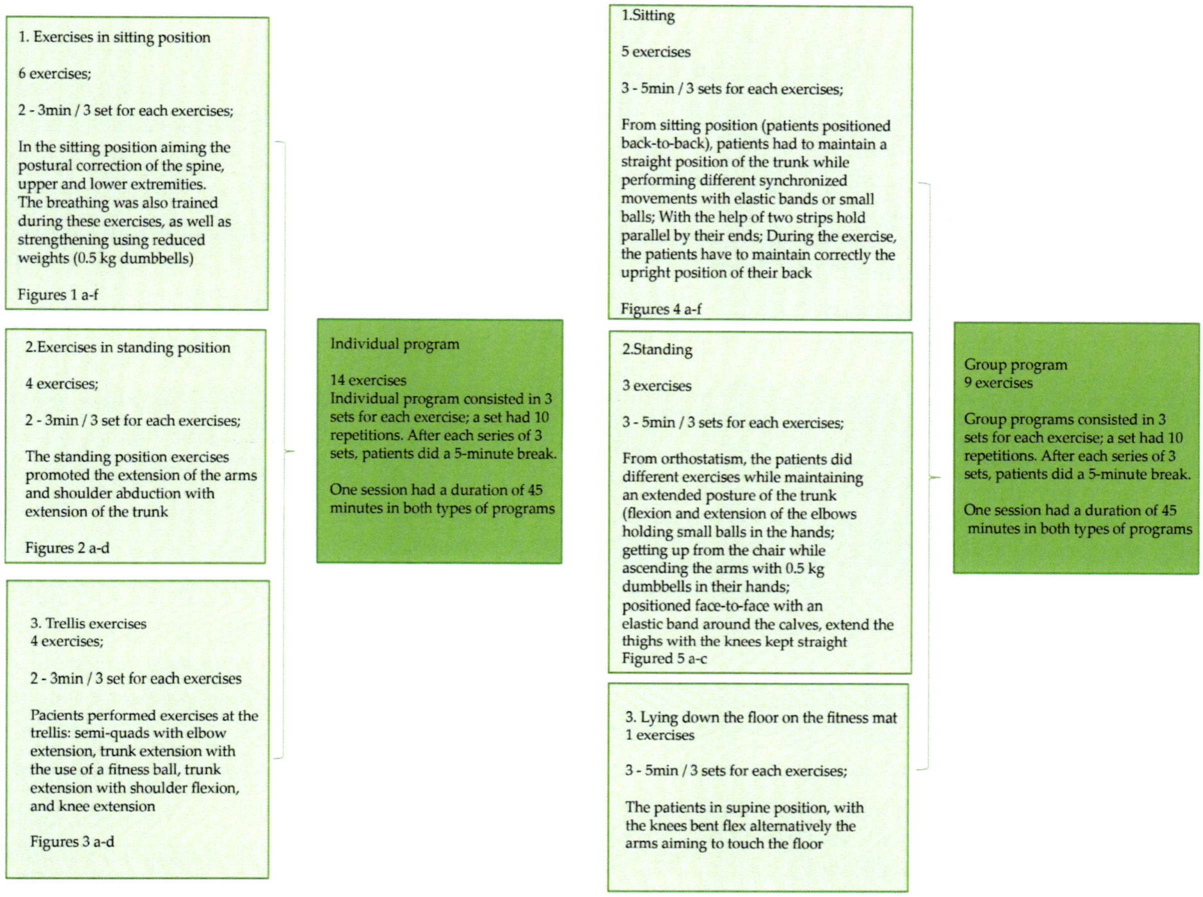

Figure 10.1. *An example report of exercises for patients with Parkinson's disease.*

Source: Zippenfening HA, Amaricai E, Raducan MR. Assessment of Individualized and Group Physical Exercise Programs in Patients with Parkinson's Disease: A Pilot Study. Applied Sciences. 2023; 13(15):8962. https://doi.org/10.3390/app13158962.

10.4.1. Yoga for the Motor Symptoms in Patients with Parkinson's Disease

Regular yoga or mindfulness sessions have been compared to non-exercising controls in three randomized, controlled trials. While all three noted improvements over baseline in a number of motor function and balance measures, only one demonstrated a statistically significant improvement when compared to the non-exercising controls.

If there are any benefits unique to this physical practice, three more studies have compared control groups engaged in active exercise with yoga interventions. In one such study, power training and yoga were compared to non-exercise controls. It was discovered that both groups significantly outperformed the controls on tests of muscle strength, balance, gait, and motor function, but not each other. In a different analysis, the yoga group did show decreased bradykinesia and rigidity along with increased muscle strength and power when specifically compared to the non-exercise controls.

An 8-week study involving 138 patients and a separate study of 17 patients evaluated after 12 weeks compared yoga to resistance training and found improvements in motor function and balance measures (mUPDRS, TUG test, BBS) in all exercise groups post-intervention, though these were not different between groups again.

10.4.2. Yoga for Non-Motor Symptoms in Patients with Parkinson's Disease

The Hospital Anxiety and Depression Scale (HADS) was used in a large study by Kwok and colleagues to compare the effects of yoga to resistance training on anxiety and depression. Apart from the aforementioned motor benefits, they observed a noteworthy interaction effect favoring the yoga intervention on the HADS (anxiety and depression scores), specific subscales on the Holistic Well-being Scale (HWS), and PDQ-8.

A follow-up examination of a previously reported study revealed improvements in quality of life on the PDQ-8 and fatigue on the 16-item Parkinson's Disease Fatigue Scale (PFS-16) when compared to baseline, but not for controls. Bega and Stein's study demonstrated a significant improvement over resistance training in terms of anxiety and emotional dysregulation on the Quality of Life in Neurological Disorders (Neuro-QoL) scale (Walteret a, 2019). Results are otherwise mixed as to the benefits of yoga on non-motor symptoms; however, many of these studies are not specifically powered to detect change in these outcomes.

10.4.3. The Effects of Yoga on Imaging and Biomarkers

There is little information available about how yoga interventions affect the body's chemical and radiographic alterations. In order to assess the impact of a mindfulness-based intervention on brain structure using magnetic resonance imaging (MRI), Pickut and colleagues carried out a randomized, controlled trial.

When compared to non-exercise controls, patients who had completed eight weeks of mindfulness showed increased gray matter density in prespecified regions of interest in both the bilateral hippocampi and the right amygdala.

Large clusters of activity in the right and left caudates, respectively, were identified by whole-brain analysis as regions involved in the pathophysiology of Parkinson's disease. Although oxidative stress markers did not differ between the intervention and control groups, Cheung et al published a randomized trial that included an outcome measure that assessed changes in these markers.

10.5. Massage Therapy

Massage therapy involves the manipulation of soft tissues, including muscles, tendons, ligaments, and fascia, using various techniques such as stroking, kneading, compression, and stretching.

These techniques can be applied with the hands, fingers, elbows, forearms, or specialized tools, depending on the therapist's training and the client's needs. Massage therapy promotes physical relaxation, improves circulation, enhances lymphatic drainage, and reduces stress by stimulating the body's natural relaxation response and releasing endorphins, the body's natural painkillers.

10.5.1. Benefits of Massage Therapy in Parkinson's Disease

1. **Muscle Relaxation and Pain Relief:** Rigidity and muscle stiffness are common symptoms of Parkinson's disease due to the loss of dopamine-producing neurons in the brain. Massage therapy can help relax tight muscles, improve flexibility, and alleviate pain and discomfort associated with muscle rigidity.
2. **Improving Range of Motion and Flexibility:** Massage techniques such as stretching, mobilization, and myofascial release can help improve joint mobility, increase range of motion, and enhance flexibility, allowing individuals with Parkinson's disease to move more freely and perform activities of daily living with greater ease.
3. **Enhancing Circulation and Lymphatic Drainage:** Massage therapy improves blood circulation and lymphatic drainage, facilitating the delivery of oxygen and nutrients to tissues and organs while removing metabolic waste products and toxins. Improved circulation can help reduce swelling, edema, and inflammation, promoting tissue healing and recovery.
4. **Alleviating Non-Motor Symptoms:** In addition to its physical benefits, massage therapy can address non-motor symptoms such as anxiety, depression, and sleep disturbances commonly experienced by individuals with Parkinson's disease. The relaxation response induced by massage promotes mental and emotional well-being, reduces stress and anxiety levels, and improves sleep quality and duration.
5. **Enhancing Body Awareness and Mindfulness:** Massage therapy encourages individuals with Parkinson's disease to become more aware of their bodies, sensations, and movement patterns. By focusing attention on the present moment and cultivating mindfulness, massage promotes body awareness, self-regulation, and stress management skills, empowering individuals to better cope with the challenges of living with a chronic condition.
6. **Improving Quality of Life:** Ultimately, massage therapy contributes to improving the overall quality of life for individuals with Parkinson's disease by addressing physical discomfort, enhancing functional mobility, reducing psychological distress, and promoting relaxation and well-being. Integrating regular massage sessions into the treatment regimen can help individuals with Parkinson's disease maintain a higher quality of life and better manage their symptoms over time.

10.5.2. Types of Massage Therapy Techniques

1. **Swedish Massage:** Swedish massage is a gentle, relaxing form of massage therapy that involves long, flowing strokes, kneading, and circular movements to promote relaxation, improve circulation, and alleviate muscle tension. It is suitable for individuals with Parkinson's disease who may have sensitive skin or prefer lighter pressure.

2. **Deep Tissue Massage:** Deep tissue massage targets deeper layers of muscle and connective tissue to release chronic tension, adhesions, and knots. It involves firm pressure, slow strokes, and focused techniques to address specific areas of tightness and discomfort. Deep tissue massage can help relieve muscle stiffness and pain associated with Parkinson's disease.
3. **Myofascial Release:** Myofascial release focuses on releasing restrictions in the fascia, the connective tissue that surrounds muscles, bones, and organs. It involves gentle, sustained pressure and stretching to release adhesions and restore mobility and flexibility. Myofascial release can be particularly beneficial for individuals with Parkinson's disease who experience fascial restrictions and movement limitations.
4. **Trigger Point Therapy:** Trigger point therapy targets specific areas of muscle tension, known as trigger points or muscle knots, that refer pain to other parts of the body. It involves applying pressure to trigger points to release tension, improve circulation, and alleviate pain and discomfort. Trigger point therapy can help reduce muscle stiffness and improve mobility in individuals with Parkinson's disease.
5. **Passive Range of Motion (ROM) Exercises:** Passive ROM exercises involve gently moving the limbs and joints through their full range of motion without the individual's active participation. Massage therapists can perform passive ROM exercises during massage sessions to improve joint mobility, increase flexibility, and reduce stiffness in individuals with Parkinson's disease.

10.5.3. Considerations for Massage Therapy in Parkinson's Disease

1. **Individualized Approach:** Massage therapy should be tailored to the individual needs, preferences, and limitations of each client with Parkinson's disease. Therapists should take into account the severity of motor symptoms, presence of co-morbidities, medication regimen, and any contraindications or precautions related to massage therapy.
2. **Communication and Feedback:** Open communication between the client and the massage therapist is essential to ensure a safe and effective massage experience. Clients should communicate their preferences, concerns, and goals for the session, while therapists should provide clear explanations, obtain informed consent, and solicit feedback throughout the session.
3. **Gentle Techniques and Modifications:** Massage therapists should use gentle techniques and modifications to accommodate the unique needs and sensitivities of individuals with Parkinson's disease. This may include adjusting pressure, pace, and positioning, providing additional support and cushions, and avoiding vigorous or abrupt movements that may trigger discomfort or exacerbate symptoms.

4. **Safety Precautions:** Massage therapists should be aware of potential safety concerns and contraindications associated with Parkinson's disease, such as orthostatic hypotension, dyskinesias, skin fragility, and cognitive impairment. They should modify their approach accordingly and prioritize client safety and comfort at all times.
5. **Collaboration with Healthcare Team:** Massage therapists should collaborate with the client's healthcare team, including physicians, physical therapists, and other allied health professionals, to ensure coordinated care and optimize treatment outcomes. They should communicate any relevant findings, observations, or recommendations from massage sessions to facilitate continuity of care and mutual understanding.

10.6. Dietary Supplements

Dietary supplements are widely used by individuals with PD as a complementary approach to managing symptoms and supporting overall health and well-being. While medications remain the cornerstone of PD treatment, some individuals turn to dietary supplements to address nutritional deficiencies, alleviate symptoms, and potentially slow disease progression. Here, we'll explore common dietary supplements used in PD management, their potential benefits, and considerations for their use:

1. **Coenzyme Q10 (CoQ10):**

- **Potential Benefits**: CoQ10 is a powerful antioxidant that plays a role in cellular energy production and mitochondrial function. Some studies suggest that CoQ10 supplementation may help protect against oxidative stress, mitochondrial dysfunction, and neurodegeneration in PD. It may also improve motor symptoms and quality of life in some individuals.
- **Considerations**: While early studies showed promising results, more recent clinical trials have yielded mixed findings regarding the efficacy of CoQ10 in PD. Further research is needed to determine optimal dosages, treatment durations, and potential interactions with other medications.

2. **Vitamin B12:**

- **Potential Benefits**: Vitamin B12 is essential for nerve function and DNA synthesis, and deficiency has been implicated in neurological disorders, including PD. Supplementing with vitamin B12 may help maintain nerve health, reduce homocysteine levels (a marker of inflammation), and alleviate cognitive impairment and neuropathy associated with PD.
- **Considerations**: Vitamin B12 deficiency is more common in older adults and individuals with gastrointestinal disorders or malabsorption issues. It's important to monitor vitamin B12 levels and supplement if deficient. High doses of vitamin B12 may interact with certain medications or exacerbate existing health conditions.

3. **Vitamin D:**

- **Potential Benefits**: Vitamin D is crucial for bone health, immune function, and neuroprotection.

Low vitamin D levels have been associated with an increased risk of PD and disease progression. Supplementing with vitamin D may help reduce inflammation, protect dopaminergic neurons, and improve motor function and quality of life in PD.

- **Considerations**: Vitamin D deficiency is common, especially in regions with limited sunlight exposure or among individuals with restricted mobility. Regular monitoring of vitamin D levels is recommended, and supplementation should be tailored to individual needs to avoid toxicity.

4. **Omega-3 Fatty Acids:**

- **Potential Benefits**: Omega-3 fatty acids, particularly eicosapentaenoic acid (EPA) and docosahexaenoic acid (DHA), have anti-inflammatory and neuroprotective properties. Some studies suggest that omega-3 supplementation may help reduce inflammation, oxidative stress, and neurodegeneration in PD, potentially improving motor and non-motor symptoms.
- **Considerations**: Omega-3 fatty acids are found in fatty fish, flaxseeds, walnuts, and other plant-based sources. Supplementation may be beneficial for individuals with low dietary intake or those who cannot tolerate fish oil due to taste or gastrointestinal issues.

5. **Antioxidants (Vitamin E, Vitamin C, Selenium):**

- **Potential Benefits**: Antioxidants help neutralize free radicals and reduce oxidative damage to cells and tissues. Some studies suggest that antioxidants such as vitamin E, vitamin C, and selenium may help protect against oxidative stress, mitochondrial dysfunction, and neurodegeneration in PD, potentially slowing disease progression.
- **Considerations**: High-dose antioxidant supplementation may not be beneficial and could even be harmful in some cases. It's important to obtain antioxidants from a balanced diet rich in fruits, vegetables, whole grains, and nuts rather than relying solely on supplements.

6. **Multivitamins and Mineral Supplements:**

- **Potential Benefits**: Multivitamins and mineral supplements provide a convenient way to ensure adequate intake of essential nutrients, especially in individuals with poor dietary habits or malabsorption issues. They may help address nutritional deficiencies, support overall health, and enhance energy levels and vitality.
- **Considerations**: Not all individuals require multivitamin supplementation, and excessive intake of certain vitamins and minerals may have adverse effects. It's important to consult with a healthcare provider before starting any new supplement regimen, especially in individuals with pre-existing medical conditions or those taking multiple medications.

Mindfulness-Based Stress Reduction (MBSR) has emerged as a promising complementary approach for individuals living with PD, offering a holistic framework for managing symptoms and improving overall well-being. Developed by Dr. Jon Kabat-Zinn in the late 1970s, MBSR combines mindfulness meditation, yoga, and awareness practices to cultivate present-moment awareness and reduce stress reactivity. In the context of PD, MBSR aims to help individuals cope with the physical, emotional, and psychological challenges of living with a chronic neurodegenerative condition. By cultivating mindfulness, individuals with PD can develop greater acceptance, resilience, and self-regulation skills, enabling them to navigate the ups and downs of the disease with greater ease and equanimity.

A Closer Look

Mindfulness-Based Stress Reduction (MBSR)

Research suggests that MBSR can have beneficial effects on both motor and non-motor symptoms of PD, as well as on overall quality of life. Mindfulness practices such as mindful breathing, body scans, and mindful movement can help individuals with PD become more attuned to their bodies, sensations, and movement patterns, facilitating greater awareness of symptoms and improved self-care. By learning to respond skillfully to physical discomfort and emotional distress, individuals with PD may experience reduced anxiety, depression, and perceived stress, leading to enhanced emotional well-being and quality of life.

Moreover, MBSR may contribute to neuroplasticity and neuroprotection in PD by promoting adaptive changes in brain structure and function. Neuroimaging studies have shown that mindfulness meditation can modulate brain activity in regions involved in emotion regulation, attention, and self-awareness, potentially mitigating the impact of neurodegeneration on cognitive and affective processes. Additionally, by reducing stress and inflammation, MBSR may help slow disease progression and preserve motor function in individuals with PD.

Despite its potential benefits, MBSR may pose challenges for individuals with PD, including physical limitations, cognitive impairments, and communication difficulties. Modifications and adaptations may be necessary to accommodate the unique needs and abilities of individuals with PD, such as offering seated meditation practices, providing additional support and guidance, and incorporating assistive devices or props. Moreover, integrating MBSR into PD care requires collaboration between healthcare professionals, mindfulness instructors, and individuals with PD and their caregivers to ensure safety, accessibility, and effectiveness.

Summary

- Acupuncture is a form of ancient Chinese medicine whereby thin needles are inserted into the skin at precise points (acupoints) to balance the flow of energy (*qi*) throughout the body. It is based on a theory that many different meridians run throughout the body and represent different organ systems, connected by these points.
- Tai Chi, or *taiji quan*, is a traditional Chinese martial art practice that has been utilized for centuries to address physical and mental well-being. The term refers to the concept of yin and yang, which incorporates complex and disciplined movements to achieve dynamic balance, along with breathing and meditation.
- Similar to Tai Chi, Qi Gong is a traditional Chinese practice that combines movement, posture, breathing, and meditation to enhance the flow of *qi*. Though less common in Western culture, Qi Gong has been practiced for nearly 5000 years in China and predates the study of Tai Chi. Though few studies have been conducted to evaluate its effect on PD, there seems to be a growing interest reflected by the recency of randomized clinical trials.
- Yoga is an ancient Indian meditative and spiritual practice that has evolved in recent years to become a popular physical fitness and relaxation exercise. It involves a series of movements coordinated to breath and meditation, focusing on the mind–body connection.
- Massage therapy involves the manipulation of soft tissues, including muscles, tendons, ligaments, and fascia, using various techniques such as stroking, kneading, compression, and stretching. These techniques can be applied with the hands, fingers, elbows, forearms, or specialized tools, depending on the therapist's training and the client's needs.
- Dietary supplements are widely used by individuals with PD as a complementary approach to managing symptoms and supporting overall health and well-being. While medications remain the cornerstone of PD treatment, some individuals turn to dietary supplements to address nutritional deficiencies, alleviate symptoms, and potentially slow disease progression.

References

1. Aroxa, F. H., Gondim, I. T., Santos, E. L., Coriolano, M. D., Asano, A. G., & Asano, N. M. (2017). Acupuncture as adjuvant therapy for sleep disorders in Parkinson's disease. *Journal of Acupuncture and Meridian Studies, 10*(1), 33–38. https://doi.org/10.1016/j.jams.2016.06.006.
2. Cho, S. Y., Lee, Y. E., Doo, K. H., Lee, J. H., Jung, W. S., Moon, S. K., et al. (2018). Efficacy of combined treatment with acupuncture and bee venom acupuncture as an adjunctive treatment for Parkinson's disease. *Journal of Alternative and Complementary Medicine, 24*(1), 25–32. https://doi.org/10.1089/acm.2017.0151.
3. Cho, S. Y., Shim, S. R., Rhee, H. Y., Park, H. J., Jung, W. S., Moon, S. K., et al. (2012). Effectiveness of acupuncture and bee venom acupuncture in idiopathic Parkinson's disease. *Parkinsonism & Related Disorders, 18*(8), 948–952. https://doi.org/10.1016/j.parkreldis.2012.05.015.
4. Cristian, A., Katz, M., Cutrone, E., & Walker, R. H. (2005). Evaluation of acupuncture in the treatment of Parkinson's disease: A double-blind pilot study. *Movement Disorders, 20*(9), 1185–1188. https://doi.org/10.1002/mds.20530.

5. Dimitrova, A., Murchison, C., & Oken, B. (2017). Acupuncture for the treatment of peripheral neuropathy: A systematic review and meta-analysis. *Journal of Alternative and Complementary Medicine, 23*(3), 164–179. https://doi.org/10.1089/acm.2016.0294.

6. Donley, S., McGregor, S., Wielinski, C., & Nance, M. (2019). Use and perceived effectiveness of complementary therapies in Parkinson's disease. *Parkinsonism & Related Disorders, 58*, 46–49. https://doi.org/10.1016/j.parkreldis.2018.07.007.

7. Doo, K. H., Lee, J. H., Cho, S. Y., Jung, W. S., Moon, S. K., Park, J. M., et al. (2015). A prospective open-label study of combined treatment for idiopathic Parkinson's disease using acupuncture and bee venom acupuncture as an adjunctive treatment. *Journal of Alternative and Complementary Medicine, 21*(10), 598–603. https://doi.org/10.1089/acm.2014.0223.

8. Dorsey, E. R., Constantinescu, R., Thompson, J. P., Biglan, K. M., Holloway, R. G., Kieburtz, K., et al. (2007). Projected number of people with Parkinson's disease in the most populous nations, 2005 through 2030. *Neurology, 68*(5), 384–386. https://doi.org/10.1212/01.wnl.0000247740.47667.03.

9. Eng, M. L., Lyons, K. E., Greene, M. S., & Pahwa, R. (2006). Open-label trial regarding the use of acupuncture and yin tui na in Parkinson's disease outpatients: A pilot study on efficacy, tolerability, and quality of life. *Journal of Alternative and Complementary Medicine, 12*(4), 395–399. https://doi.org/10.1089/acm.2006.12.395.

10. Finseth, T. A., Hedeman, J. L., Brown, R. P., 2nd, Johnson, K. I., Binder, M. S., & Kluger, B. M. (2015). Self-reported efficacy of cannabis and other complementary medicine modalities by Parkinson's disease patients in Colorado. *Evidence-Based Complementary and Alternative Medicine, 2015*, Article 874849. https://doi.org/10.1155/2015/874849.

11. Fukuda, S., Kuriyama, N., & Egawa, M. (2015). Acupuncture for gait disturbance in Parkinson's disease: Immediate effects of acupuncture treatment. *Journal of the American Geriatrics Society, 63*(10), 2189–2190. https://doi.org/10.1111/jgs.13657.

12. Hackney, M. E., & Earhart, G. M. (2008). Tai Chi improves balance and mobility in people with Parkinson's disease. *Gait & Posture, 28*(3), 456–460. https://doi.org/10.1016/j.gaitpost.2008.02.005.

13. Hall, E., Verheyden, G., & Ashburn, A. (2011). Effect of a yoga programme on an individual with Parkinson's disease: A single-subject design. *Disability and Rehabilitation, 33*(15–16), 1483–1489. https://doi.org/10.3109/09638288.2010.525192.

14. Wang, H., Guo, J., Zhang, Y., Fang, J., Qiu, S., He, Y., et al. (2023). Efficacy of scalp acupuncture with the long-stay method on motor dysfunction in patients with acute ischemic stroke: A randomized controlled trial. *Neurology, 19*, 1273–1283.

15. Hinnell, C., Hurt, C. S., Landau, S., Brown, R. G., Samuel, M., & Group P-PS. (2012). Nonmotor versus motor symptoms: How much do they matter to health status in Parkinson's disease? *Movement Disorders, 27*(2), 236–241. https://doi.org/10.1002/mds.24006.

16. Kluger, B. M., Rakowski, D., Christian, M., Cedar, D., Wong, B., Crawford, J., et al. (2016). Randomized, controlled trial of acupuncture for fatigue in Parkinson's disease. *Movement Disorders, 31*(7), 1027–1032. https://doi.org/10.1002/mds.26631.

17. Kong, K. H., Ng, H. L., Li, W., Ng, D. W., Tan, S. I., Tay, K. Y., et al. (2018). Acupuncture in the treatment of fatigue in Parkinson's disease: A pilot, randomized, controlled study. *Brain and Behavior, 8*(1), e00897. https://doi.org/10.1002/brb3.897.

18. Lei, H., Toosizadeh, N., Schwenk, M., Sherman, S., Karp, S., Sternberg, E., et al. (2016). A pilot clinical trial to objectively assess the efficacy of electroacupuncture on gait in patients with Parkinson's disease using body worn sensors. *PLoS One, 11*(5), e0155613. https://doi.org/10.1371/journal.pone.0155613.

19. Lei, S., Liu, Q., Leong, I., Fan, J., Tsang, Y., Liu, X., et al. (2024). Acupuncture therapy for Parkinson's disease: A case report demonstrating symptomatic improvement without medication. *Frontiers in Neurology, 14*, Article 1330054. https://doi.org/10.3389/fneur.2023.1330054.

20. Li, Z., Chen, J., Cheng, J., Huang, S., Hu, Y., Wu, Y., et al. (2018). Acupuncture modulates the cerebello-thalamo-cortical circuit and cognitive brain regions in patients of Parkinson's disease with tremor. *Frontiers in Aging Neuroscience, 10*, Article 206. https://doi.org/10.3389/fnagi.2018.00206.

21. Longhurst, J. C. (2010). Defining meridians: A modern basis of understanding. *Journal of Acupuncture and Meridian Studies, 3*(2), 67–74. https://doi.org/10.1016/S2005-2901(10)60018-3.

22. Ray Chaudhuri, K., Poewe, W., & Brooks, D. (2018). Motor and nonmotor complications of levodopa: Phenomenology, risk factors, and imaging features. *Movement Disorders, 33*(6), 909–919. https://doi.org/10.1002/mds.27386.

23. Ren, X. M. (2008). Fifty cases of Parkinson's disease treated by acupuncture combined with madopar. *Journal of Traditional Chinese Medicine, 28*(4), 255–257.

24. Santos-Garcia, D., & de la Fuente-Fernandez, R. (2013). Impact of non-motor symptoms on health-related and perceived quality of life in Parkinson's disease. *Journal of the Neurological Sciences, 332*(1–2), 136–140. https://doi.org/10.1016/j.jns.2013.06.011.

25. Schiapparelli, P., Allais, G., Rolando, S., Airola, G., Borgogno, P., Terzi, M. G., et al. (2011). Acupuncture in primary headache treatment. *Neurological Sciences, 32*(Suppl 1), S15–S18. https://doi.org/10.1007/s10072-011-0530-3.

26. Shin, J. Y., Pohlig, R. T., & Habermann, B. (2017). Use of complementary health approaches in individuals with Parkinson's disease. *Journal of Gerontological Nursing, 43*(2), 46–54. https://doi.org/10.3928/00989134-20170110-01.

27. Shulman, L. M., Wen, X., Weiner, W. J., Bateman, D., Minagar, A., Duncan, R., et al. (2002). Acupuncture therapy for the symptoms of Parkinson's disease. *Movement Disorders, 17*(4), 799–802. https://doi.org/10.1002/mds.10098.

28. Suchowersky, O., Gronseth, G., Perlmutter, J., Reich, S., Zesiewicz, T., & Weiner, W. J. (2006). Practice parameter: Neuroprotective strategies and alternative therapies for Parkinson's disease (an evidence-based review). *Neurology, 66*, 976–982. https://doi.org/10.1212/01.wnl.0000206363.57955.1f.

29. Toosizadeh, N., Lei, H., Schwenk, M., Sherman, S. J., Sternberg, E., Mohler, J., et al. (2015). Does integrative medicine enhance balance in aging adults? Proof of concept for the benefit of electroacupuncture therapy in Parkinson's disease. *Gerontology, 61*(1), 3–14. https://doi.org/10.1159/000371933.

30. Walter, A. A., Adams, E. V., Van Puymbroeck, M., Crowe, B. M., Urrea-Mendoza, E., Hawkins, B. L., et al. (2019). Changes in nonmotor symptoms following an 8-week yoga intervention for people with Parkinson's disease. *International Journal of Yoga Therapy, 29*(1), 91–99. https://doi.org/10.17761/2020-00019.

31. Wang, Y., Xie, C. L., Wang, W. W., Lu, L., Fu, D. L., Wang, X. T., et al. (2013). Epidemiology of complementary and alternative medicine use in patients with Parkinson's disease. *Journal of Clinical Neuroscience, 20*(8), 1062–1067. https://doi.org/10.1016/j.jocn.2012.10.012.

32. Wells, R. E., Baute, V., & Wahbeh, H. (2017). Complementary and integrative medicine for neurologic conditions. *Medical Clinics of North America, 101*(5), 881–893. https://doi.org/10.1016/j.mcna.2017.05.006.

33. Xiao, C., Zhuang, Y., & Kang, Y. (2016). Effect of Health Qigong Baduanjin on fall prevention in individuals with Parkinson's disease. *Journal of the American Geriatrics Society, 64*(11), e227–e228. https://doi.org/10.1111/jgs.14408.

34. Yu, S. W., Lin, S. H., Tsai, C. C., Chaudhuri, K. R., Huang, Y. C., Chen, Y. S., et al. (2019). Acupuncture effect and mechanism for treating pain in patients with Parkinson's disease. *Frontiers in Neurology, 10*, Article 1114. https://doi.org/10.3389/fneur.2019.01114.

35. Zhou, W., & Benharash, P. (2014). Effects and mechanisms of acupuncture based on the principle of meridians. *Journal of Acupuncture and Meridian Studies, 7*(4), 190–193. https://doi.org/10.1016/j.jams.2014.05.002.

INDEX

FSC
www.fsc.org
MIX
Papier | Fördert gute Waldnutzung
FSC® C083411

Kolibri 360 GmbH
Ferdinand-Jühlke-Straße 7
99095 Erfurt, Deutschland
produktsicherheit@kolibri360.de